Pharmacology I for Medications

in Nuclear Medicine and Medical Imaging

Geoffrey Currie,
BPharm, MMedRadSc (NucMed), MAppMngt (Health), MBA, PhD, AM

Pharmacology Primer for Medications

in Nuclear Medicine and Medical Imaging

Geoffrey Currie
BPharm, MMedRadSc (NucMed), MAppMngt (Health), MBA, PhD, AM
Professor in Nuclear Medicine
School of Dentistry and Health Sciences
Charles Sturt University, Wagga Wagga, Australia

International Consulting Editor of the *Journal of Nuclear Medicine Technology*

Published by
Society of Nuclear Medicine and Molecular Imaging

10-digit: 0-932004-97-0

13-digit: 978-0-932004-97-0

Society of Nuclear Medicine & Molecular Imaging, Inc.
1850 Samuel Morse Drive, Reston, VA 20190–5316

© 2020 Society of Nuclear Medicine & Molecular Imaging, Inc. All rights reserved.

This book is protected by copyright. No part of it may be reproduced, stored in a retrieval system or transmitted in any form or by any means, electronic, mechanical, photocopying, recording, or otherwise, without the prior written permission of the publisher.

Made in the United States of America.

Library of Congress Control Number: 2020945953

DEDICATION

This book is dedicated to:

- My colleagues in nuclear medicine and medical radiation technology in Australia, New Zealand, the United States, Canada, Europe, Asia, and across the globe who are advancing our profession and patient care through a deeper understanding of pharmacology.

- The Society of Nuclear Medicine and Molecular Imaging Technologist Section and the *Journal of Nuclear Medicine Technology* for supporting this book and Kathy Thomas for her enthusiasm and drive to get pharmacology on the continuing education and continuing professional development map.

- Charles Sturt University and the Rural Alliance in Nuclear Scintigraphy for supporting me in the development of this and related work and activities.

- Most important, my children, Hugo and Josie, who are patient and supportive of the many hours I spend writing and developing educational resources for my colleagues across the globe. They are my motivation and inspiration. They bring joy to so many aspects of my life, including writing this book. Without their support and enthusiasm, this book would not have happened.

PREFACE

The Society of Nuclear Medicine and Molecular Imaging Technologist Section (SNMMI-TS) scope of practice for a nuclear medicine technologist in the United States defines interventional (imaging) medications as those medications used to evoke a specific physiological or biochemical response used in conjunction with diagnostic imaging or therapeutic procedures. The same document defines adjunctive medications as those medications used to respond to a patient's condition during a nuclear medicine procedure. Patients presenting to nuclear medicine may be taking medication that can interfere with the nuclear medicine procedure. These medications represent cessation medications. The SNMMI-TS scope of practice for a nuclear medicine technologist requires that nuclear medicine technologists display a thorough understanding and working knowledge of indications, contraindications, warnings, precautions, proper use, drug interactions, and adverse reactions for each medication to be used. That knowledge development requires a foundational understanding of the principles of pharmacology.

The same scope of practice requirements are reflected in regulatory policies of the Medical Radiation Practice Board of Australia, the European Association of Nuclear Medicine, and the Canadian Association of Medical Radiation Technologists, and they apply to colleagues across the medical radiation science field, including nuclear medicine, radiography, radiation therapy, computed tomography (CT), and magnetic resonance imaging (MRI). The pharmacological understanding of principles and applications and the capability to deliver or administer medications is a minimum capability; it is not advanced practice.

While new graduates are emerging with these capabilities and knowledge, a gap remains for many practitioners with established careers. Global efforts have been made to provide education opportunities to bridge that gap, including a series that I authored in the *Journal of Nuclear Medicine Technology* (JNMT) from which many chapters in this book are drawn; a lecture series I provided at a SNMMI conference, which was recorded and subsequently released; and a course of study I developed through the Rural Alliance in Nuclear Scintigraphy (RAINS) and the Australian and New Zealand Society of Nuclear Medicine (ANZSNM) in Australia.

Scope of Practice for Nuclear Medicine Technologists				
Capability	*Australia (AHPRA), 2020*	*USA (SNMMI-TS), 2017*	*Europe (EANM), 2017*	*Canada (CAMRT), 2014*
Understand principles and applications of pharmaceuticals	Yes	Yes	Yes	Yes
Apply principles of pharmacology of pharmaceuticals	Yes	Yes	Yes	Yes
Deliver/administer pharmaceuticals	Yes	Yes	Yes	Yes

This book focuses on the theoretical needs of the medical radiation science community not captured in other pharmacology reference books. It is written from the context of and at a level for medical radiation practitioners. It is intended to provide not a deep treatment of pharmacology principles but rather a concise overview of basic principles as applied to the practice of medical radiation science. The references used in Chapter 1 are an excellent starting point for those interested in deeper pharmacology insights. I hope this text meets your educational needs.

Geoff

References

Canadian Association of Medical Radiation Technologists. (2014). *Advanced Practice in Medical Radiation Technology: A Canadian Framework* [White paper]. http://www.camrt.ca/.

European Association of Nuclear Medicine (EANM) Technologist Committee. *EANM benchmark document on nuclear medicine technologist competencies.* 2017. https://www.eanm.org/publications/technologists-publications. Accessed April 22, 2018.

Medical Radiation Practice Board of Australia (MRPBA). Professional capabilities for medical radiation practice, 2020.

SNMMI-TS Scope of Practice Task Force. Nuclear medicine technologist scope of practice and performance standards. *J Nucl Med Technol.* 2017;45(1):53–64.

LEARNING OUTCOMES

The purpose of this text is to help medical radiation practitioners develop capability in applying knowledge for safe and effective use of medicines. Clearly, this capability development must occur within the constraints of relevant regulatory and statutory requirements. To that end, specific learning outcomes include to be able to

- Apply the principles of pharmacology to the safe and effective use of medicines.
- Recognize general, patient-specific, and scenario-specific risks, precautions, and contraindications for use of medicines.
- Apply the pharmacokinetic and pharmacodynamic principles of medications to identify and explain normal and adverse reactions to medications.
- Administer medications safely, effectively, and appropriately according to procedures and within regulatory and statutory parameters.
- Monitor patients for, identify, and manage adverse reactions.

TABLE OF CONTENTS

Preface vii

Chapter 1 **Introduction to Pharmacology** 1
　　　　　Introduction 2
　　　　　Receptor Principle 3
　　　　　Receptor Action 5
　　　　　Cholinergic Pharmacology 6
　　　　　Adrenergic (Norepinephrine) Pharmacology 8
　　　　　Pharmacology of Other Important Receptors 9

Chapter 2 **Pharmacodynamics** 17
　　　　　Introduction 18
　　　　　Drug Action 18
　　　　　Drug Receptor Interactions 19
　　　　　Dose-Response Relationship 20
　　　　　Drug Interactions 23

Chapter 3 **Pharmacokinetics** 25
　　　　　Introduction 26
　　　　　Absorption 28
　　　　　Distribution 30
　　　　　Metabolism 33
　　　　　Elimination 34
　　　　　Insight 34

Chapter 4 **Dose Forms and Administration** 45
　　　　　Introduction 46
　　　　　Routes of Administration 46
　　　　　Dose Form 46
　　　　　Drug Administration 51
　　　　　Example Calculations 52
　　　　　Insight 53

Chapter 5 **Individual Variations in Pharmacology** 55
　　　　　Introduction 56
　　　　　Pharmacologic Considerations in Women 56
　　　　　Pharmacologic Considerations in Children 57
　　　　　Effects of Aging 58
　　　　　Insight 62
　　　　　Summary 65

Chapter 6	**Renal Imaging Interventions**	**67**
	Introduction	68
	Furosemide (Lasix)	68
	Captopril	71
	Enalapril	73
	Summary	73
	Insight	73
Chapter 7	**Biliary Imaging Interventions**	**75**
	Introduction	76
	Sincalide	77
	Morphine	78
	Phenobarbital	80
	Summary	80
Chapter 8	**Cardiac Imaging Interventions**	**83**
	Introduction	84
	Pharmacological Stress Testing	84
	Adenosine	84
	Dipyridamole	89
	Regadenoson	91
	Dobutamine	91
	Adjunctive Medications	92
	Aminophylline	93
	Nitroglycerin (Glyceryl Trinitrate)	95
	Salbutamol	96
	Cessation Medications	98
	Xanthines	99
	Beta-Blockers	99
	Calcium Channel Blockers	100
	Nitrates	100
	Digoxin	101
	Insight	101
Chapter 9	**Other Imaging Interventions**	**105**
	Introduction	106
	Less Common Interventional Studies	106
	Acetazolamide	106
	Cimetidine	110
	Ranitidine	112
	Omeprazole	112

Adjunctive Medications Common in General Nuclear Medicine 113
    Chloral Hydrate 113
    Diazepam 114
    Bisacodyl 115
    Heparin 115
Insight 116

Chapter 10 Iodinated CT Contrast 121
Introduction 122
CT Contrast 122
Properties of CT Contrast 122
Mechanism of Action 126
Pharmacokinetics 127
Adverse Reactions 128
Management of Adverse Reactions 132
Extravasation 133
Interactions 134
Contraindications and Precautions 134
Summary 134

Chapter 11 Gadolinium MRI Contrast 137
Introduction 138
MRI Contrast 138
Properties of Gadolinium MRI Contrast 139
Mechanism of Action 141
Pharmacokinetics 141
Contraindications and Precautions 143
Adverse Reactions 143
Nephrogenic Systemic Fibrosis 145
Management of Adverse Reactions 146
Extravasation 146
Interactions 147
Summary 147

Chapter 12 The Crash Cart/Emergency Trolley 149
Introduction 150
Medications 151
Medication Use in an Emergency 152
Emergency Medication Pharmacology 156

Chapter 13	**Pain Management**	**173**
	Introduction	174
	Pain Management with Opioid Analgesics	174
	Anti-Inflammatory Mediators in Pain Management	179
	Adjunctive Pain Medications	185
	Pain Prevention with Anesthetics	185
Chapter 14	**Chemotherapy**	**191**
	Introduction	191
	Pathogens	192
	Cancer	192
	Immunotherapy	198
	Insight	199
	Case Study	202
Chapter 15	**Issues with Over-the-Counter Medications**	**207**
	Introduction	208
	Analgesia	208
	Antipyretic (Fever)	210
	Antihistamines	211
	Gastric Acid Reducers	213
	Laxatives	214
	Antidiarrhea	216
	Bronchodilation	216
	Sympathomimetic Decongestant	218
	Cough Medicines	220
	Insight	222
Chapter 16	**Lifestyle and Sports Drugs**	**225**
	Introduction	226
	Drugs Used in Sports	227
	Lifestyle Drugs	229
Chapter 17	**Known Interactions with Radiopharmaceuticals**	**235**
	Introduction	236
	Adverse Reactions to Radiopharmaceuticals	236
	Iatrogenic Changes to Radiopharmaceutical Biodistribution	236
	Insight	238

About the Author *241*

Index *243*

CHAPTER 1

Introduction to Pharmacology

Chapter Objectives

Specific learning outcomes (page ix) of this text addressed in this chapter:

- Apply the principles of pharmacology to the safe and effective use of medicines.
- Apply the pharmacokinetic and pharmacodynamic principles of medications to identify and explain normal and adverse reactions to medications.

After reading, digesting, reflecting on, and reviewing the content of this chapter, readers should be able to

1. Demonstrate command of key pharmacology terms.
2. Demonstrate enhanced understanding of the principles associated with pharmacology.
3. Demonstrate critical thinking to effect problem solving related to the receptor principle.
4. Recognize, explain, and interpret clinical problems and evidence in relation to cholinergic and adrenergic pharmacology.
5. Demonstrate understanding of the serotonin, purine, and histamine pharmacology.
6. Apply knowledge of general pharmacology principles and concepts in a translational manner to clinical practice.

Key Terms

adrenergic	affinity	exogenous	muscarinic	potency
agonist	beta-blocker	hormesis	neurotransmitter	purine
allosteric	cholinergic	ligand	nicotinic	vasodilation
antagonist	drug	medication	pharmacodynamics	receptor
antibody	endogenous	medicine	pharmacokinetics	selectivity
antigen	efficacy	methylation	pharmacology	xanthine

Some of the text, tables, and figures in this chapter were extracted from "Pharmacology Part 1: Introduction to Pharmacology and Pharmacodynamics" by Geoff Currie (*J Nucl Med Technol.* 2018;46:81–86).

2 Pharmacology Primer for Medications

Introduction

Pharmacology is the scientific study of the action and effects of drugs on living systems and the interaction of drugs with living systems. Pharmacology includes the study of prescribed and over-the-counter medications, legal and illicit drugs, natural and synthetic compounds, *exogenous* (sourced from outside the body) and *endogenous* (produced inside the body) drugs, and drugs that produce benefit, harm, or both benefit and harm. As a general rule, pharmacology is divided into *pharmacodynamics* and *pharmacokinetics* (Fig. 1-1). It should, however, be recognized that some texts add the additional subdivisions (Table 1-1) of pharmacogenetics, pharmacogenomics, pharmacoepidemiology, pharmacoeconomics, and pharmacovigilance. A quantum shift in pharmacology has taken place since the mid-1900s with a leap from simply describing what effect a drug causes to providing an understanding of how drugs work.

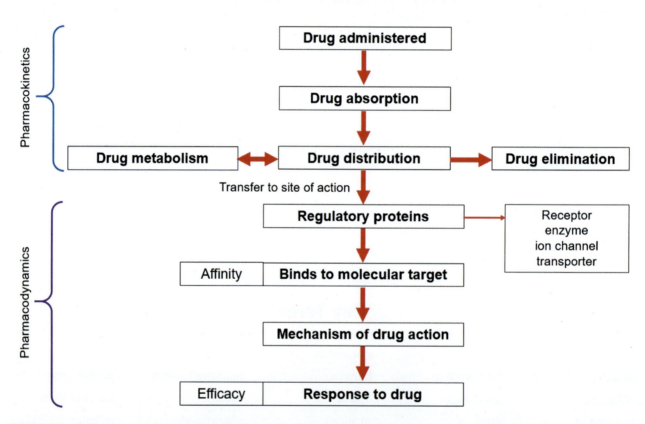

FIGURE 1-1 Schematic representation of the relationship between pharmacokinetics and pharmacodynamics.

TABLE 1-1	Definitions of Pharmacology Terms
Pharmaco-	*Is the Study of*
-dynamics	How the drug affects the living system
-kinetics	How the living system affects the drug
-genetics	Variations in drug response due to genetic influences
-genomics	Genetic factors to guide drug therapy
-epidemiology	Variability of the drug response across a population
-economics	The comparative cost:benefit ratios of treatment strategies
-vigilance	The adverse effects of drugs

A *drug* is simply a chemical or substance that causes a physiological effect when introduced to the body. Morphine is a good example of an exogenous drug that mimics endogenous morphine (endorphins). Obviously, a wide variety of everyday chemicals (e.g., water) could be classified as drugs; thus, drugs are generally defined on the basis of key parameters such as *potency* and *selectivity*. Importantly, some drugs elicit variable effects with varying doses: they may be beneficial at one dose and harmful at another (hormesis). The basic principle of toxicology was captured by Paracelsus in 1538: the dose makes the poison, or in Latin, *sola dosis facit venenum*. Thallium is an example of a chemical used for imaging in nuclear medicine, but it has also been used as a poison—as depicted in the odd black-and-white movie and, more recently, in the James Bond movie *Spectre* (2015)—because it is highly toxic, colorless, odorless, and tasteless. A medicine is a specific chemical preparation composed of one or more drugs that is administered in order to elicit a therapeutic effect (e.g., disease or symptom treatment or prevention).

Receptor Principle

Receptors are proteins (macromolecules), found on cell surfaces or inside the cell, that mediate drug activity. Receptors respond to specific neurotransmitters, hormones, antigens, chemicals, or substances. A chemical (ligand) binds to a specific site (receptor) and triggers a response (signal) in the cells. The intracellular changes initiated by the ligand-receptor complex can be through direct or indirect action; however, the ligand generally functions as either an *agonist* or an *antagonist*. An agonist mimics the endogenous ligand to produce a similar response (e.g., morphine is an agonist for opioid receptors), whereas an antagonist blocks the usual ligand and thereby inhibits the physiological response (e.g., naloxone is an antagonist for opioid receptors) (Fig. 1-2). Following is a more detailed classification of drug action:

- An agonist creates a conformation change at the site of action that mimics the physiological ligand. Potency is determined by affinity and efficacy. A full agonist has high efficacy. Dobutamine is an example of an adrenergic agonist.
- A partial agonist demonstrates both agonist and antagonist action, which produces a truncated response. The submaximal effects represent intermediate to low efficacy. Tamoxifen is a partial agonist. Although morphine is a full agonist for opioid receptors in the central nervous system (CNS), it is a partial agonist in other tissues, such as those associated with sphincter of Oddi contraction.

- An antagonist binds at the site of action but does not produce the conformational change. It does not produce a response, and it blocks an agonist from binding (zero efficacy). Beta-blockers (beta-adrenergic antagonists) and captopril (angiotensin-converting enzyme antagonism inhibitor) are examples. A competitive antagonist represents displacement of the opportunity for the ligand or agonist to bind to the site of action.

- Reversible competitive antagonism reflects antagonist affinity and propensity for dissociation with a higher-affinity ligand or agonist (or by virtue of higher concentration) being able to displace the antagonist. The use of aminophylline to "reverse" dipyridamole for cardiac stress testing is a classic example.

- Irreversible competitive antagonism results when the dissociation of the antagonist from the site of action occurs either slowly or not at all. Phenoxybenzamine is an irreversible antagonist used in pheochromocytoma patients for hypertension management.

- An inverse agonist produces a negative response and thus is more than simply antagonism. H_1 antihistamines such as loratadine may have previously been thought of as histamine antagonists; however, they act as inverse agonists, as do a number of common H_2 antihistamines, such as cimetidine and ranitidine.

- An allosteric modulator indirectly affects action; benzodiazepines are a typical example. They do not bind at the site of action but can produce an increase (allosteric agonist) or decrease (allosteric antagonist) in the action of the ligand or agonist. An allosteric antagonist may also be referred to as *noncompetitive antagonists*.

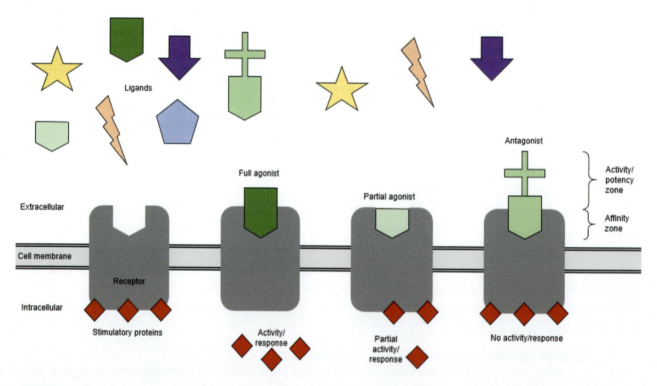

FIGURE 1-2 Schematic representation of the receptor concept. Ligands specific for a receptor may produce a response or a partial response across the cell membrane, or they may block a response.

Receptor Action

At this time, readers would find value in reviewing the anatomy and physiology of the nervous system using other resources. In brief, the nervous system is divided into the CNS and the peripheral nervous system (PNS). The CNS is further divided into the brain and the spinal cord, and the PNS is further divided into the somatic and autonomic nervous systems. The autonomic nervous system (ANS) is responsible for homeostasis, is not under conscious control, relies on autonomic reflexes, and is further divided into the parasympathetic nervous system, sympathetic nervous system, and enteric nervous system. Most organs and tissues have innervation from both parasympathetic and sympathetic nervous systems, and these generally elicit opposing actions (Table 1-2).

The key receptors for ANS action, medication targets, and adverse reactions include muscarinic and nicotinic cholinergic receptors, beta- and alpha-adrenoreceptors, and dopamine receptors. As outlined subsequently in more detail, there are 5 muscarinic receptor subtypes (M_1, M_2, M_3, M_4, and M_5), the first 3 of which are of most interest. There are 2 nicotinic receptor subtypes (N_N and N_M), 2 α-receptor subtypes ($α_1$ and $α_2$), 3 β-receptor subtypes ($β_1$, $β_2$, and $β_3$), and 4 dopamine receptor subtypes (D_1, D_2, D_3, and D_4). In terms of endogenous neurotransmitters or modulators, the key ones to keep in mind are acetylcholine, which has inhibitory effects on M_1 and M_2 and excitatory effects on N_M; the inhibitory effects of norepinephrine ($α_2$), dopamine (D_1 and D_2), serotonin (5-HT_1, 5-HT_2, and 5-HT_3), adenosine triphosphate (ATP) (P_2), and adenosine (P_1); histamine (H_3); and the excitatory effects of epinephrine ($β_2$) and angiotensin II (AT_1).

TABLE 1-2 Summary of Parasympathetic and Sympathetic Receptor Actions for the Autonomic Nervous System

Tissue	Parasympathetic		Sympathetic	
	Action	Receptor	Action	Receptor
Heart	Decreases heart rate, conduction velocity, force of contraction, and contractility	M_2	Increases heart rate, conduction velocity, force of contraction, and contractility	$β_1$ and some $β_2$
Arterioles			Constriction and dilation	$α_1$, $α_2$, $β_2$
Lung	Bronchoconstriction	M_3	Bronchodilation	$β_2$
Gastrointestinal tract	Increases motility, relaxes sphincters, increases secretion	M_3	Decreases motility	$α_2$, $β_2$
			Contracts sphincters	$α_1$
	Contracts gallbladder	M_3	Inhibits secretions	$α_2$
	Gastric acid secretion	M_1	Relaxes gallbladder	$β_2$
Eye	Contracts sphincter muscle (miosis) and ciliary muscle (near vision)	M_3	Contracts radial muscle (mydriasis)	$α_1$
			Relaxes ciliary muscle (far vision)	$β_2$
Bladder	Contracts wall and relaxes sphincter	M_3	Relaxes wall	$β_2$
			Contracts sphincter	$α_1$
Uterus	Contraction	M_3	Relaxation	$β_2$
			Contraction	$α$
Male glands	Erection	M_3	Ejaculation	$α_1$

Cholinergic Pharmacology

Acetylcholine (ACh) is the main neurotransmitter of the parasympathetic nervous system (Fig. 1-3), but it should be kept in mind that it is also associated with neurotransmission in the sympathetic and somatic nervous systems and has receptor action in the CNS. Medications that modulate cholinergic neurotransmission can potentially produce a wide range of effects; however, selectivity can be achieved by using medications specific for muscarinic or nicotinic receptors (or their subtypes). Nicotinic receptors are found in the sympathetic and parasympathetic nervous systems. Muscarinic receptors are activated by ACh released by parasympathetic nerves and also mediate the actions of the sympathetic cholinergic nerves (e.g., sweating).

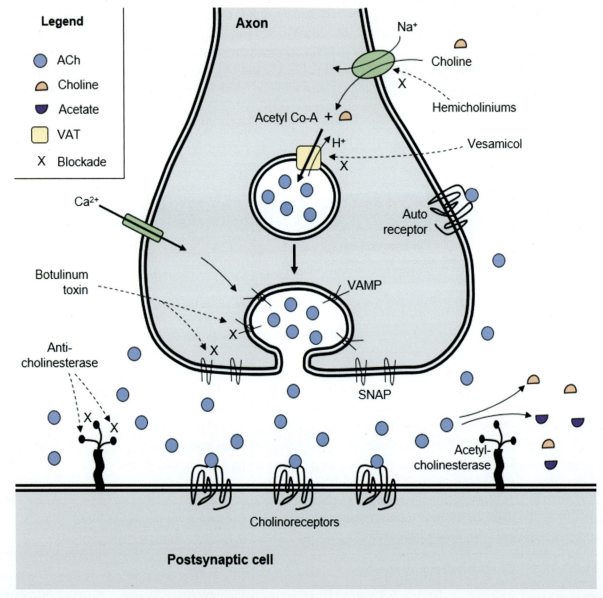

FIGURE 1-3 Schematic representation of cholinergic pharmacology. Choline transport into the presynaptic nerve can be inhibited through the sodium dependent transporter by hemicholinium medications. ACh is synthesized from choline and acetyl coenzyme A and is transported into the vesicle through the vesicle-associated transporter (VAT). This can be blocked by vesamicol. Release of ACh from the vesicle is dependent on calcium and modulation by synaptosome-associated proteins (SNAPs) and vesicle-associated membrane proteins (VAMPs). Vesicle release of ACh can be inhibited by botulinum toxin at SNAPs and VAMPs. Anticholinesterase can block synaptic breakdown of ACh to choline and acetate.

ACh activation of muscarinic receptors (G protein–coupled receptors) produce a range of actions. M_1 receptor activation tends to be neural, M_2 is cardiac and presynaptic, and M_3 is glands and smooth muscle. M_4 and M_5 act on CNS neurons and are similar in action to M_2 and M_1, respectively. Endogenous ACh produces decreased heart rate, decreased cardiac output, vasodilation, hypotension, arrhythmias, smooth muscle contraction (gut, bladder, bronchi), increased exocrine secretion (sweat, tears, saliva, etc.), pupil constriction (miosis), decreased intraocular pressure, and reduced ocular focal length (lens bulge). Muscarinic agonists (parasympathomimetics) are not widely used in clinical practice but have some roles in decreasing ocular pressure; they include bethanechol, pilocarpine, carbachol, methacholine, exogenous ACh (all as nonselective M_1, M_2, and M_3 agonists), and oxotremorine (selective M_1 agonist). Like muscarinic agonists, muscarinic antagonists are not widely used clinically, but they can be used as antispasmodics, muscle relaxants, bronchodilators, sedatives, and to treat urinary urgency and/or incontinence, dilate the pupil, treat peptic ulcer, or prevent motion sickness. Muscarinic antagonists (parasympatholytics) include belladonna alkaloids (atropine and scopolamine) and synthetic atropine substitutes. The effects include increased heart rate, vasoconstriction, hypertension, smooth muscle relaxation (gut, bladder, bronchi), bronchodilation, decreased exocrine secretion (sweat, tears, saliva, etc.), pupil dilation (mydriasis), increased intraocular pressure, cycloplegia, depression, restlessness, agitation, hyperactivity, and increased body temperature. Pirenzepine is selective for M_1, gallamine for M_2, and ipratropium bromide and darifenacin for M_3. Tolterodine is nonselective (M_2 and M_3), and nonselective medications for M_1, M_2, and M_3 receptors include atropine, scopolamine, and propantheline. Atropine is the most widely known muscarinic antagonist and is used intravenously to treat sinus bradycardia (Chapter 12), as a preanesthetic, as a low and long-lasting sedative, to treat tremor and rigidity in Parkinson disease, to treat motion sickness, as an antispasmodic, and as a mydriatic to counter miosis. Scopolamine is also known as hyoscine, which is used widely for motion sickness and nausea.

Nicotinic receptors are also cholinergic G protein–coupled receptors that respond to ACh. Nicotinic receptors are found in the CNS, PNS, and numerous tissues throughout the body. The name, as it suggests, comes from the action of nicotine, which does not act on muscarinic receptors. The N_N receptor subtype is associated with the neuronal autonomic ganglia, while the N_M receptor subtype is associated with the neuromuscular junction. ACh is an endogenous agonist of N_M, causing muscle contraction, and of N_N, causing increased postganglionic activation. Nicotinic agonists (parasympathomimetics) include nicotine (N_N and N_M), lobeline (N_M and N_N), carbachol (N_N), and anticholinesterases (cholinesterases break ACh into choline and acetate). Nicotinic antagonists (parasympatholytics) are sometimes referred to as *ganglion blockers* and *neuromuscular blockers*. Trimethaphan and mecamylamine are N_N antagonists used for hypertension treatment, while gallamine and vecuronium are N_M antagonists used as muscle relaxants.

Anticholinesterase medications (parasympathomimetics) are an interesting group of drugs (or chemicals). They can be short acting (2–3 min), medium acting (0.5–6 h) (carbamates), or irreversible (100+ h) (organophosphates). Organophosphates function at the neuromuscular junction, have CNS effects, and are used as insecticides and herbicides; their dangers as a toxin are widely reported. The sporadic and highly energized activity of an insect after being sprayed with insecticide (e.g., fly with fly spray) provides an insight into why organophosphates as nerve gas agents (sarin and tabun) are so devastating. Other than organophosphates and physostigmine, anticholinesterase medications do not have CNS effects. Cholinesterases inactivate ACh by breaking it down into choline and acetate (Fig. 1-3). The effects of anticholinesterases are to inhibit that breakdown and increase ACh, which leads to increased exocrine secretion, bradycardia, hypotension, smooth muscle contraction, pupil constriction, muscle fasciculation, and increased twitch tension. CNS excitation, convulsions, and respiratory failure occur with physostigmine, and peripheral nerve demyelination occurs with organophosphates. It should be noted that cholinesterase inactivated by organophosphates can be reactivated with pralidoxime. The main therapeutic applications of anticholinesterase medications are to treat myasthenia gravis (edrophonium, neostigmine, and pyridostigmine), as eye drops in glaucoma (physostigmine and ecothiopate), and to reverse neuromuscular-blocking drugs (neostigmine). If neostigmine is given intravenously, atropine can be used to block N_M receptors in the heart to prevent cardiac depression.

8 Pharmacology Primer for Medications

Nicotinic receptors can also be inhibited or blocked at the ganglion (N_N) with ganglion-blocking medications (parasympatholytics) that inhibit ACh release (Fig. 1-3). The results of this inhibition include decreased arterial pressure, decreased cardiac output, vasodilation, decreased gut motility, urine retention, postural hypotension, and impotence. The key medications in this class include botulinum toxin (Botox), which inhibits ACh release; hemicholinium, which inhibits ACh formation by blocking choline uptake; and vesamicol, which inhibits the vesicle-associated transporter to block release.

Adrenergic (Norepinephrine) Pharmacology

Endogenous *catecholamines* include norepinephrine (noradrenaline), epinephrine (adrenaline), and dopamine, which is the precursor for norepinephrine (NE) synthesis (Fig. 1-4). Epinephrine is released from the adrenal gland and circulates systemically, while NE is released from sympathetic nerve terminals. As previously outlined, NE acts as a neurotransmitter via activation of α- and β-adrenoreceptors. In terms of potency for receptors, NE has the greatest potency for α agonism, followed by epinephrine and then isoprenaline. In contrast, potency of β-agonism is greatest for isoprenaline, followed by epinephrine and then NE. Whereas NE and epinephrine are endogenous catecholamines, ephedrine and amphetamine are noncatechol agonists.

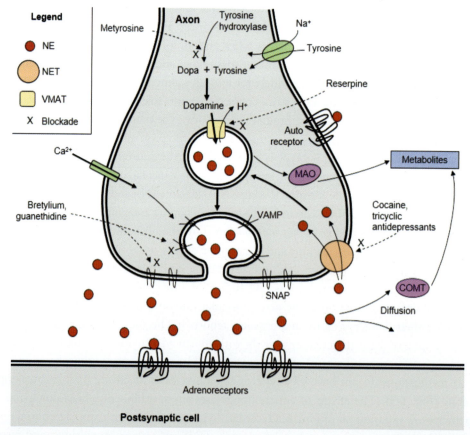

FIGURE 1-4 Schematic representation of adrenergic pharmacology. Tyrosine is transported into the presynaptic nerve, where it is synthesized with dopa into dopamine, but this process can be inhibited by metyrosine blockade of tyrosine hydroxylase. NE is synthesized from dopamine inside the vesicle. Dopamine is transported into the vesicle through the vesicular monoamine transporter (VMAT). This can be blocked by reserpine. Release of NE from the vesicle is dependent on calcium and modulation by synaptosome-associated proteins (SNAP) and vesicle-associated membrane proteins (VAMP). Vesicle release of NE can be inhibited by bretylium and guanethidine at SNAPs and VAMPs. Cocaine and tricyclic antidepressants can inhibit reuptake of NE into the presynaptic nerve via the NE transporter (NET). NE is diffused and either undergoes reuptake (NET) or is metabolized by catechol-O-methyltransferase (COMT). NE can also be metabolized within the presynaptic neuron by monoamine oxidase (MAO).

Agonism of α-adrenoreceptors inhibits smooth muscle contraction in the gut, whereas $α_1$ activation specifically contracts smooth muscle (except the gut) and stimulates glycolysis in the liver. Agonism of $α_2$ inhibits ACh and NE release from nerve terminals (Figs. 1-3 and 1-4). Selective $α_1$-agonist medications tend to be used as decongestants and include phenylephrine, oxymetazoline, naphazoline, and xylometazoline. Selective $α_2$-agonist medications tend to be used for hypertension, migraine, and withdrawal from drugs of addiction with clonidine being the main medication in this class. NE (treats severe hypotension), epinephrine (treats bronchospasm, glaucoma, and anaphylaxis), and methoxamine (decongestant and hypotensive) are direct-acting, nonselective α-agonists. Ephedrine is a nonselective, indirect α- and β-agonist that is used as a decongestant and for asthma, incontinence, and hypotension. Amphetamine is a nonselective, indirect α- and β-agonist that is used for attention deficit hyperactivity disorder (ADHD), fatigue, narcolepsy, and obesity with the methamphetamine variation exhibiting greater CNS potency (see discussion in Chapter 15).

Antagonists of the α-adrenoreceptor cause vasodilation, decreased arterial pressure, and hypotension. Prazosin and indoramin are selective $α_1$-antagonists and are useful for essential hypertension, and tamsulosin is selective for $α_{1A}$-antagonism and has been used in benign prostate hypertrophy. Yohimbine is a selective $α_2$-antagonist that has aphrodisiac properties. Nonselective α-antagonists include phenoxybenzamine, phentolamine, and tolazoline and may be useful for hypertension, pheochromocytoma, and Raynaud syndrome. Labetalol is better known as a β-blocker but also has nonselective α antagonism.

A more detailed discussion of β-adrenoreceptors is provided in Chapter 8. Agonism of $β_1$-receptors increases the heart rate, cardiac contraction force, cardiac output, and myocardial oxygen use but can cause arrhythmia. Agonism of $β_2$-receptors relaxes smooth muscle (bronchodilation, vasodilation), increases glycolysis in liver and muscle, and decreases histamine release. Agonism of $β_3$-receptors releases fatty acids (lipolysis). Dobutamine is a selective $β_1$-receptor agonist that is used in nuclear medicine for stress testing (see Chapter 8). Salbutamol, terbutaline, salmeterol, and metaproterenol are all selective $β_2$-receptor agonists largely used as bronchodilators. Epinephrine, isoprenaline, and dopexamine are nonselective β-receptor agonists.

As previously outlined, there are 3 subtypes for β-adrenergic receptors. The following 2 are of interest:

- $β_1$-receptors are found in the heart and kidneys with responsibility for increasing the rate and force of cardiac contraction and renin secretion respectively (Fig. 1-5).
- $β_2$-receptors are found in the lungs, liver, and skeletal muscle, causing vasodilation, bronchodilation, glycogenolysis, and glucagon release (Fig. 1-6).

Antagonists of the β-adrenergic receptors are referred to as *β-blockers* and function by competitive blockade of the actions of catecholamines. β-Blockers can be selective for either $β_1$ (atenolol, bisoprolol, esmolol, and metoprolol) or $β_2$ (butaxamine); however, it is common for β-blockers to be nonselective (propranolol, sotalol, oxprenolol, and pindolol) or nonselective for α and β receptors (labetalol and carvedilol), although they do not generally act on $β_3$. Antagonism of the β-adrenoreceptor results in decreased heart rate, decreased contraction force, decreased oxygen demand, peripheral vasoconstriction, bronchospasm, glycogenolysis inhibition, decreased lipolysis, decreased high-density lipoprotein (HDL), and decreased intraocular pressure. Consequently, selective and nonselective β-blockers are used to treat hypertension, arrhythmia, angina, and glaucoma.

Pharmacology of Other Important Receptors

Serotonin, or 5-hydroxytryptamine (5-HT), is a monoamine neurotransmitter produced primarily in the wall of the intestine (90%) with some CNS production. 5-HT is stored in platelets and is released in response to vasoconstriction and stress. The actions of 5-HT include increased smooth muscle contraction (bronchi, gut, uterus), vasoconstriction in large vessels, vasodilation in arterioles, increased microvascular permeability, platelet aggregation, stimulation of peripheral nociceptive nerve endings (pain), and CNS excitation. Increased 5-HT can cause migraine; carcinoid syndrome produces increased 5-HT secretion; and depression can be associated with lower levels of 5-HT. 5-HT agonists include selective serotonin reuptake inhibitors (SSRIs) that are used to treat depression; 5-HT$_1$ agonists such as buspirone, sumatriptan, and naratriptan that are used for vasoconstriction in migraine (and contraindicated in coronary artery disease); 5-HT$_2$ agonists such as dexfenfluramine that are used for appetite suppression; and 5-HT$_4$ agonists such as metoclopramide that are used for anxiety, memory, and gut motility or cisapride used for gastroesophageal reflux and gastroparesis.

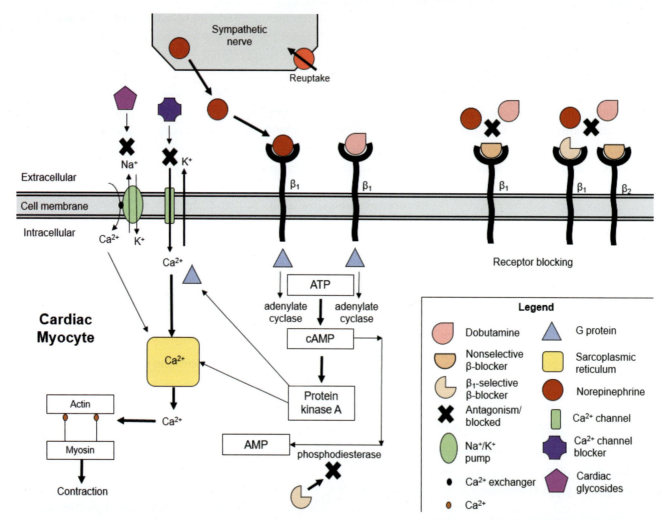

FIGURE 1-5 Schematic representation of the action of inotropic and chronotropic agents in a cardiac myocyte. Endogenous norepinephrine is released from the sympathetic nerve. Note that in a re-uptake mechanism failure (e.g., heart failure), excess norepinephrine is available for beta-1 (β$_1$) activation. In the extracellular space, endogenous norepinephrine and exogenous dobutamine can couple with β$_1$-receptors. Receptor β$_1$ couples with an adenylate cyclase–stimulating G protein to drive increased intracellular calcium, which facilitates formation of actin-myosin cross-bridges and produces an increased force and rate of contraction. This response can be antagonized by a β-blocker either nonselective (e.g., propranolol) or selective for β$_1$ (e.g., atenolol). Calcium channel blockers act to antagonize the voltage-dependent calcium channel to block the inotropic and chronotropic contraction response. Likewise, cardiac glycosides such as digoxin antagonize the sodium-potassium pump to increase intracellular calcium via the calcium exchanger, increasing the force of contraction.

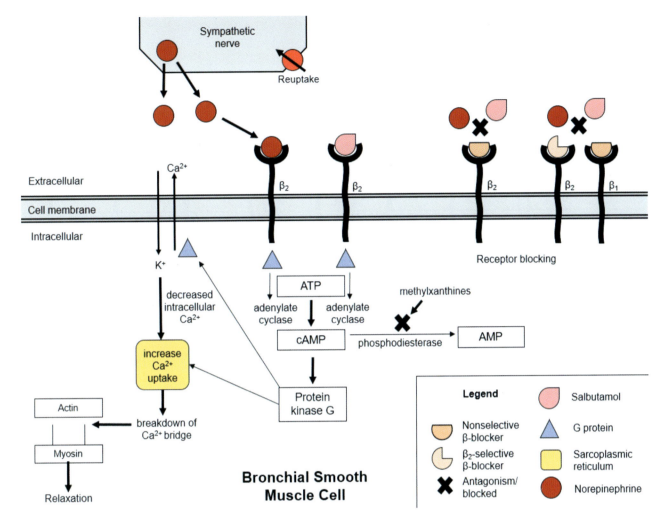

FIGURE 1-6 Schematic representation of the action of β-agonism in a bronchial smooth muscle. Endogenous NE is released from the sympathetic nerve. In the extracellular space, endogenous NE and exogenous salbutamol can couple with $β_2$-receptors. Receptor $β_2$ couples with an adenylate cyclase–stimulating G protein to produce decreased intracellular calcium through calcium efflux and uptake in the sarcoplasmic reticulum, leading a reduction in actin-myosin cross-bridge formation, and producing smooth muscle relaxation and bronchodilation. Inhibition of phosphodiesterase conversion of cyclic adenosine monophosphate (cAMP) to adenosine monophosphate (AMP) by methylxanthines (e.g., caffeine, theobromine, theophylline) further decreases intracellular calcium. This response can be antagonized by a β-blocker, either nonselective (e.g., labetalol) or selective for $β_2$ (e.g., butoxamine).

5-HT antagonists block synthesis, block storage, block receptors, and have some nonspecific activity. Cyproheptadine and methysergide block $5HT_2$ to inhibit gut smooth muscle activity in carcinoid syndrome. Ketanserin blocks $5HT_2$ and $5HT_{1C}$ to inhibit platelet aggregation and treat hypertension. Ondansetron blocks $5HT_3$ to prevent nausea. Ergot alkaloids target α-, D-, and 5HT-receptors with the most common being ergometrine (post-partum hemorrhage), methysergide (migraine), and ergotamine (treats migraine and nausea).

Purine pharmacology is discussed further in Chapter 8. Adenosine is a natural regulator of blood flow and coronary demand, acting directly on adenosine cell surface receptors (Fig. 1-7). Adenosine also modulates sympathetic neurotransmission. There are 4 main adenosine receptor subtypes. A_1 blocks AV conduction, reduces the force of cardiac contraction (negative inotropic and chronotropic action), decreases glomerular filtration rate, causes cardiac depression, produces renal vasoconstriction, decreases CNS activity, and causes bronchoconstriction. A_{2A} is responsible for the anti-inflammatory response, vasodilation, decreased blood pressure, decreased

12 Pharmacology Primer for Medications

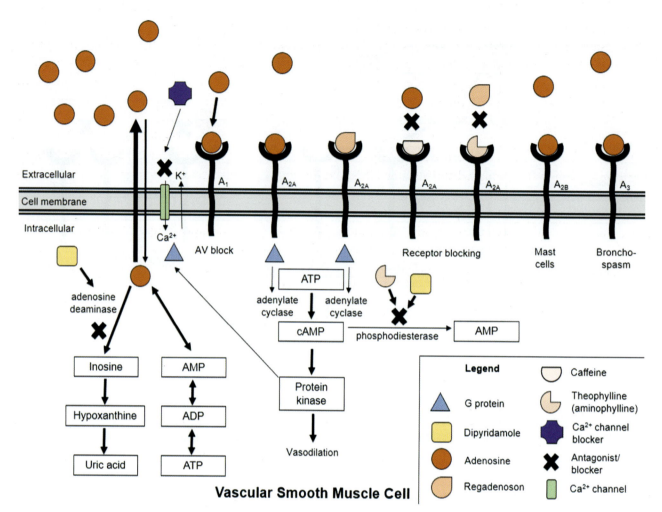

FIGURE 1-7 Schematic representation of the action of vasodilating agents in a vascular smooth muscle cell. Endogenous adenosine is produced in vascular smooth muscle cells and leaves the cell. In the extracellular space, endogenous and exogenous adenosine can couple with the 4 types of adenosine receptors. Receptor A_1 couples with an adenylate cyclase inhibitory G protein to produce atrioventricular (AV) block and some bronchoconstriction. Receptor A_3 couples with an adenylate cyclase inhibitory G protein to produce bronchoconstriction. Receptor A_{2B} couples with an adenylate cyclase–stimulating G protein to produce mast cell degranulation, peripheral vasodilation, and antiplatelet activity. Receptor A_{2A} couples with an adenylate cyclase–stimulating G protein to convert ATP to cyclic adenosine monophosphate (cAMP) and to produce coronary and peripheral vasodilation. Regadenoson is selective for receptor A_{2A} to produce vasodilation. Caffeine has greater selectivity for receptors A_1 and A_{2A} to antagonize those actions. Theophylline (aminophylline and tea) has 3 to 5 times higher potency than caffeine in antagonizing receptors A_1 and A_{2A}, whereas theobromine (typical of chocolate) has lower potency than caffeine. Dipyridamole antagonizes adenosine deaminase, which reduces adenosine metabolism and thus increases availability of adenosine in the extracellular space. Dipyridamole is also a phosphodiesterase inhibitor, so it blocks conversion of cAMP to AMP, further increasing vasodilation. Calcium channel blockers act to antagonize the voltage-dependent calcium channel to block vasodilation.

CNS activity, inhibition of platelet aggregation, and bronchodilation. A_{2B} stimulates phospholipase activity and release of mast cell mediators, and it has actions on the colon and bladder (also contributes to bronchoconstriction). A_3 stimulates phospholipase activity and release of mast cell mediators (also contributes to bronchoconstriction). Endogenous adenosine is produced in vascular smooth muscle cells and leaves the cell. In the extracellular space, endogenous and exogenous adenosine can couple with the 4 types of adenosine receptors. The principle agonists include the neurotransmitter adenosine and the adenosine phosphates adenosine monophosphate (AMP), adenosine diphosphate (ADP), ATP, and the A_{2A} selective Regadenoson. Dipyridamole is an indirect agonist that blocks adenosine metabolism, thereby increasing bioavailability of adenosine. Xanthines are purines found throughout the body that structurally resemble the adenine portion of adenosine; this similarity allows antagonism of adenosine. *Methylation* (CH_3) of the xanthine produces a number of methylxanthines, including caffeine, theobromine, and theophylline. Caffeine is typically found in coffee, tea, guarana, and yerba mate; theobromine in chocolate and yerba mate; and theophylline mostly in tea (and the medication aminophylline).

Histamine is an amine that has wide dispersion in the body, particularly in mast cells of the lung, skin, and gut. Histamine release from the mast cell is mediated by an interaction between the antigen and the IgE antibody (Fig. 1-8) or in response to substance P. There are 4 histamine receptors; however, the main 2 are H_1 and H_2. H_1 acts on smooth muscle, endothelial tissue, the CNS, and the heart to increase vascular permeability, cause vasodilation, cause smooth muscle contraction (e.g., bronchoconstriction), and stimulate nerve endings to produce pain and itch. H_2 acts on the gastric parietal cells (refer to Chapter 9), neutrophils, the CNS, and the heart, with the main action being the secretion of gastric acid and increased heart rate and cardiac output. H_3 acts on the CNS and intestines to inhibit histamine release, and H_4 acts on the immune system. Histamine has been implicated in 3 common conditions: peptic ulcer associated with H_2, H_1-mediated type 1 sensitivity (urticaria, hay fever), and asthma (bronchoconstriction).

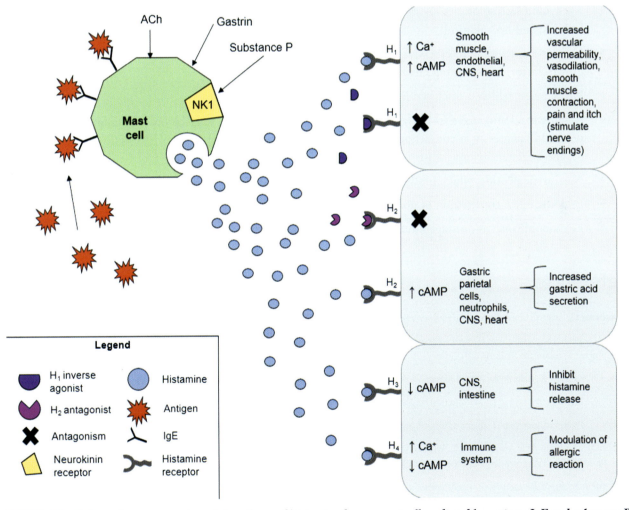

FIGURE 1-8 Schematic representation of the release of histamine from a mast cell mediated by antigen-IgE and substance P activity.

Histamine antagonists are generally referred to as *antihistamines*, but it is important to get the pharmacological classification correct. A histamine antagonist refers to H_2 antagonism by medications such as ranitidine and cimetidine, which are used to treat peptic ulcer and are discussed in more detail in Chapter 9. Antihistamine refers to H_1 medications that, rather than being antagonists of the receptor, are inverse agonists of the H_1 receptor. That is, antihistamines not only block the receptor but also produce an effect that opposes the normal histamine agonistic effect. First-generation antihistamines such as dimenhydrinate, diphenhydramine (Benadryl), and promethazine (Phenergan) are often referred to as *sedating antihistamines* because they typically have H_1 inverse agonist activity in conjunction with ACh receptor antagonism and some agonism on α and 5-HT receptors (1). Second-generation antihistamines such as loratadine, cetirizine, and fexofenadine are erroneously referred to as *nonsedating antihistamines* when they are technically *less*-sedating antihistamines. Both first- and second-generation antihistamines are used for allergic reactions, and first-generation antihistamines are also used for motion sickness and for sedation.

A number of other important classes of medications that act on receptors warrant brief mention:

- Peptides such as vasopressin, oxytocin, and cyclosporine
- Bradykinin, which acts on $β_1$- and $β_2$-receptors
- Tachykinin acting on neurokinin receptors 1, 2, and 3 (NK_1, NK_2, NK_3), including substance P, neurokinin A, and neurokinin B
- Cytokines, including interleukins 1 through 10, interferons, tumor necrosis factor (TNF), platelet-derived growth factor, transforming growth factor B, and chemokines
- Nitric oxide, which is discussed in more detail in Chapter 8
- Angiotensin I and angiotensin II, which encapsulate renin blockers (e.g., clonidine), renin inhibitors (e.g., pepstatin), angiotensin-converting enzyme (ACE) inhibitors (e.g., captopril, which is discussed in Chapter 6), and angiotensin antagonists (e.g., losartan)
- Natriuretic peptide, which inhibits renin, angiotensin, and vasopressin secretion
- Endothelin for constriction of nonvascular smooth muscle
- Eicosanoids such as prostaglandins, thromboxanes, leukotrienes, and platelet-activating factor

References

Asperheim K, Favaro J. *Introduction to Pharmacology*. 12th ed. St Louis, MO: Elsevier; 2012.

Block JH, Beale JM. *Wilson and Gisvold's Textbook of Organic Medicinal and Pharmaceutical Chemistry*. 12th ed. Philadelphia, PA: Lippincott Williams & Wilkins; 2011.

Bryant B, Knights K, Salerno E. *Pharmacology for Health Professionals*. 2nd ed. Sydney, Australia: Mosby Elsevier; 2007.

Currie G. Pharmacology part 1: introduction to pharmacodynamics. *J Nucl Med Technol*. 2018;46:81–86.

Currie G. Pharmacology part 2: introduction to pharmacokinetics. *J Nucl Med Technol*. 2018;46:221–230.

Golan DE, Tashjian AH, Armstrong EJ, Armstrong AW. *Principles of Pharmacology: The Pathophysiologic Basis of Drug Therapy*. 3rd ed. Philadelphia, PA: Lippincott Williams & Wilkins; 2012.

Greenstein B. *Rapid Revision in Clinical Pharmacology*. New York, NY: Radcliffe Publishing; 2008.

Hacker M, Messer W, Bachmann K. *Pharmacology: Principles and Practice*. London, England: Elsevier; 2009.

Jambhekar SS, Breen PJ. *Basic Pharmacokinetics*. London, England: Pharmaceutical Press; 2009.

Katzung BG, Masters SB, Trevor AJ. *Basic and Clinical Pharmacology.* 12th ed. New York, NY: McGraw Hill; 2012.

Rang H, Dale M, Ritter J, Flower R. *Rang and Dale's Pharmacology.* 6th ed. London, England: Churchill Livingston; 2008.

Stumpf WE. The dose makes the medicine. *Drug Discov Today.* 2006;11(11–12):550–555.

Waller D, Renwick A, Hillier K. *Medical Pharmacology and Therapeutics.* 2nd ed. London, England: Elsevier; 2006.

CHAPTER 2

Pharmacodynamics

Chapter Objectives

Specific learning outcomes (page ix) of this text addressed in this chapter:

- Apply the principles of pharmacology to the safe and effective use of medicines.
- Recognize general, patient-specific, and scenario-specific risks, precautions, and contraindications for use of medicines.
- Apply the pharmacokinetic and pharmacodynamic principles of medications to identify and explain normal and adverse reactions to medications.

After reading, digesting, reflecting on, and reviewing the content of this chapter, readers should be able to

1. Demonstrate command of key pharmacodynamic terms.
2. Demonstrate enhanced understanding of the principles associated with pharmacodynamics.
3. Demonstrate critical thinking to effect problem solving related to drug receptor interactions and dose-response relationships.
4. Recognize, explain, and interpret clinical problems and evidence in relation to drug interactions.
5. Apply knowledge of the general pharmacodynamic principles and concepts in a translational manner to clinical practice.

Key Terms

agonist	bioavailability	endogenous	pharmacokinetics	specificity
antagonist	dissociation	efficacy	potency	therapeutic index
antibody	dose-response	LD_{50}	receptor	therapeutic window
antigen	drug	ligand	selectivity	tolerance
affinity	ED_{50}	pharmacodynamics	sensitization	toxicity

Some of the text, tables, and figures in this chapter were extracted from "Pharmacology Part 1: Introduction to Pharmacology and Pharmacodynamics" by Geoff Currie (*J Nucl Med Technol.* 2018;46:81–86).

Introduction

Pharmacodynamics is the study of how a medication affects the body—the physiological effects of the medication. These effects can relate to the intended therapeutic action of the medication and also to unwanted adverse reactions. Radiopharmaceuticals in particular, but also contrast media used in computed tomography (CT) and magnetic resonance imaging (MRI), are intended to be as physiologically benign as possible. The tracer principle in radiopharmacy limits the pharmacodynamic action of radiopharmaceuticals. This is clearly important to ensure the integrity of the physiological process being investigated. In contrast, therapeutic medications, including interventional medications used in imaging and medical oncology, are designed to generate a physiological response. It is important to understand pharmacodynamic principles from the context of interventional medications used in practice, adjunctive medications that may be needed to respond to a patients' condition, interfering medications that could alter the biodistribution of radiopharmaceuticals and contrast agents, and cessation medications that may alter the physiological process being investigated.

Drug Action

A number of other important terms need to be understood to characterize drugs. *Specificity* is the measure of a receptor's ability to respond to a single ligand. Low specificity generally results in physiological responses not targeted or intended by the drug, and side effects provide a good example. It is not uncommon for a drug to be developed for a theoretical action, but poor specificity for that action undermines efficacy, while a side effect may emerge as the new targeted role. A classic example is sildenafil (Viagra), which was developed to treat hypertension and angina. It was not particularly effective, but an observed side effect has become the new targeted role of the drug. *Selectivity* defines the ability of the receptor to distinguish between drugs and has the same implications as specificity; the terms are often used interchangeably. Adenosine is nonselective (4 adenosine receptors with different actions) and consequently has the unwanted effect of potential bronchospasm (A_1 receptor), while Regadenoson is selective for A_{2A} receptor (vasodilation and bronchodilation).

Affinity defines the strength of attraction between the drug and its receptor. A high affinity is generally associated with a lower dose requirement (compared to low affinity for the same receptor). *Potency* describes the relationship between the drug dose and the magnitude of the effect. High potency induces a strong effect with a low drug dose. *Efficacy* is the in vivo potency, the maximum response achieved from a drug. The interaction (e.g., absorption, metabolism, excretion) of the drug in the body may alter the relative *bioavailability* and thereby change the theoretical effect of the drug. Rapid metabolism of a high-potency drug, for example, may render it low efficacy, whereas rapid absorption, minimal first-pass metabolism, and delayed excretion may see higher efficacy despite much lower potency.

Generally speaking, the ideal drug would be easily administered and fully absorbed; would not be plasma bound; would have rapid onset, useful duration of action, chemical stability, high selectivity and specificity, high affinity, high potency, and high efficacy; would have no interactions; would undergo spontaneous elimination; and would show high *therapeutic index* (no adverse effects). Unfortunately, there are no examples of synthetic or natural drugs that satisfy all of these criteria. Furthermore, there may be circumstances in which these ideal properties are not wanted. For example, high affinity can also cause a prolonged action, which may not be desirable (e.g., dipyridamole vs. adenosine). High potency is not always desirable, and poor selectivity might provide a good case example; that is, a drug that has nonselective biodistribution will have a poorer safety profile (compared to a less potent alternative) if it is also highly potent.

Drug Receptor Interactions

Human receptors are generally proteins, so it is worth reviewing protein structure. Nonetheless, receptors are not the only targets for drug binding. Other targets include ion channels, enzymes, and transporters. While there are about 300 amino acids present in various animals, plants, and microbial systems, only 20 amino acids are coded by DNA to appear in proteins in humans. Cells produce proteins with different properties and activities by joining the 20 amino acids in many different combinations and sequences. The properties of proteins are determined by the physical and chemical properties of the amino acids. Proteins can be large molecules with complex 3-dimensional shapes and structures. Protein structure is best considered in terms of primary, secondary, tertiary, and quaternary structures. The primary structure simply relates to the protein configuration associated with the amino acid sequence—the order of amino acids in the polypeptide chain (peptide bonds). The secondary structure relates to the way the polypeptide chain is folded (hydrogen bonds), creating pleated sheets and helices. The tertiary structure relates to the interactions between amino acid side chains (hydrogen bonds, disulfide binds, ionic binds, and hydrophobic interactions). The quaternary structure relates to interactions between different polypeptide chains within the same protein. Perhaps a simple way to consider protein structure would be that primary structure is an array of letters, secondary structure is creation of words from the letters, tertiary structure is a sentence from the words, and quaternary structure is a paragraph of multiple sentences woven together. From an imaging context, beta-amyloid plaque associated with dementia arises from a folding error (secondary structure) that results in cleavage of the protein.

All types of bonding are involved in drug receptor interactions. Figure 2-1 uses physical characteristics to schematically represent receptors, but note that each drug-binding site has a unique chemical characteristic that is largely defined by the amino acids at the binding site. How the drug and receptor interact (structure, shape, and reactivity) determines how tightly they bind. A short duration of action for a drug is generally associated with weaker bonds, whereas stronger bonds produce drug-receptor interactions of longer duration (potentially irreversible). In decreasing strength, the binding forces associated with *drug-receptor binding* include the following:

- Covalent bonds
- Ionic interactions
- Hydrogen bonds
- Hydrophobic effects
- Van der Waals forces

In most cases, a combination for these interactions is involved for each drug-receptor interaction.

When considering the drug-receptor binding, the rate at which the association between drug and receptor occurs relative to the rate of dissociation defines affinity, or the strength of attraction. Low affinity, and thus higher dose requirements, is associated with drugs in which the rate of dissociation is appreciably higher than the rate of association. Conversely, high-affinity drugs requiring lower doses for effect tend to be associated with a rate of association (k_1) well in excess of the rate of dissociation (k_2). The dissociation constant (k_d) is simply the ratio k_2/k_1 (smaller means higher affinity) and provides an insight into both the drug effect and the half maximal effect.

$$k_d = k_2 \div k_1$$

20 Pharmacology Primer for Medications

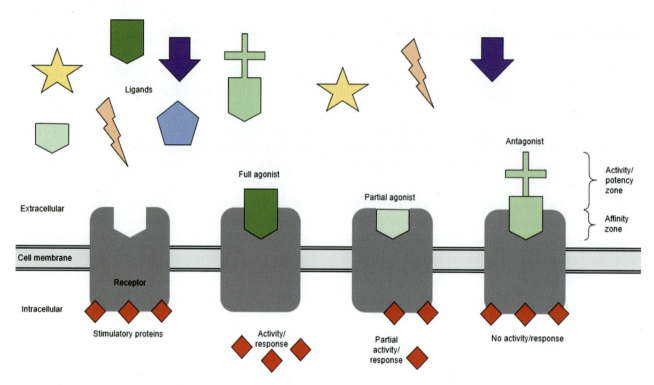

FIGURE 2-1 Schematic representation of the receptor concept. Ligands specific for a receptor may produce a response or partial response across the cell membrane, or they may block a response.

Dose-Response Relationship

The effect of a drug is a product of the concentration of the drug at the binding site; however, specific responses to drug concentrations are typically nonlinear, and considering that drug effect is a function of dose and time, a significant level of complexity exists. To simplify this concept, *dose-response curves* are generated using a logarithmic x-axis scale for drug dose and a linear y-axis for effect at a specific time point (e.g., equilibrium [i.e., steady state], or at maximum effect) (Fig. 2-2). The time to steady state is influenced by a number of factors, including the rate of dissociation (k_2). It should be kept in mind that the drug-response curve varies among individuals for the same drug and dose across gender, weight, race, and age demographics and for an individual (e.g., level of hydration, blood pressure, and self-limiting illness). Thus, a drug-response curve represents a mean response that can be generally applied to a population. The dose-response curve provides a valuable insight into drug characteristics and allows understanding of specific pharmacodynamic concepts:

- Dose response, slope of the curve, maximal effect (Fig. 2-2)
- Potency and efficacy (Fig. 2-3A)
- ED_{50} (50% effective dose), LD_{50} (50% lethal dose) therapeutic window (TW), and therapeutic index (TI) (Fig. 2-3B)
- *Tolerance* (Fig. 2-4A)
- *Sensitization* (Fig. 2-4B)
- Activation and antagonism (Fig. 2-5) including allosteric regulation (enzyme regulation through binding to an effector site other than the enzymes active site)

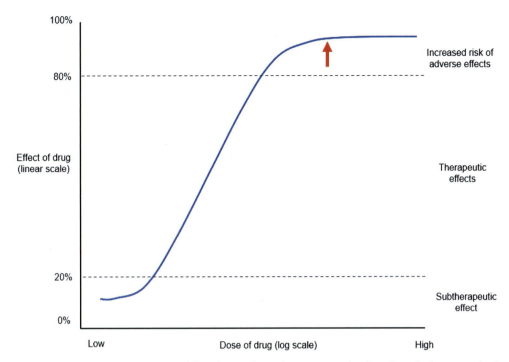

FIGURE 2-2 Steady-state dose-response curve. The plateau (arrow) represents the dose for which maximal effect is achieved and above which additional dosage does not change the effect. There is also a drug dose below which no noticeable effect will be observed. The slope of the line provides an indication of how small (steep) or large (flat) a change in dose is required to observe increased effects.

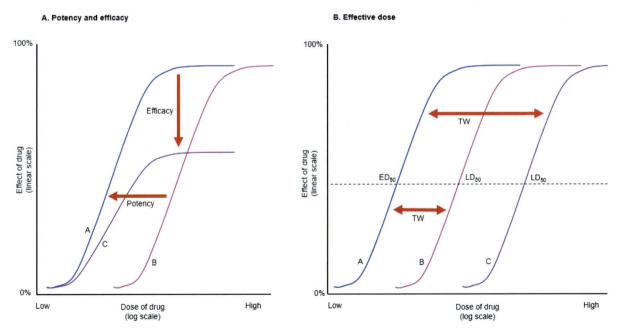

FIGURE 2-3 Dose-response curve representing the concepts of potency and efficacy (A). High potency (drug A) is represented by a shift to the left from drug B, strong effect with low dose. Submaximal effect (drug C) despite increasing dose demonstrates lower efficacy compared to drug A. The dose-response curve can also be used to represent the same drug but with different outcomes (B). Curve A represents the targeted therapeutic effect and ED_{50} is a dose that produces an effect in 50% of the population. Curve C represents the same drug but more dire effects, and LD_{50} is a dose that produces death in 50% of the population. The difference between curves A and C is the TW, or the margin of safety, and can be represented as the TI by expressing the ratio LD_{50}/ED_{50}. Curve B provides an example of a drug that would have a narrow TW, or lower TI.

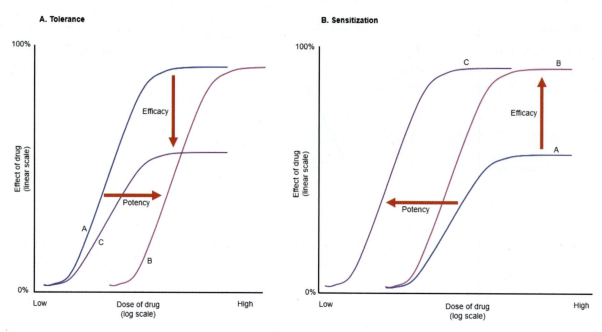

FIGURE 2-4 Following repeated doses of a drug, a patient may develop tolerance (A), which means the patient needs higher doses to generate the same effect (move from curve A to B) or has lower effects from the same dose (curve A to C). It should be noted that an individual may develop tolerance to the targeted effect of a drug without developing tolerance to side effects, which changes the TI. Following repeated doses of a drug, a patient may also develop sensitization (B), which means the patient generates greater effects from the same dose (move from curve A to B) or experiences the same effects from a lower dose (curve A to C). It should be noted that an individual may develop sensitization to one effect of a drug without developing sensitization to other effects.

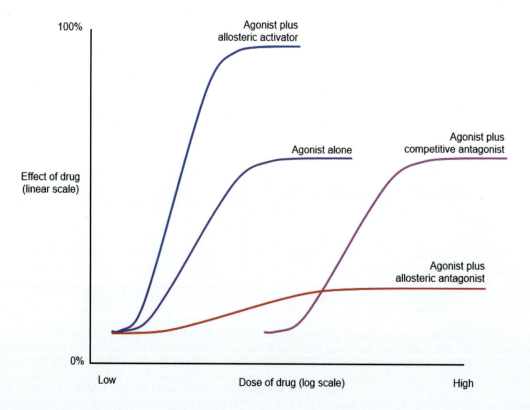

FIGURE 2-5 Agonist activity at a receptor may be altered by an antagonist, potentiated by allosteric activation of other receptors, or inhibited by allosteric inhibition at other receptors.

Drug Interactions

Drug interactions can cause harm due to either increased drug effect (*toxicity*) or decreased drug effect leading to therapeutic failure. A number of strategies can be used to reduce the impact of drug interactions. The most appropriate for those in the medical radiation sciences include the following:

* Recognizing potential interactions between drugs (e.g., assessing patient medication history prior to administration of interventional medication)
* Recognizing factors that might potentiate drug interaction (e.g., age, diet, hydration level, comorbidity, environmental factors)
* Recognizing drugs with a narrow TI

Interactions between drugs (*drug-drug interaction*) are an important cause of patient harm. Interactions are particularly important to consider in medical imaging or radiation therapy patients because the mean age of patients exceeds 60 years, and both *polypharmacy* (concurrent use of multiple medications) and the degenerative effects of aging on organ function increase the risk of interaction. Pharmacokinetic drug-drug interactions are discussed in Chapter 3. Pharmacodynamic drug-drug interactions result in cumulative (e.g., angiotensin-converting enzyme [ACE] inhibitors act on potassium-sparing diuretics to lead to hyperkalemia), additive (e.g., ACE inhibitors and loop diuretics reduce blood pressure), synergistic (e.g., alcohol and sedatives have an effect greater than the sum of the individual drugs), or antagonistic effects (e.g., nonsteroidal anti-inflammatory reduce the effect of ACE inhibitors on blood pressure) (Fig. 2-6).

While dose-response curves provide some translational principles to therapeutic nuclear medicine and medical oncology, the tracer principle associated with radiopharmaceuticals generally relegates pharmacodynamics to the periphery. *Pharmacodynamics* is the study of how the drug affects the body, and by design, radiopharmaceuticals should have little or no effect on the body. Nonetheless, pharmacodynamics provides essential insights into the effects of contrast media, interventional medications, and adjunctive medications on patients. Furthermore, understanding of pharmacodynamic principles provides the tools to mitigate drug interactions between adjunctive and interventional medications and medications the patient may have prescribed or self-prescribed.

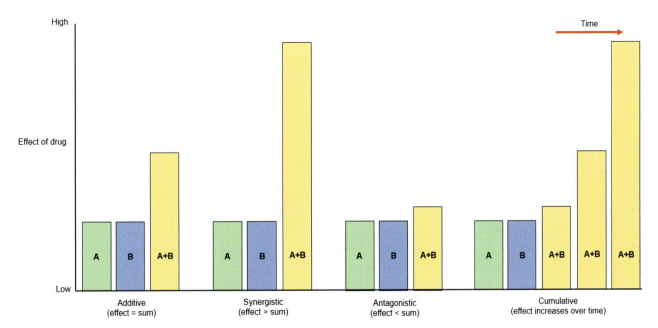

FIGURE 2-6 Schematic representation of pharmacodynamic drug-drug interactions.

References

Asperheim K, Favaro J. *Introduction to Pharmacology*. 12th ed. St Louis, MO: Elsevier; 2012.

Block JH, Beale JM. *Wilson and Gisvold's Textbook of Organic Medicinal and Pharmaceutical Chemistry*. 12th ed. Philadelphia, PA: Lippincott Williams & Wilkins; 2011.

Bryant B, Knights K, Salerno E. *Pharmacology for Health Professionals*. 2nd ed. Sydney, Australia: Mosby Elsevier; 2007.

Currie G. Pharmacology part 1: introduction to pharmacodynamics. *J Nucl Med Technol*. 2018;46:81–86.

Currie G. Pharmacology part 2: introduction to pharmacokinetics. *J Nucl Med Technol*. 2018;46:221–230.

Golan DE, Tashjian AH, Armstrong EJ, Armstrong AW. *Principles of Pharmacology: The Pathophysiologic Basis of Drug Therapy*. 3rd ed. Philadelphia, PA: Lippincott Williams & Wilkins; 2012.

Greenstein B. *Rapid Revision in Clinical Pharmacology*. New York, NY: Radcliffe Publishing; 2008.

Hacker M, Messer W, Bachmann K. *Pharmacology: Principles and Practice*. London, England: Elsevier; 2009.

Jambhekar SS, Breen PJ. *Basic Pharmacokinetics*. London, England: Pharmaceutical Press; 2009.

Katzung BG, Masters SB, Trevor AJ. *Basic and Clinical Pharmacology*. 12th ed. New York, NY: McGraw Hill; 2012.

Rang H, Dale M, Ritter J, Flower R. *Rang and Dale's Pharmacology*. 6th ed. London, England: Churchill Livingston; 2008.

Waller D, Renwick A, Hillier K. *Medical Pharmacology and Therapeutics*. 2nd ed. London, England: Elsevier; 2006.

CHAPTER 3

Pharmacokinetics

Chapter Objectives

Specific learning outcomes (page ix) of this text addressed in this chapter:

- Apply the principles of pharmacology to the safe and effective use of medicines.
- Recognize general, patient-specific, and scenario-specific risks, precautions, and contraindications for use of medicines.
- Apply the pharmacokinetic and pharmacodynamic principles of medications to identify and explain normal and adverse reactions to medications.

After reading, digesting, reflecting on, and reviewing the content of this chapter, readers should be able to

1. Demonstrate command of key pharmacokinetics terms.
2. Demonstrate enhanced understanding of the principles associated with pharmacokinetics.
3. Demonstrate critical thinking to effect problem solving related to absorption, distribution, metabolism, and excretion (ADME).
4. Recognize, explain, and interpret clinical problems and evidence in relation to ADME.
5. Solve rudimentary pharmacokinetic problems.
6. Apply knowledge of the general principles and concepts in a translational manner to clinical practice.

Key Terms

ADME	conjugation	first-pass metabolism	parenteral	reduction
ADMET	curve stripping	half clearance	pharmacokinetics	steady state
bioavailability	enteral	half-life	pharmacology	therapeutic range
biotransform	efficacy	hydrolysis	prodrug	toxicity
clearance	equilibrium	metabolism	protein binding	volume of distribution
compartment model	first-order kinetics	oxidation	rate constant	zero-order kinetics

Some of the text, tables, and figures in this chapter were extracted from "Pharmacology Part 2: Introduction to Pharmacology and Pharmacodynamics" by Geoff Currie (*J Nucl Med Technol*. 2018;46:221–230).

Introduction

As previously outlined, pharmacology is the scientific study of the action and effects of drugs on living systems and the interaction of drugs with living systems. For general purposes, pharmacology is divided into pharmacodynamics and pharmacokinetics (Fig. 3-1). The principle of *pharmacokinetics* is captured by the philosophy of Paracelsus (medieval alchemist): "All things are poison and nothing is without poison; only the dose makes a thing not a poison" (commonly shortened to "the dose makes the poison.") Therapeutic benefits are gained from a drug within a window below which there is no therapeutic benefit and above which there are harmful effects (toxicity). The narrow *therapeutic range* of some drugs means that only small variations in blood concentration are necessary to result in toxicity (or no effect). Key to maintaining drug concentrations within the therapeutic range is bioavailability, and factors that may influence bioavailability are an essential aspect of pharmacokinetics. Pharmacokinetics provides a valuable insight into the biological behavior of interventional and adjunctive medications for medical radiation patients and for the radiopharmaceuticals and contrast agents administered to them. The biological behavior of medications is especially important to consider because both age (the mean age of medical imaging and radiation therapy patients tends to exceed 60 years) and disease can have a significant impact on drug, contrast agent, and radiopharmaceutical bioavailability, pharmacological response, drug sensitivity, and drug interactions.

Except in the case of intravenous or intra-arterial administration, for a drug to have an effect, it must navigate at least one membrane (Fig. 3-2). First, a drug must enter general circulation from the site of administration, and second, it must get to the site of action. A drug may need to overcome physical, chemical, and biological barriers, such as the blood-brain barrier. Drugs are transported across a biological membrane by different mechanisms that need to be considered:

- Passive (simple) diffusion requires a degree of lipid solubility to cross the phospholipid bilayer, and the drug moves using the concentration gradient until equilibrium is reached.
- Facilitated diffusion requires no energy, nor can it move against a concentration gradient, but the drug sufficiently resembles the natural ligand to bind to the carrier macromolecule and traverse the membrane.
- Active transport also capitalizes on the drug's resemblance to the natural ligand, allowing it to bind to carrier macromolecules; however, this process uses energy to transport a drug against the concentration gradient.
- Other carrier-mediated transport mechanisms exist that are nonspecific drug transporters, such as P-glycoprotein.
- Pinocytosis incorporates the drug into a lipid vesicle for carrier-mediated transport into the cell cytoplasm.
- Transport through pores or ion channels can occur with the concentration gradient for small water-soluble drugs.

Pharmacokinetics is essentially the study of the absorption, distribution, metabolism, and excretion (ADME) of drugs, how the body affects the drug (Fig. 3-3). It is, however, also the study of associated *toxicity* (ADMET). Pharmacokinetics does not limit its scope to healthy or normal subjects but rather includes variations in bioavailability, physiological or pathological conditions, disease-related dose adjustment, and drug interactions. Combined, these aspects of pharmacokinetics allow customization of drug dosage regimes to enhance outcomes.

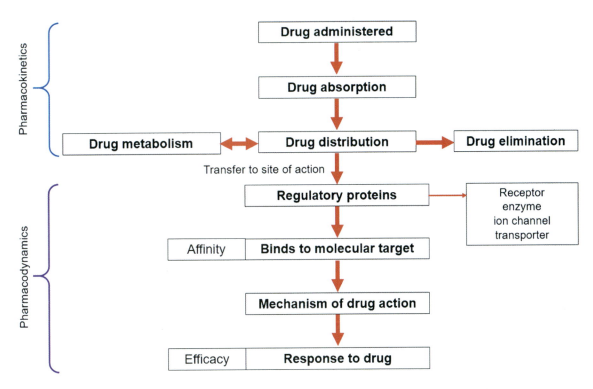

FIGURE 3-1 Schematic representation of the relationship between pharmacokinetics and pharmacodynamics.

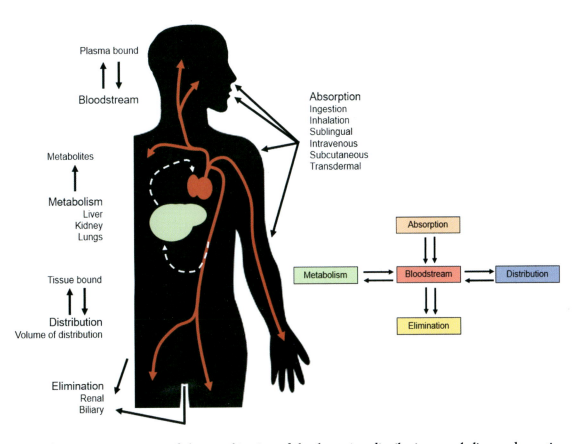

FIGURE 3-2 Schematic representation of pharmacokinetics and the absorption, distribution, metabolism, and excretion concept.

28 Pharmacology Primer for Medications

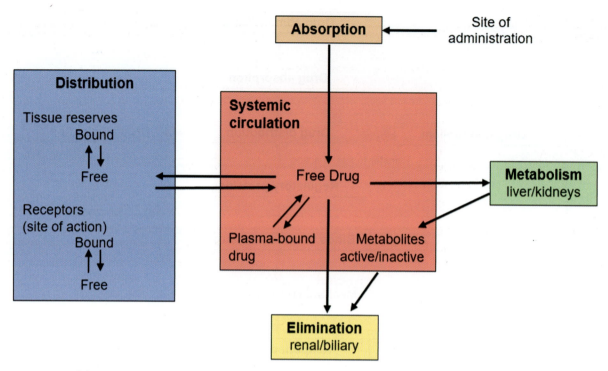

FIGURE 3-3 Schematic representation of pharmacokinetics and the ADME concept highlighting the interplay among free and bound drugs and the pathway from site of administration to site of action.

Absorption

Absorption is the transportation of a drug from the site of administration to the general circulation. Absorption and the factors that may impede absorption of the drug directly affect drug bioavailability. *Bioavailability* in the context of pharmacokinetics is the fraction of the administered drug that reaches the systemic circulation. Clearly, intravenous and intra-arterial injections transfer the drug directly into the general circulation and provides 100% bioavailability. This assumes drugs reach the site of action directly from systemic circulation. Drugs requiring metabolism prior to action, even with intravenous administration, may have less than 100% bioavailability. The oral (enteral) route is the most common drug administration route. Oral medications are the simplest to administer but may have variable bioavailability depending on many factors that influence drug absorption, including the following:

- Molecular size of the drug
- Lipid solubility of the drug
- Degree of ionization of the drug
- Dosage form (e.g., tablet, solution)
- Chemical nature of the drug
- Whether there is complex formation
- Pharmacological effect of the drug
- Dose and concentration of the drug
- Blood flow (at site of administration)
- Site of absorption
- Route of administration (Table 3-1)

TABLE 3-1	Characteristics of Various Routes of Administration of Drugs	
Route	*Advantages*	*Disadvantages*
Intranasal (e.g., antihistamine)	Rapid delivery and immediate effect. High bioavailability. No first-pass metabolism. Avoids gastric environment.	Local irritation. Limited to small doses and small range of drugs.
Sublingual (e.g., nitroglycerin)	Easy and convenient delivery. Rapid delivery and immediate effect. High bioavailability. No first-pass metabolism. Avoids gastric environment. Self-administration.	Changes in absorption if swallowed, chewed, or following emesis.
Oral/enteral (e.g., captopril)	Easy, reliable, economic, convenient, painless, no infection risk. Self-administration.	First-pass metabolism or elimination decreases bioavailability. Slow delivery and onset of action. Dose form needs to accommodate gastric environment (e.g., transit stomach intact for small bowel absorption). Bioavailability can be influenced by changes in gut status (e.g., emesis, diarrhea, constipation).
Rectal (e.g., laxatives)	Rapid delivery and immediate effect. High bioavailability. No first-pass metabolism. Avoids gastric environment. Suitable for patients with emesis or otherwise inappropriate oral route.	Unpleasant form of administration with bacteremia risk for the immunocompromised. Altered absorption in diarrhea and constipation.
Inhalation (e.g., albuterol [Ventolin])	Rapid delivery and immediate effect. High bioavailability. No first-pass metabolism. Avoids gastric environment. Direct delivery to affected tissues. Self-administration.	Local irritation. Limited to small doses and small range of drugs. May require special equipment and decreased efficacy with incorrect use.
Intramuscular (e.g., morphine)	Intermediate onset of action. Suitable for oil-based drugs. Less skill required to administer than for intravenous.	Local edema, irritation, or pain. Slower onset of action. Infection risk.
Intravenous (e.g., furosemide [Lasix])	Rapid delivery and immediate effect. Bioavailability is 100%. No first-pass metabolism. Avoids gastric environment. Controlled drug delivery.	Irritation or pain. Risk of infection. Solution must be dissolved well. Risk of embolism. Action not easily reversed. Rapid onset of toxicity.
Subcutaneous (e.g., insulin)	Slower absorption and onset of action. Suitable for oil-based drugs.	Local edema, irritation or pain. Small volumes. Slow onset of action. Infection risk.
Transdermal (e.g., fentanyl)	Easy, reliable, economic, convenient, painless. Enables slow and prolonged drug delivery. No first-pass metabolism. Avoids gastric environment. Self-administration.	Slow onset of action. Local skin reactions can occur. Needs highly lipophilic drugs.
Percutaneous (e.g., diclofenac [Voltaren gel])	Easy, reliable, economic, convenient, painless. Suitable for local effect.	Slow onset of action. Local skin reactions can occur.

Generally speaking, the common routes of administration of drugs can be categorized as follows:

- Oral (enteral) administration is simple, convenient, and painless, allowing self-administration of drugs in easily handled drug forms. Gastrointestinal absorption means that the drug is transported via the portal system to the liver and undergoes first-pass metabolism. First-pass metabolism may render some of the drug inactive, decreasing bioavailability.

- Mucous membranes are highly vascular, which allows rapid entry of the drug to the systemic circulation. This route avoids first-pass metabolism and the hostile gut environment. In some cases, the drug can be delivered directly to the site of action (e.g., lungs). The drug may be delivered in a dissolvable form (suppository, pessary), mist, aerosol, or liquid to any number of sites, including sublingual, ocular, lung, intranasal, rectal, and vaginal.

- Injection (parenteral) of drugs directly into tissue (e.g., systemic circulation, cerebrospinal fluid, tissue) avoids first-pass metabolism and provides rapid delivery to the site of action. The degree of vascularity impacts the rate of onset of action with slow onset from subcutaneous administration, intermediate onset from intramuscular administration, and rapid onset from intravenous administration. Parenteral administration affords the greatest control over drug delivery and includes intravenous, intra-arterial, intramuscular, subcutaneous, intraperitoneal, and intrathecal.

- Transdermal and percutaneous administration require passive diffusion of highly lipophilic drugs across the skin. This approach provides slow onset of action and potential for slow, continuous drug delivery (e.g., nicotine patches).

Distribution

Distribution refers to the movement of the drug from the systemic circulation to tissues. The drug needs to be distributed to the site of action in sufficient concentration to generate the therapeutic action. Distribution essentially involves the circulatory system (including some minor lymphatic involvement), which distributes drugs to all tissues except brain and testes (due to membrane barriers). Consequently, relative blood flow to tissues influences the drug dose required. Using simple diffusion following intravenous injection as an example, the initial high plasma concentration reaches equilibrium following rapid entry into cells with high perfusion. Poorly perfused tissues continue to concentrate the drug, which decreases plasma concentrations. In turn, the high concentrations of the drug in well-perfused tissues decreases to reach equilibrium across the membranes (Fig. 3-4). This is a principle exploited in thallium-201-based stress and redistribution myocardial perfusion studies. Given tissue concentration of a drug is difficult to measure, plasma concentration is used to estimate tissue concentration. Major factors that affect the distribution of drugs include the following:

- Diffusion rate
- Affinity of the drug to the tissues
- Blood flow (perfusion)
- Binding to plasma proteins

An important concept to understand when discussing pharmacokinetics, and one that surfaces in radiopharmacy, is protein binding. Within the blood, a drug may have an affinity to plasma proteins, typically, intracellular proteins, albumin, and glycoproteins. The *plasma protein binding* of drugs (mostly albumin) has low specificity and has no action (no potency) but forms drug-protein complexes in a similar fashion to drug-receptor complexes previously discussed (Chapter 2). Most drug-protein binding in plasma is reversible and can act as a reservoir, releasing free drug when unbound concentrations of free drug decline (Fig. 3-3). For drugs with a large amount of plasma protein

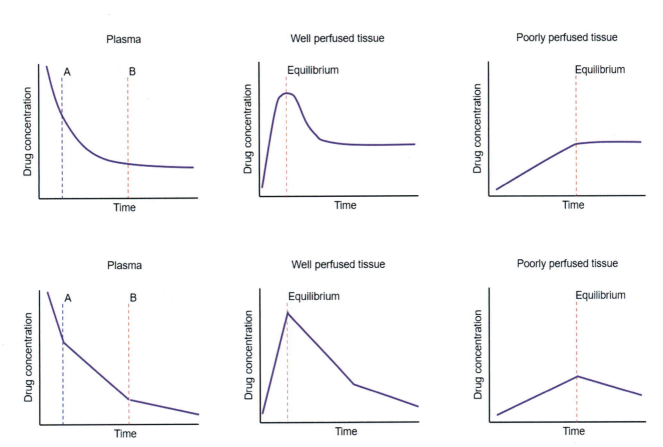

FIGURE 3-4 Schematic representation of equilibrium between drug concentration and plasma, well-perfused tissue, and poorly perfused tissue. Top: The three graphs in the top row do not incorporate the effects of metabolism or elimination but illustrate early equilibrium in well-perfused tissue (A) followed by a period of concentration in poorly perfused tissues (A to B) before reaching equilibrium in all tissues and plasma (B). Bottom: The three graphs in the bottom row provide the phases as discrete intervals (straight line) and illustrate the impact of elimination.

binding (e.g., ibuprofen), equilibrium may occur between tissues and plasma with a small fraction of the actual drug (free drug) in the body. The vast reserves of plasma protein–bound drug can provide prolonged effects through sustained release of the drug. There is, however, competition for plasma binding that can have significant implications for drug effects. Ibuprofen, for example, if displaced through competition, would result in significantly higher free drug in tissue and blood. Co-administration of aspirin and warfarin compete for the same plasma protein–binding sites and thus potentiate the effects of each drug. A small number of drugs may bind irreversibly to plasma proteins via covalent bonding. As a result, bound drug is not released in response to decreasing plasma and/or tissue concentrations. The radiopharmaceutical technetium-99m (^{99m}Tc) diethylenetriaminepentaacetic acid (DTPA) has about 10% plasma protein binding, which has a minor influence on half clearance and glomerular filtration rate (GFR) calculations. Conversely, ^{99m}Tc gluconate has high protein binding (>50%), which truncates pharmacokinetics. ^{99m}Tc mercaptoacetyltriglycine (MAG3) has as much as 90% plasma protein binding and so relies on tubular secretion and effective plasma renal flow (rather than GFR). When a drug is highly plasma protein bound, it typically has a lower volume of distribution.

The *volume of distribution* (V) is an important concept for pharmacokinetic principles and calculations. The volume of distribution is the amount of drug administered divided by the plasma concentration of the drug. It represents the distribution of the drug between plasma and tissue compartments. Most of the time, the volume of distribution does not actually equal the real volume of the compartments; it is simply a model to help elucidate drug behavior. For example, a 70 kg person might be expected to have less than 70 L of volume throughout his or her body, yet a volume of distribution for a given drug might exceed several hundred liters. A volume of several hundred liters is clearly not possible in a 70 kg person, but the model allows a theoretical understanding of drug behavior. When the volume of distribution is high, it reflects a relatively low drug concentration in plasma (minimal plasma protein binding) and extensive distribution through body tissues. It really represents an apparent volume of distribution or the fluid volume that would be required at steady state (equilibrium) to contain the plasma concentration equivalent to the total drug amount in the body. The volume of distribution is used as a principle for compartment modeling and in pharmacokinetic calculations, but it is not an actual physical volume.

Compartment modeling is used in pharmacokinetics to explain the relationship between drugs (or contrast agents or radiopharmaceuticals) and their distribution within the body. The body might be considered to comprise four liquid compartments: plasma water (5%), interstitial water (16%), intracellular water (35%), and fat (20%). A smaller fifth compartment of transcellular water (2%) is sometimes used and represents compartments partitioned by a barrier, such as the blood-brain barrier and testes. In each compartment, a drug may be present in either bound or free forms, and it is the free form that can move from one compartment to another. Movement between compartments can be measured and expressed as a rate constant (*k*). For simplicity and depending on what is being modeled, compartment modeling may use one-, two-, or multiple-compartment models (Fig. 3-5).

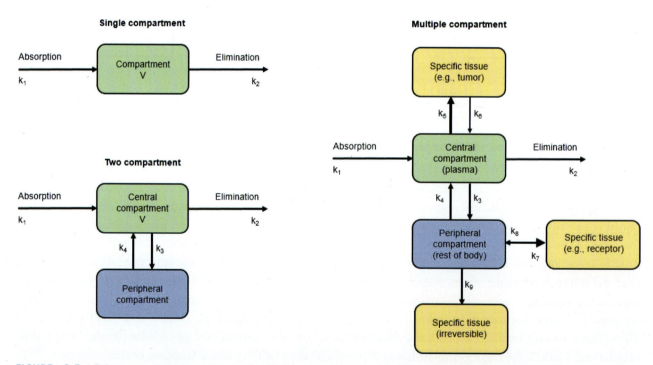

FIGURE 3-5 Schematic representation of single-compartment model, two-compartment model, and multiple-compartment model. The rate constant (k) reflects the movement from one compartment or volume of distribution (V) to the other and can be calculated numerically. Schematically, the rate constant may be represented in several ways. On the multiple-compartment model, k_5 and k_6 have arrows with different sizes, which indicates greater movement of drug to the tissue compartment than from it. Likewise, for k_7 and k_8, a single arrow might be used with a different-sized arrowhead representing the relative k values. When drug transport between compartments is not reversible, a single arrow is used (k_9). Note that multiple methods would not be used on a single schematic, as is done here.

Metabolism

Drug *metabolism* largely occurs in the liver but can also occur in the kidneys, lungs, skin, and gastrointestinal tract. Metabolism involves enzymes that modify the drug in various cells, such as hepatocytes in the liver. Most drugs are lipid soluble to allow them to cross the phospholipid bilayer membranes and be suitable for oral absorption. Lipid-soluble drugs are also reabsorbed from urine before elimination, so metabolism of lipid-soluble drugs to water-soluble structures is necessary for effective renal elimination. A *prodrug* is an inactive drug that is metabolized into an active form. Most angiotensin-converting enzyme (ACE) inhibitors are prodrugs (e.g., inactive enalapril biotransforms to enalaprilat), but captopril is already in its active form.

Conversely, metabolism of active drugs relates to enzymic modification of the drug structure to render it less active (e.g., aspirin becomes salicylic acid), inactive (e.g., morphine becomes inactive morphine-3-glucuronide, although a second metabolite, morphine-6-glucuronide, is more active), or for most drugs (e.g., paracetamol or acetaminophen in Fig. 3-6), more susceptible to elimination. Some drug metabolites, however, can have their own activity and, in some cases, be more active (e.g., nitroglycerin becomes the more active nitric oxide).

Modifications to drugs and prodrugs are called *biotransformations* and can be categorized as follows:

- Phase I—oxidative, reduction, and hydrolysis reactions—may be referred to as preconjugation. Oxidation generally adds a polar group to the chemical structure of a drug by adding an oxygen. Reduction tends to add a hydrogen while hydrolysis adds water to the drug structure.

- Phase II—conjugation reactions—generally facilitates attachment of the drug to a polar molecule. Either the drug or the metabolite from phase I metabolism is covalently bonded to a substrate. Some examples include glucuronidation, methylation, acetylation, and sulfation.

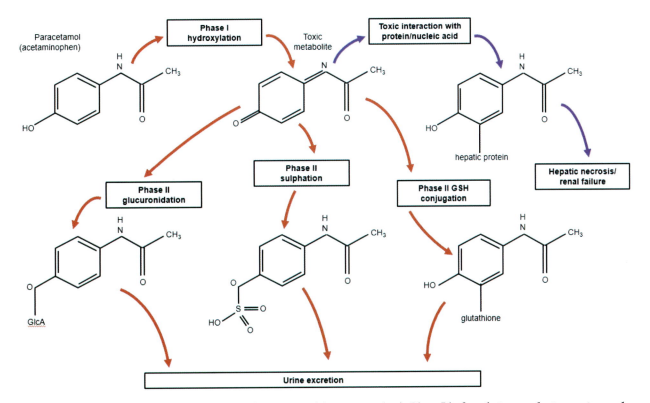

FIGURE 3-6 Phase I and phase II metabolism of paracetamol (acetaminophen). Phase I hydroxylation results in a toxic metabolite with three forms of phase II metabolism converting the metabolite to a form for urine excretion. Toxic interaction can occur, leading to liver necrosis and potentially to renal failure, especially with depleted hepatic glutathione (GSH).

Most drugs undergo both phase I and phase II metabolism, but some drugs only undergo either phase I or phase II metabolism. While a detailed discussion of the mechanisms of metabolism are beyond the scope of this discussion, Figure 3-6 provides a summary insight into the process.

Elimination

Drugs and their metabolites can be eliminated from the body through a number of mechanisms and in several forms. Some drugs can have fractional *elimination* via several routes. Liquid elimination includes renal and biliary (urine and bile) excretion primarily but also sweat, tears, saliva, and breast milk. Paracetamol (acetaminophen) is excreted via the kidneys, while salicylic acid (metabolite of aspirin) can be excreted via sweat. Lidocaine is excreted via the biliary system. Caffeine and theophylline (metabolite of prodrug aminophylline) are partially excreted in saliva. People can be tested for drug use using urine and saliva samples. Solid excretion occurs via the gastrointestinal tract (feces) and in hair. Differentiating fecally eliminated drugs can be confounded by biliary excretion that transits the colon and, for drugs administered orally, that which remains unabsorbed. Nonetheless, digoxin is an example of excretion in feces via colonic lumen secretion. Drugs eliminated via the hair can be incorporated into the hair structure (e.g., codeine and morphine) or secreted onto the hair by sebum or sweat. Volatile drugs may be eliminated via gases in the lungs, with alcohol being the most common example.

Renal excretion via glomeruli filtration may be followed by tubular reabsorption. The purpose of reabsorption is to retain key nutrients and other substances (e.g., amino acids and vitamins). Some drugs may also pass back into circulation via reabsorption. Similarly, drugs eliminated via the biliary system may be reabsorbed from the intestines and returned via the hepatic portal vein (enterohepatic cycle). In both circumstances, the effective duration of effect of drugs is prolonged.

Elimination of drugs from the plasma introduces four important quantitative concepts:

- Clearance (CL) is the rate of elimination of the drug from the body and is the product of the elimination rate constant (k) and the volume of distribution (V).
- Half-life ($T_{0.5}$) is the time required for the amount of drug present to be reduced by 50%. This can be a measure of plasma half-life or total body half-life.
- First-order kinetics is when a constant fraction (exponential) of drug is eliminated per unit of time and is similar in concept to radioactive decay (Fig. 3-7). In theory, the amount of drug present never reaches zero.
- Zero-order kinetics is when there is a constant rate (linear) of drug elimination, and this means the rate of elimination is independent of drug concentration. Unlike first-order kinetics, a constant amount of drug is eliminated per unit of time, and drug present will reach zero (Fig. 3-7).

Insight

Perhaps the best way to demonstrate an understanding of pharmacokinetics is mathematically. These are simple calculations for those in medical radiation science, as there are parallels with a number of other equations used (e.g., radioactive decay and attenuation coefficient). The scenarios presented in Table 3-2 are designed to highlight application of pharmacokinetic calculations. Of course, these applications are examples, and the methods of calculation can be readily adapted for other scenarios.

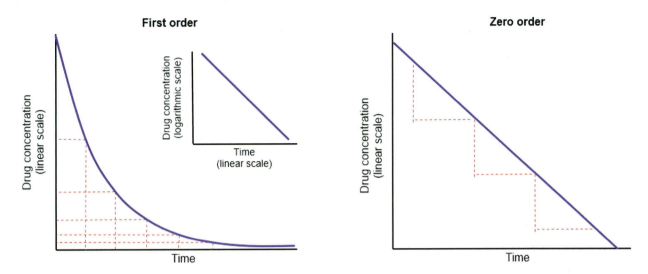

FIGURE 3-7 Schematic representation of first-order and zero-order elimination. First order-elimination follows an exponential trend and can be displayed with a logarithmic y-axis to generate a straight line (inset). Zero-order elimination eliminates a constant amount of drug per unit time.

TABLE 3-2 Summary of Useful Formulae and Definitions in Pharmacokinetics

Use	Equation	Definitions
Drug concentration	$C = C_0 e^{-kt}$	C = Drug concentration at time t after C_0 C_0 = Drug concentration at reference time k = Elimination rate constant t = Time between C and C_0
Elimination rate constant	$k = \ln 2 \div T_{0.5}$	k = Elimination rate constant $\ln 2 = 0.693$ $T_{0.5}$ = Half clearance time
Volume of distribution	V = amount in body (µg)/actual C_0	V = Volume of distribution actual C_0 = Concentration at the time of administration
Area under the curve	$AUC_{0-\infty} = (F \times D) \div (V \times k)$	$AUC_{0-\infty}$ = Area under the curve (total drug dose) from time zero to infinity F = Fraction of drug absorbed D = Dose V = Volume of distribution k = Rate constant
Clearance	$CL = k \times V$	CL = Clearance k = Elimination rate constant V = Volume of distribution
Time to maximum concentration	$T_{max} = (1 \div [k_a - k]) \ln(k_a \div k)$	T_{max} = Time to maximum concentration k_a = Absorption rate constant k = Elimination rate constant

TABLE 3-3	Data for First Scenario
Time (h)	*Plasma Concentration (µg/L)*
2	139
4	65.6
6	31.1
8	14.6

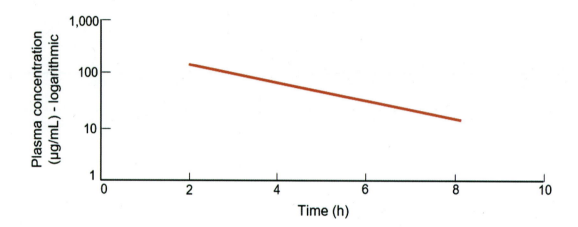

FIGURE 3-8 Logarithmic-linear plot confirming a single-compartment monoexponential curve.

Consider a patient weighing 70 kg who is given an intravenous bolus injection of 25 mg of a drug. If plasma concentrations after injection are as given in Table 3-3, the elimination rate constant and half-life can be readily calculated. The first step is to plot the data on semi-logarithmic scales to demonstrate a straight line (confirming first-order kinetics). Rather than use the slope of the line (Fig. 3-8) for subjective calculations (or estimates), it is easier to use the following equation, where C is the drug concentration at a given time, C_0 is the drug concentration at the reference time, k is the elimination rate constant, and t is time between C and C_0:

$$C = C_0\, e^{-kt}$$

$$14.6 = 139\, e^{-k.6}$$

$$14.6 \div 139 = e^{-k.6}$$

$$\ln 0.1057 = -k.6$$

$$k = 0.3745\ h^{-1}$$

With the elimination rate constant now determined, the half clearance time can also be calculated:

$$k = \ln 2 \div T_{0.5}$$

$$T_{0.5} = \ln 2 \div k$$

$$T_{0.5} = 0.693 \div 0.3745$$

$$T_{0.5} = 1.85\ h$$

The volume of distribution in liters can be calculated as

$$V = \text{amount of drug in body (ug)} \div \text{actual } C_0$$

Convert milligrams to micrograms

While the origin (actual C_0) can be estimated to determine the theoretical blood concentration at the point of drug administration by reading off the plot, it is more accurate, given k has been determined, to simply calculate it:

$$C = C_0 e^{-kt}$$

$$139 = C_0 e^{-0.3745 \times 2}$$

$$139 = C_0 \times 0.4728$$

$$C_0 = 139 \div 0.4728$$

$$\mathbf{C_0 = 294 \text{ mg/L}}$$

Thus

$$V = 25,000 \div 294$$

$$\mathbf{V = 85 \text{ L}}$$

The area under the curve (AUC) from the time of administration to infinity ($AUC_{0-\infty}$) can be used to calculate total drug burden, where F is the fraction of the drug absorbed (100% for intravenous administration) and D is the dose (in micrograms):

$$AUC_{0-\infty} = FD \div Vk$$

$$AUC_{0-\infty} = 25,000 \text{ μg} \div (85 \times 0.3745)$$

$$AUC_{0-\infty} = 25,000 \div 31.8325$$

$$\mathbf{AUC_{0-\infty} = 785.36 \text{ μg or } 0.785 \text{ mg/h/L}}$$

Clearance (CL) can be readily calculated as

$$CL = k \times V$$

$$CL = 0.3745 \times 85$$

$$\mathbf{CL = 31.83 \text{ L/h}}$$

The second scenario considers a more complex problem. Drug concentrations of interest may include other tissues (besides the plasma compartment) or plasma concentrations but without the advantage of immediate absorption associated with an intravenous administration (e.g., oral). In these cases, both absorption and the absorption rate constant, rather than just the elimination rate constant, need to be considered. Consider the plasma concentrations in arbitrary units (U) of an orally administered drug in Table 3-4. Graphing this data does not yield the monoexponential curve expected of first-order kinetics, and this represents the overlapping influence of absorption and elimination (Fig. 3-9). The logarithmic plot, however, demonstrates a late section with a straight line from 7 hours

38 Pharmacology Primer for Medications

onward. This section has minimal impact from absorption, so it can be used to determine the elimination rate constant and half clearance time.

TABLE 3-4 Data for Second Scenario	
Time (min)	Plasma Concentration (U/L)
0	0
1	31.3
2	49.3
3	58.6
4	62.5
5	62.8
7	58.1
10	50.6
16	36.1
24	25.3

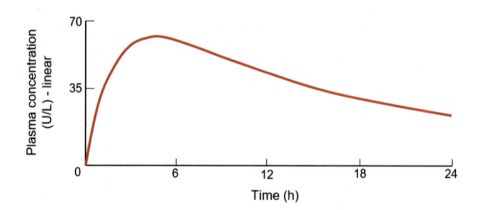

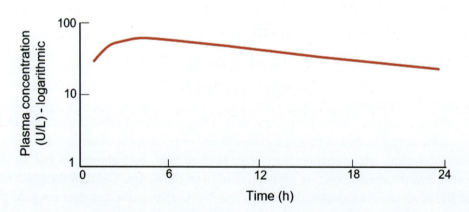

FIGURE 3-9 Linear-linear and logarithmic-linear plots demonstrating interplay between absorption and elimination for second scenario.

$$C = C_0 e^{-kt}$$
$$25.3 = 58.1 e^{-k \times 17}$$
$$25.3 \div 58.1 = e^{-k \times 17}$$
$$\ln 0.4355 = -k \times 17$$
$$\mathbf{k = 0.0489 \text{ min}^{-1}}$$

$$k = \ln 2 \div T_{0.5}$$
$$T_{0.5} = \ln 2 \div k$$
$$T_{0.5} = 0.693 \div 0.0489$$
$$\mathbf{T_{0.5} = 14.17 \text{ min}}$$

To determine the absorption rate constant, a process known as *curve stripping* is required. Using the elimination rate constant determined above and the data from 7 hours onward (Table 3-5), the equation can be used to determine the value for each time interval projected back along the elimination line (bold figures in Table 3-5), in effect stripping away the influence of absorption. For example, times 1, 3, and 5 hours can be calculated respectively as

$$C = C_t e^{-kt}$$
$$25.3 = C_1 e^{-0.0489 \times 23}$$
$$25.3 = C_1 \times 0.3247$$
$$\mathbf{C_1 = 77.92}$$

$$C = C_t e^{-kt}$$
$$25.3 = C_3 e^{-0.0489 \times 21}$$
$$25.3 = C_3 \times 0.3581$$
$$\mathbf{C_3 = 70.65}$$

$$C = C_t e^{-kt}$$
$$25.3 = C_5 e^{-0.0489 \times 19}$$
$$25.3 = C_5 \times 0.3949$$
$$\mathbf{C_5 = 64.06}$$

Subtraction of the plasma values from the elimination curve values generates a value, R, which can be added to the table of data (Table 3-5). Graphing R on a logarithmic-linear plot (Fig. 3-10) generates an absorption rate. It is worth noting that the absorption line may not be a straight line representing a second compartment associated with distribution (e.g., vascular and extra vascular). While one should not assume a straight line for absorption in calculations, it offers a practical approach. In this particular case, there is a straight-line relationship between time zero and 3 hours that can be used for accurate calculations. Thus, the absorption rate constant (k_a) can be determined as

$$C = C_0 e^{-k_a \times t}$$
$$12.1 = 46.6 e^{-k_a \times 2}$$
$$12.1 \div 46.6 = e^{-k_a \times 2}$$
$$\ln 0.2596 = -k_a \times 2$$
$$\mathbf{k_a = 0.6742 \text{ min}^{-1}}$$

With both the elimination and absorption rate constants now calculated, the time to peak concentration (T_{max}) can be calculated as

$$T_{max} = (1 \div [k_a - k]) \ln(k_a \div k)$$
$$T_{max} = (1 \div [0.6742 - 0.0489]) \ln(0.6742 \div 0.0489)$$
$$T_{max} = (1 \div [0.6742 - 0.0489]) \ln(13.8)$$
$$T_{max} = 1.6 \times 2.6$$
$$\mathbf{T_{max} = 4.2 \text{ min}}$$

TABLE 3-5 Data for the stable elimination period (7–24 h) are used to calculate the elimination rate constant (k) and backproject the elimination curve by calculating the earlier values for the elimination confounded by absorption (bold). Simple subtraction of the plasma concentration from the elimination values generates R, which can be plotted to determine absorption.

Time (h)	Plasma Concentration (U/L)	Elimination Curve Concentration	R (Elimination – Plasma)
0	0	**81.8**	81.8
1	31.3	**77.9**	46.6
2	49.3	**74.0**	24.7
3	58.6	**70.7**	12.1
4	62.5	**67.1**	4.6
5	62.8	**64.1**	1.3
7	58.1	58.1	
10	50.6	50.6	
16	36.1	36.1	
24	25.3	25.3	

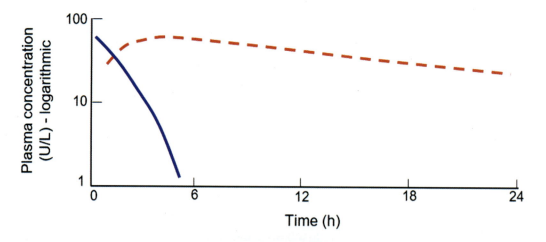

FIGURE 3-10 Logarithmic-linear plots for raw data (dashed) and for R.

A third scenario provides an opportunity to incorporate AUC calculations in a more complex scenario. Consider the data in Table 3-6. After subcutaneous injection of a drug with a dose of 7.5 mg/kg, plasma concentrations in blood were monitored (in µg/mL). The data can be plotted (Fig. 3-11) and the straight-line portion of the logarithmic curve used to determine both the elimination rate constant and subsequently the backprojected values for the elimination curve, as demonstrated in the second scenario (Table 3-7). The elimination rate constant (k) is calculated as

$$C = C_0 \, e^{-kt} \qquad\qquad T_{0.5} = \ln 2 \div k$$

$$3.2 = 11 \, e^{-k \times 4} \qquad\qquad T_{0.5} = \ln 2 \div 0.3087$$

$$k = 0.3087 \text{ h}^{-1} \qquad\qquad T_{0.5} = 2.25 \text{ h}$$

TABLE 3-6	Data for Third Scenario
Time (h)	Plasma Concentration (µg/mL)
0	0
0.5	16
1	22
1.5	22
2	19
4	11
6	5.6
8	3.2

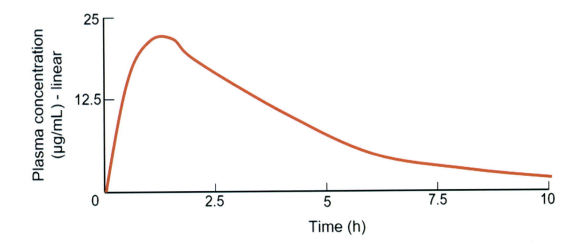

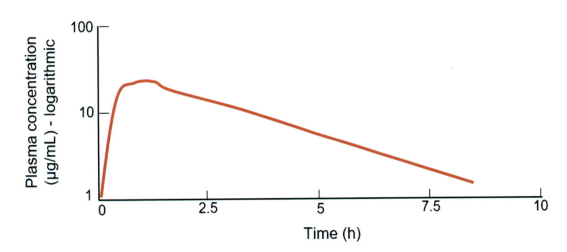

FIGURE 3-11 Linear-linear (top) and logarithmic-linear (bottom) plots demonstrating interplay between absorption and elimination for the third scenario.

42 Pharmacology Primer for Medications

TABLE 3-7	Data for the Stable Elimination Period (2–8 h)*		
Time (h)	Plasma Concentration (µg/mL)	Elimination	R
0	0	**37.8**	**37.8**
0.5	16	**32.4**	**16.4**
1	22	**27.8**	**5.8**
1.5	22		
2	19	19	
4	11	11	
6	5.6	5.6	
8	3.2	3.2	

*Data are used to calculate the elimination rate constant (k) and backproject the elimination curve by calculating the earlier values for the elimination confounded by absorption (bold). Simple subtraction of the plasma concentration from the elimination values generates R, which can be plotted to determine absorption.

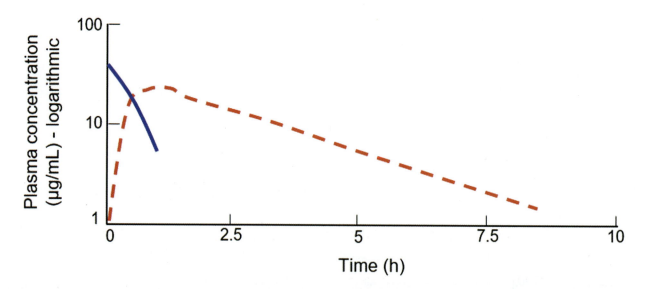

FIGURE 3-12 Logarithmic-linear plots for raw data (dashed) and for the elimination curve minus the plasma curve (R) (solid line).

Subtraction of the plasma values from the elimination curve values generates the previously introduced value, R, which can be added to the table of data (Table 3-7). Graphing R on a logarithmic-linear plot (Fig. 3-12) generates an absorption curve. Thus, the absorption rate constant (k_a) can be determined as

$$C = C_0\ e^{-k_a \cdot t}$$

$$5.8 = 37.8\ e^{-k_a \times 1}$$

$$k_a = 1.8744\ h^{-1}$$

As previously discussed, AUC is a valuable metric in pharmacokinetics. A number of methods are employed to determine the total AUC when absorption and elimination phases need to be accommodated; most tend to be unnecessarily complex or inaccurate due to estimation errors. The total AUC represents the total drug dose, or drug burden. An understanding of mathematics provides both greater accuracy and simplification. This method relies on an accurate determination of k_a. It also assumes accurate calculation of k and then C_0 (plasma). The preceding mathematics indicate that the AUC is simply the area prescribed by k_a subtracted from the area prescribed by k. Thus, AUC can be calculated as

$$AUC = [C_0 \div k] - [C_0 \div k_a]$$

$$AUC = [37.8 \div 0.3087] - [37.8 \div 1.8744]$$

$$AUC = 122.45 - 20.17$$

$$\mathbf{AUC = 102.28\ \mu g}$$

These tools have a raft of applications to problem solve or to better understand drug (or contrast agent and radiopharmaceutical) behavior. To avoid duplication, not all parameters were calculated in each scenario; however, they could be if appropriate. One may also note parallels between these calculations and those used to problem solve in radiopharmacy.

References

Asperheim K, Favaro J. *Introduction to Pharmacology*. 12th ed. St Louis, MO: Elsevier; 2012.

Block JH, Beale JM. *Wilson and Gisvold's Textbook of Organic Medicinal and Pharmaceutical Chemistry*. 12th ed. Philadelphia, PA: Lippincott Williams & Wilkins; 2011.

Bryant B, Knights K, Salerno E. *Pharmacology for Health Professionals*. 2nd ed. Sydney, Australia: Mosby Elsevier; 2007.

Currie G. Pharmacology part 1: introduction to pharmacodynamics. *J Nucl Med Technol*. 2018;46:81–86.

Currie G. Pharmacology part 2: introduction to pharmacokinetics. *J Nucl Med Technol*. 2018;46:221–230.

Currie G, Kiat H, Wheat J. Pharmacokinetic considerations for digoxin in older people. *TOCMJ*. 2011;5:130–135.

Cusack BJ. Pharmacokinetics in older persons. *Am J Geriatr Pharmacother*. 2004;2:274–302.

Delafuente JC. Pharmacokinetic and pharmacodynamic alterations in the geriatric patient. *Consult Pharm*. 2008;23:324–334.

El Desoky ES. Pharmacokinetic-pharmacodynamic crisis in the elderly. *Am J Ther*. 2007;14:488–498.

Golan DE, Tashjian AH, Armstrong EJ, Armstrong AW. *Principles of Pharmacology: The Pathophysiologic Basis of Drug Therapy*. 3rd ed. Philadelphia, PA: Lippincott Williams & Wilkins; 2012.

Greenstein B. *Rapid Revision in Clinical Pharmacology*. New York, NY: Radcliffe Publishing; 2008.

Hacker M, Messer W, Bachmann K. *Pharmacology: Principles and Practice*. London, England: Elsevier; 2009.

Heard K. Acetylcysteine for acetaminophen poisoning. *N Engl J Med*. 2008;359(3):285–292.

Jambhekar SS, Breen PJ. *Basic Pharmacokinetics*. London, England: Pharmaceutical Press; 2009.

Katzung BG, Masters SB, Trevor AJ. *Basic and Clinical Pharmacology*. 12th ed. New York, NY: McGraw Hill; 2012.

Rang H, Dale M, Ritter J, Flower R. *Rang and Dale's Pharmacology*. 6th ed. London, England: Churchill Livingston; 2008.

Stumpf WE. The dose makes the medicine, *Drug Discov Today*. 2006;11(11-12):550–555.

Waller D, Renwick A, Hillier K. *Medical Pharmacology and Therapeutics*. 2nd ed. London, England: Elsevier; 2006.

CHAPTER 4

Dose Forms and Administration

Chapter Objectives

Specific learning outcomes (page ix) of this text addressed in this chapter:

- Apply the principles of pharmacology to the safe and effective use of medicines.
- Administer medications safely, effectively, and appropriately according to procedures and within regulatory and statutory parameters.

After reading, digesting, reflecting on, and reviewing the content of this chapter, readers should be able to

1. Demonstrate command of key terms.
2. Demonstrate enhanced understanding of the principles associated with routes of administration and dose forms.
3. Demonstrate critical thinking to effect problem solving related to drug administration.
4. Recognize, explain, and interpret clinical problems and evidence in relation to drug administration.
5. Apply knowledge of the general principles and concepts in a translational manner to clinical practice.

Key Terms

bioavailability	dose form	intramuscular	site of action	suspension
buccal	enteral	intravenous	solution	sustained release
capsule	enteric coated	parenteral	subcutaneous	tablet
compliance	intra-arterial	pessary	sublingual	topical
controlled release	intradermal	prodrug	suppository	transdermal

Introduction

The *dose form* is the means by which a medication is delivered to a cellular site of action. This is relevant to radiopharmaceuticals used for diagnosis or therapy and to contrast agents and medications. The purpose of the dose form is primarily to ensure the dose is accurately delivered to the site of action. That might mean a route of administration, or dose form, that protects the medication from hostile or incompatible environments. The dose form may also be optimized for sustained or controlled release of the medication, controlling the therapeutic window of the medication. At times, the dose form allows the medication a vehicle for entry into the body, whether via an orifice, intracavity, or transdermal. Finally, the dose form may be chosen simply to overcome an unpleasant taste, smell, or texture. Dose forms can be described on the basis of either their routes of administration or their physical form. Many drugs are available in more than one dose form, and the decision on which dose form to use may depend on patient age, comorbidity, compliance or consciousness, patient preference, expected time to response, expected duration of effect, whether a local or systemic effect is desired or tolerable, and the medication itself. For example, the bronchodilator salbutamol can be given by inhalation or intravenous routes, with the latter being more appropriate in life-threatening situations. Opioid analgesia can be given intravenously, orally, or in controlled release transdermal patches.

Routes of Administration

The *route of administration* of a medication is simply the method by which it is introduced to the body. In nuclear medicine and radiology, the most common route of administration is parenteral. Parenteral includes intravenous, intramuscular, subcutaneous, intra-arterial, and intradermal. For medications, the most common route of administration is oral. The specific dose form can be variable, as discussed shortly. It is, however, important to understand all routes of administration (Table 4-1), as interventional or adjunctive medications in the medical imaging or radiation oncology department have a wide range of routes of administration (Fig. 4-1).

Enteral refers to medications intended to be taken into the gastrointestinal tract: swallowed, inserted rectally, or delivered via an enteral feeding tube. Medications designed for other means of delivery, such as sublingual or buccal administration, are meant for dissolution in the mouth and therefore are not considered enteric drugs. A small number of oral medications are designed to have a direct action in the gastrointestinal tract; however, the vast majority are designed to be absorbed from the gastrointestinal tract into the systemic circulation. Oral administration of medications is simple, safe, and convenient, but it comes with variability of absorption (inter- and intra-individuals) and the challenge of optimizing the dose form to traverse the gastrointestinal tract and dissolve for absorption in the correct location. Clearly, absorption properties affect drug bioavailability, which can vary with oral administration. For example, for absorption in the stomach, the medication should be compounded to dissolve in an acidic solution, whereas for absorption in the intestine, it should be compounded to resist dissolution in acidic environments of the stomach and to dissolve in the basic environment of the intestine. For this reason, crushing or chewing enteric-coated tablets to make oral administration easier can undermine medication effectiveness. Conversely, some medications can be crushed or chewed (or capsules opened) for more rapid oral absorption and more immediate effects.

Dose Form

Solutions allow the medication to be dissolved in liquid (often water or syrups) and rapidly absorbed after oral administration. Some medications do not dissolve well and are more effective when administered orally as a suspension. These medications should be mixed before measuring the dose. Medications may come as a suspension or may be made into a suspension from powder at the time of use. Some tablet or capsule dose forms can be administered as a suspension, but one should be aware that the tablet or capsule form may be masking an unpleasant taste that will be unveiled by a suspension. Flavor is often added to commercial medications sold as a suspension.

TABLE 4-1 Summary of Dose Forms with Common Examples of Medications Administered in Each Form

Route of Administration	Dose Form	Example
Oral (enteral)	Tablet Capsule Solution Syrup Elixir Suspension Gel Fast-dissolving tablet or powder	Captopril Celecoxib Ibuprofen Amoxicillin Butabarbital Nystatin Miconazole Aspirin
Sublingual, buccal	Tablet Lozenge Gum Film	Lorazepam Nitroglycerin
Parenteral (by injection)	Solution Suspension	Morphine Frusemide
Topical	Ointment Cream Paste Powder Lotion Solution Patch	Hydrocortisone Fentanyl Salicylic acid EMLA (lidocaine and prilocaine mixture)
Intraocular	Ointment Solution	Chloramphenicol
Intra-aural	Suspension	Auralgan (antipyrine, benzocaine and glycerin mixture)
Intranasal	Solution Spray	Budesonide Budesonide aqua
Intrarespiratory	Aerosol Inhaler	Salmeterol Salbutamol
Rectal (also enteral)	Solution Ointment Suppository	Bisacodyl
Vaginal	Solution Ointment Emulsion foam Tablet Pessary	Clotrimazole
Urethral	Solution Suppository	Alprostadil

48 Pharmacology Primer for Medications

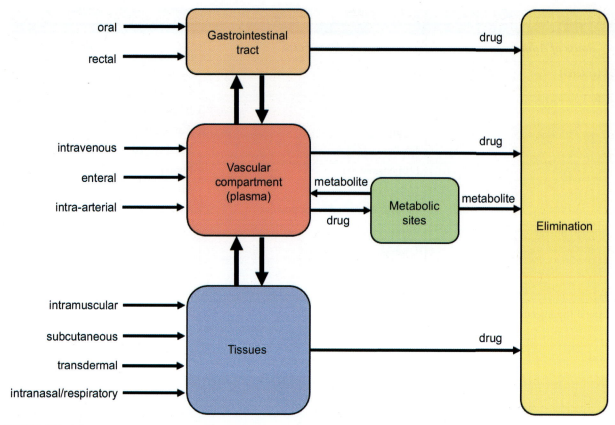

FIGURE 4-1 The basic compartment model for various common routes of administration.

Tablets are a form of the medication compressed into a solid shape. The medication in powder form is typically mixed with other ingredients, such as flavors, colors, fillers, agents to help disintegrate the tablet under the right conditions, and coatings that help the tablet resist disintegration under the wrong conditions. Over and above the internal environment, tablets may be coated to protect medication from light and humidity. For commercially manufactured tablets, every tablet has a unique design (shape, color, size, markings) that makes it identifiable. Tablets may also be scored (Fig. 4-2) in half or quarters to facilitate breaking into smaller units for ease of swallowing or to provide lower doses. Scored medications provide some indication that the medication is designed for disintegration in the stomach and could be crushed or suspended if required.

Capsules generally have similar ingredients to a tablet, but instead of being compressed into a solid form, the powder is sealed in a gelatin capsule. Capsules can also contain a liquid. Gelatin capsules can be hard or soft depending on whether sugar is added to the capsule composition. Capsules, like tablets, come in a variety of colors, sizes, and shapes to help identify medications (along with unique codes and monographs). Because the medication is not compressed, the rapid dissolving of the capsule means the medication is more rapidly absorbed to give a more immediate effect. Capsule sizes range from 000 (approximately 26.1 mm by 9.6 mm with a volume of 1.37 mL) to size 5 (approximately 11.1 mm by 4.7 mm with a volume of 0.13 mL).

Parenteral administration simply means administered by injection, including intravenous, intramuscular, subcutaneous, intra-arterial, and intradermal injection (Fig. 4-3). While it offers a rapid administration method that avoids variations in bioavailability associated with medication absorption or first-pass metabolism, parenteral administration introduces risk and requirements for sterility. Nonetheless, some medications are either degraded in the gut or have poor solubility, making parenteral the most effective route of administration. Parenteral administration also provides a rapid onset of action for the medication, which is convenient in an emergency (Chapter 12).

Chapter 4 | Dose Forms and Administration 49

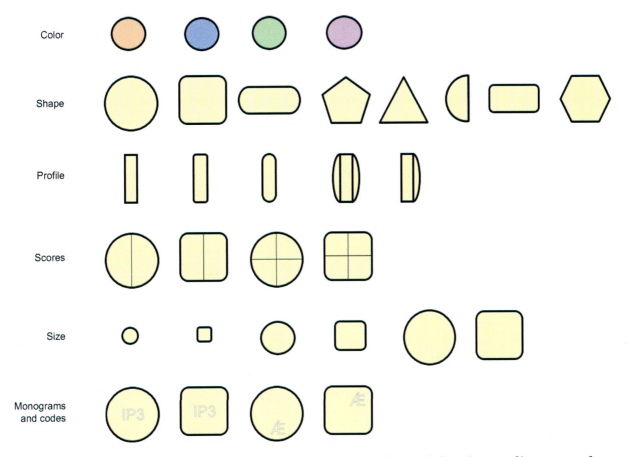

FIGURE 4-2 Characteristics that help identify specific medications in tablet form, including shape, profile, presence of scores, size, monograms or codes, and tablet color.

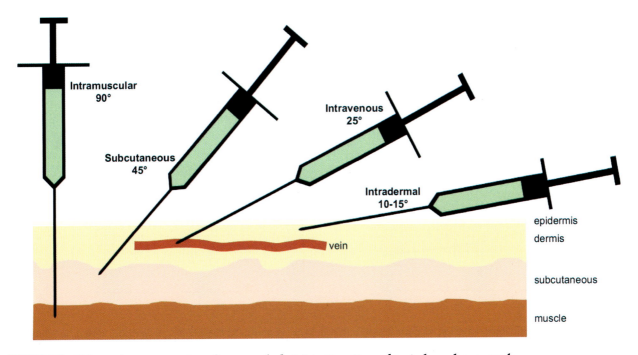

FIGURE 4-3 Schematic representation of parenteral administration sites and typical angular approach.

Topical medications are usually delivered via the skin in the form of creams, gels, lotions, and pastes. Generally, they serve 2 roles: the dose form that has an effect (e.g., skin lubricant or protectant) and the medicinal effect (e.g., antibacterial). These types of medication have a very broad array of effects, which range from surface and local effects after absorption into the dermis to systemic effects after penetration to the subcutaneous tissues. When percutaneous absorption is the goal of medication delivery (i.e., delivery to systemic circulation via the skin), the rate of absorption requires a degree of control, and the vehicle designed to do that is a transdermal device. An advantage of transdermal delivery of medications is the slow, controlled release that maintains fairly uniform medication levels (Fig. 4-4).

The purpose of delivering a medication into the rectum, vagina, or urethra is generally to address local symptoms; however, soluble drugs are readily and rapidly absorbed in the colon, so this may be a means of systemic delivery. The hostility of the stomach may mean the rectum is a preferred delivery method of some systemic medications susceptible to degradation in the acid environment. While solutions, gels, foams, and ointments might be used in rectal, vaginal, or urethral medication administration, suppositories are the main dose form. A suppository is a solid form that softens and melts once through the orifice to deliver local therapeutic effects. The formulation can be modified to alter the medication release rate. In the vagina, a suppository is referred to as a *pessary*. Topical medications can also be applied to the eyes, ears, or nasal cavity in the form of ointments, suspensions, and solutions for local effects. Nasal sprays can be absorbed into systemic circulation, offering a rapid and convenient alternative method of systemic drug delivery that avoids gut and first-pass metabolism. Nonetheless, most respiratory-delivered medications (e.g., aerosols and dry powder inhalation) produce a local effect. Table 4-1 lists a number of other dose forms used less commonly.

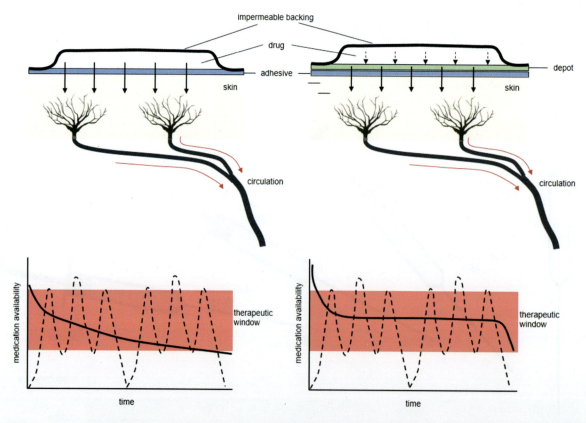

FIGURE 4-4 Schematic representation of transdermal patch delivery system. On the left is a monolithic system in which the release rate of the medication decreases over time. On the right is the depot system in which the drug transfers into a membrane-bound reservoir to allow constant rate of medication release. The corresponding plots represent the transdermal dose delivery in the solid line and the oral or parenteral profile in dashed lines.

Drug Administration

Basic rules must be followed prior to administration of medications, and these rules apply equally to radiopharmaceuticals and contrast media. It is essential, prior to administration, that we are certain of

- Correct patient
- Correct dose (drug amount, volume, concentration)
- Correct route of administration
- Correct form for that route
- Correct drug (or radiopharmaceutical or contrast agent)
- Correct preparation of drug (reconstitution, temperature, volume)
- Correct documentation

In addition, medications used therapeutically and therapeutic radiopharmaceuticals require

- Correct time and date
- Correct frequency

Two very important capabilities associated with drug administration should be second nature in medical radiation science. Nonetheless, they warrant discussion:

1. Variation to dose associated with patient age or weight
2. Accurate calculation of drug doses and concentration

Radiopharmaceutical doses (megabecquerels [MBq] or millicuries [mCi]) and medications (drug content in milligrams) are frequently adjusted on the basis of age or weight. This is important because the critical organs (radiation dose or toxicity) have different physiological activity and tolerance in children and with weight changes. If, for example, a 6-year-old child weighed 75 kg, would that constitute an adult dose? In terms of distribution (drug efficacy or radiopharmaceutical count density), the answer would be yes. But physiologically, despite being of adult weight, the child's liver or kidneys may be anatomically or physiologically well behind adulthood. As a result, drug metabolism and toxicity, or radiation dose burden for a radiopharmaceutical, are altered with potential harmful consequences. Recall, the dose makes the poison. Conversely, an adult of low weight with normal liver function may metabolize a drug quickly and yield poor therapeutic response if the drug is adjusted down on the basis of weight. While a one-size-fits-all approach should not be adopted (instead, considering the individual medication and patient characteristics or properties), a number of generic methods for dose adjustment are used in adults (children are discussed in Chapter 5). Perhaps the most common is adjustment according to body surface area. Body surface area is calculated as a function of height and weight and has been shown to correlate in adults with a number of physiological processes. This offers a fairly generic approach with no consideration for specific organ function. It may, in medications metabolized in a specific organ, be better to assess specific organ function and adjust the dose on the basis of those findings. Liver function tests, for example, might be used to customize doses of medications metabolized in the liver. Consider that a normally functioning liver might more rapidly decrease concentrations of a drug or increase concentrations of active metabolites. Conversely, decreased liver function may prolong clearance and increase dose effects or delay efficacy of a prodrug (active metabolites). Perhaps in medical radiation sciences, a more familiar approach is the use of creatinine clearance levels to adjust doses or make decisions (e.g., computed tomography [CT] contrast). Kidney function significantly influences the clearance, and thus bioavailability, of a large number of medications (and radiopharmaceuticals and contrast agents). Drugs can rapidly fall outside the therapeutic window, leading to either toxicity or lack of efficacy. Creatinine clearance can be used as a proxy for renal function and used to adjust medications or, importantly, identify patients in whom the medication (or contrast agent) should not be administered. While creatinine serum analysis is considered quick and simple, glomerular filtration rate is more accurate and also simply calculated in nuclear medicine.

Example Calculations

Calculating drug doses and concentrations is simple but important, and it is easy to make a mistake. A simple mistake of one order of magnitude could be catastrophic for the patient. The basic mathematics is undertaken routinely for radiopharmaceutical reconstitution and dose preparation and in contrast preparation but warrants a refresher from the context of medications. The first operation is to simply determine what volume of a drug is required to be drawn for an administration of a specific dose. If 35 mg of a drug is required, and that drug is contained as 200 mg in a volume of 10 mL, then the volume needed is

$$\text{Volume} = (35 \times 10) \div 200 = 1.75 \text{ mL}$$

Concentration is an important concept and an essential part of drug reconstitution. Some drugs are more stable in powdered form and are reconstituted prior to use. Nuclear medicine cold kits are an example, as are medications such as some antibiotics. The concentration changes the volume of each dose. For example, if a container contained 2,000,000 μg of drug, how much diluent (e.g., saline, water for injections) should be added if the end product should be 50,000 μg/mL?

$$\text{Volume} = (2,000,000 \times 1) \div 50,000 = 40 \text{ mL}$$

If the patient were required to take 250 mg of the above medication once a day, what volume would the patient need to take?

$$\text{Volume} = (250,000 \times 40) \div 2,000,000 = (250,000 \times 1) \div 50,000 = 5 \text{ mL}$$

Finally, some medications are required to be administered over a period of time. For example, a patient requires an infusion but the drug cannot be delivered at more than 35 g per hour. The medication is diluted in a 2 L saline bag containing 100 g of the medication. What is the maximum rate the medication can be administered?

$$\text{Volume for 35 g} = (2,000 \times 35) \div 100 = 700 \text{ mL/h}$$

The recommended dose of dipyridamole is 0.142 mg/kg/min infused over 4 minutes. The 50 mg of dipyridamole is contained in 10 mL of single-use vial. The total drug volume should be diluted at least 1:2 with saline with a final dose range of 20 mL to 50 mL. For an 80 kg patient,

$$\text{Dose} = 0.142 \times 80 \times 4 = 45.44 \text{ mg (single vial)}$$

$$\text{Volume} = (10 \times 45.44) \div 50 = 9.01 \text{ mL}$$

$$\text{Diluent} = 20 - 9.01 = 10.99 \text{ mL}$$

$$\text{Rate} = 20 \div 4 = 5 \text{ mL/min}$$

For a 120 kg patient,

$$\text{Dose} = 0.142 \times 120 \times 4 = 68.16 \text{ mg (2 vials)}$$

$$\text{Volume} = (10 \times 68.2) \div 50 = 13.6 \text{ mL}$$

$$\text{Diluent} = 13.6 \times 2 = 27.2 \text{ mL (round to 30)}$$

$$\text{Rate} = 30 \div 4 = 7.5 \text{ mL/min}$$

Insight

There are a number of classification systems around the world, and several are summarized in Table 4-2. Generally, they share common criteria around accepted medical use, safety risk, and abuse risk. The regulations around each schedule of drug should be understood for the jurisdiction in which the drug is being used.

TABLE 4-2 Drug Schedules and Criteria for the United States, Roughly Translated to Schedules for the United Kingdom, Canada, and Australia						
U.S. Schedule	Potential for Abuse	Accepted Medical Use	Abuse Could Lead to Injury	U.K. Schedules	Canadian Schedules	Australian Schedules
I	High	No	No data	1		9 (prohibited substances)
II	High	Yes	Severe	2	I	8 (controlled drug)
III	Moderate	Yes	Moderate	2	I	7 (dangerous poison)
						6 (poison)
						5 (caution)
IV	Low	Yes	Low	3		4 (prescription only)
V	Very low	Yes	Very low	4	II	3 (pharmacist only)
	Negligible	Yes	Negligible	5	III	2 (pharmacy medicine)

References

Asperheim K, Favaro J. *Introduction to Pharmacology*. 12th ed. St Louis, MO: Elsevier; 2012.

Aulton M. *Aulton's Pharmaceutics: The Design and Manufacture of Medicine*. 3rd ed. London, England: Churchill Livingston; 2007.

Bryant B, Knights K, Salerno E. *Pharmacology for Health Professionals*. 2nd ed. Sydney, Australia: Mosby Elsevier; 2007.

Hacker M, Messer W, Bachmann K. *Pharmacology: Principles and Practice*. London, England: Elsevier; 2009.

CHAPTER 5

Individual Variations in Pharmacology

Chapter Objectives

Specific learning outcomes (page ix) of this text addressed in this chapter:

- Apply the principles of pharmacology to the safe and effective use of medicines.
- Recognize general, patient-specific, and scenario-specific risks, precautions, and contraindications for use of medicines.
- Apply the pharmacokinetic and pharmacodynamic principles of medications to identify and explain normal and adverse reactions to medications.
- Administer medications safely, effectively, and appropriately according to procedures and within regulatory and statutory parameters.
- Monitor patients for, identify, and manage adverse reactions.

After reading, digesting, reflecting on, and reviewing the content of this chapter, readers should be able to

1. Demonstrate command of key pharmacology terms.
2. Demonstrate enhanced understanding of the principles associated with pharmacology in women, children, and the elderly.
3. Demonstrate critical thinking to effect problem solving related to changes in pharmacology associated with age and gender.
4. Recognize, explain, and interpret clinical problems and evidence in relation to altered pharmacology in women, children, and older people.
5. Demonstrate understanding of the effects of aging on pharmacokinetics.
6. Demonstrate understanding of the specific content of the chapter.
7. Apply knowledge of the general principles and concepts in a translational manner to clinical practice.

Key Terms

adverse reaction	concentration	elimination	metabolism	teratogenic
bioavailability	concordance	half-life	neonate	therapeutic index
comorbidity	dose adjustment	inotropic	polypharmacy	therapeutic range
compliance	dose form	loading dose	prodrug	toxicity

Introduction

The basic principles of pharmacology are strongly influenced by variations in individual characteristics, organ development, health, and other factors. It is important to consider how the standard modeling of pharmacology might change under different conditions. While all permeations cannot be covered, a broad examination of the following population subgroups is designed to provider deeper insight into pharmacology and the capability to manage our patients:

- Women
- Children
- The elderly

Given the disproportionate representation of elderly patients in the medical imaging department, a greater focus is placed on this subgroup.

Pharmacologic Considerations in Women

Women require specific attention when it comes to medication and pharmacology. One issue is that human modeling is often based on a 70 kg man, and the mean surface area used (1.73 m^2) in some calculations is an average of that for men (1.9 m^2) and women (1.6 m^2) and could result in unfavorable pharmacology. Furthermore, many drugs readily cross the placenta in a pregnant woman and have potential deleterious effects on the fetus. While a detailed discussion of the potential *teratogenic* effects of various medications is beyond the scope of this text, it is essential that any medication administered is done so with an understanding of the patients' pregnancy status and the teratogenic risk classification for the drug. From a medical imaging context, the following classes of medications are known to pose teratogenic risk: angiotensin-converting enzyme (ACE) inhibitors, diazepam, iodide, and warfarin. When administering a medication to a patient who is pregnant, it is important to understand the following:

- Potential for the medication to produce harmful effects on the fetus
- Gestational age of the fetus
- Other medications or chemicals being used
- Dosage of the drug

In addition, women's altered physiology during pregnancy can have a significant impact on medication action. During pregnancy, gastric motility can decrease and may delay absorption of some medications, altering bioavailability. Nausea leading to vomiting could eliminate oral medications and nullify the effect. The *volume of distribution* (V) alters with the change in body mass and fluid distribution, which alters medication distribution. During different stages of pregnancy, enzymes responsible for liver metabolism of drugs can increase or decrease to produce opposing effects on drug bioavailability. *Bioavailability* can also be altered with changes to renal function, increasing glomerular filtration rate (GFR) and drug elimination. It is also noteworthy that some drugs undergo metabolism in the placenta as a protection mechanism for the fetus, which may affect bioavailability in the woman. Furthermore, fetal metabolism is lower than the metabolism of a developed fetus or adult, and consequently, medications crossing the placenta could have a more significant effect on the fetus even with equivalent dose per body mass.

Similarly, most drugs administered to women who are lactating will appear in breast milk. This language is important because some reports use the misleading language "concentrate" in breast milk. If the latter were true, it would pose a significant risk of toxicity to the feeding child. In reality, most medications have very low concentrations in breast milk, well short of therapeutic effects. Nonetheless, it is important to understand the characteristics of the individual medication. There are three factors to consider:

1. The half-life of the medication allows doses to be taken immediately after feeding, leaving extended time for clearance when half-lives are short (<4–6 h). The long half-life of diazepam leaves a child susceptible to sedation from breast milk, while sedation following chloral hydrate can be avoided by feeding immediately prior to administration.
2. Concentration in breast milk determines whether the medication is of sufficient quantity to elicit a pharmacological effect in the infant. Accumulation in breast tissue needs to be delineated from elimination in breast milk. In nuclear medicine, accumulation in tissue irradiates the child at feeding time by proximity, while elimination in milk creates internal contamination. For medications, consumption through milk elimination is the only issue. Fat soluble medications have higher concentrations in milk at the end of the feeding.
3. Severity of potential effects of the medication is the second half of the risk analysis (probability and severity). Regardless of the probability or level of medication elimination in breast milk, if the potential of adverse effects in the child are severe, then breast-feeding and the medication use should not be concurrent. Diazepam provides a good example because not only does it have a long half-life but accumulation can occur in newborns, leading to potential toxicity.

Pharmacologic Considerations in Children

While the general principles of pharmacology in children mirror those of pharmacology in adults, there are several important considerations. Drug absorption may be affected, particularly in neonates. In neonates, blood flow, muscle mass, gastric pH, gastric empty times, and peristalsis may all cause altered drug absorption and irregular bioavailability. Furthermore, the dose form may need to be varied in neonates and children, and this may impact bioavailability. The variations in body composition across the span from neonate to adolescent produces substantial differences in drug biodistribution, and this is especially critical to consider for water-soluble medications. Children are more susceptible to toxicity, even when plasma concentrations are normal. Drug metabolism (liver) is also generally stunted for neonates while enzyme development occurs, increasing the half clearance time and bioavailability for some drugs. By the time a child reaches toddler status, the metabolic rate is generally higher than that in adults, resulting in decreased bioavailability. Confounding these effects are similar delays in excretion for neonates with decreased GFR.

Except for in the neonate, pediatric pharmacology is not complex. Perhaps the two major issues are dose form and dose adjustment. Adults are generally compliant with taking medications, whereas children confront difficulties associated with taste, swallowing whole tablets, and injections. Care needs to be taken that the dose form is not changed in a manner that alters its pharmacology. Crushing tablets can result in more rapid absorption. Opening capsules can circumvent the mechanism designed to deliver the drug to the site of absorption. Other times, the dose form needs to be changed. An elixir is convenient and does not require mixing before use but contains alcohol; therefore, the child equivalent is a suspension requiring mixing before use. Of course, in the medical radiation sciences, we encounter children (and some adults) who have a fear of needles, which makes injections of contrast or radiopharmaceuticals challenging. It is important to note that some intravenous medications can be administered intramuscularly. While this route may delay time to onset of action, it offers a convenient option in an emergency (e.g., frusemide in hypertension).

As previously discussed, calculating the optimal dose for a child is challenging because a child's age or weight does not provide an accurate marker of organ function and development. Childhood obesity in western countries has exacerbated this issue. There are, however, a number of methods for determining the dose of a medication for children.

- Young's rule is based on the child's age:

$$\text{Child dose} = (\text{age} \times \text{adult dose}) \div (\text{age} + 12)$$

- Clark's rule is based on the child's weight:

$$\text{Child dose} = (\text{weight in lb} \times \text{adult dose}) \div 150$$

$$\text{Child dose} = (\text{weight in kg} \times \text{adult dose}) \div 70$$

- Cowling's rule is based on the child's age:

$$\text{Child dose} = ([\text{age in y} + 1] \times \text{adult dose}) \div 24$$

- Fried's rule is also age based:

$$\text{Child dose} = (\text{age in mo} \times \text{adult dose}) \div 150$$

- Body surface area:

$$\text{Child dose} = (\text{child's surface area} \times \text{adult dose}) \div 1.73$$

A critical factor in children is the potential for calculation error. In an adult, the dose is standard and well entrenched in protocol and procedure. Adjusting an adult dose for pediatric use requires mathematics and potential for error. A single misplaced decimal point creates an order of magnitude error. All calculations should be double checked.

Effects of Aging

As humans age, organ systems function less efficiently, tissue repair is slower, and lifestyle modifications are required for assimilation. There are four characteristics of aging:

- Universality: It happens to everyone.
- Intrinsicality: It starts with the embryo.
- Progressiveness: It continues until death.
- Deleterious: It weakens body tissues.

Medical and pharmaceutical advances (e.g., medication, lifestyle changes, nutrition, surgery) have enabled slowing of progression; deleterious changes can be accommodated (e.g., medication, surgery) and even reversed (e.g., organ or joint transplantation); and while universality remains, cosmetic intervention can make it appear that age discriminates.

One characteristic of old age is the prevalence of coexisting disease and disorder. One dysfunction may lead to another, causing a cascade of age-related dysfunction. Unfortunately, older age also results in crucial organ dysfunction (Table 5-1), particularly impairment of renal and liver function, which can have a profound effect on pharmacokinetics. This is further confounded by the protracted recovery typical in the older person that may require longer-term use of medications.

TABLE 5-1 Age-Related Changes to Organ Function

Organ	Age-Related Change
Heart	◆ Major cardiovascular changes ◆ Reduced elasticity and compliance of the aorta and great arteries ◆ Higher systolic arterial pressure ◆ Increased impedance to left ventricular ejection ◆ Left ventricular hypertrophy ◆ Interstitial fibrosis ◆ Decrease in the rate of myocardial relaxation ◆ Isotonic contraction is prolonged, and isotonic velocity is reduced ◆ Reduced intrinsic heart rate and increased sinoatrial node conduction time response to postural changes differs from increased heart rate in the young to increased stroke volume in the old ◆ During exercise, the tachycardic response is reduced
Renal	◆ Renal mass decreases ◆ Reduced number of nephrons ◆ Reduced blood flow in the afferent arterioles ◆ Both renal plasma flow and GFR decline ◆ No concomitant increase in plasma creatinine because of age-related loss of muscle mass ◆ Acid-base balance is reduced response to stress ◆ Ability to concentrate the urine during water deprivation is reduced ◆ Response to water loading is also impaired ◆ Delay in balancing salt losses
Gastrointestinal tract	◆ Decreased secretion of hydrochloric acid and pepsin ◆ Reduced absorption of several substances (e.g., sugar, calcium, iron) ◆ Progressive reduction in liver volume and liver blood flow
Neuroendocrine responses	◆ Changes in neuroendocrine responses to psychosocial or physical stress ◆ Excessive hypothalamic-pituitary-adrenal (HPA) activation and hypersecretion of glucocorticoids can lead to dendritic atrophy in neurons in the hippocampus, resulting in learning and memory impairment
Body composition	◆ Significant changes in body composition occur with advancing age ◆ Progressive reduction in total body water and lean body mass ◆ Relative increase in body fat

Changes in physiology occur with disease and aging and can affect drug pharmacology. Older people can also have altered responses to the drugs due to changes in mechanical responses, receptor mechanisms, homeostasis, and CNS function. It is worth considering that older patients are disproportionately represented in the nuclear medicine patient cohort and that older patients also have a higher use of medications, particularly the use of multiple and concurrent medications (*polypharmacy*). Older patients and those with disease (or older patients with

60 Pharmacology Primer for Medications

disease) have a less homogenous response to medications, which makes responses difficult to predict. The following can be expected with aging and disease (Fig. 5-1):

- Altered absorption (e.g., slower gut absorption of captopril)
- Changed biodistribution (e.g., diazepam volume of distribution doubles)
- Altered metabolism, especially with liver function changes or disease (e.g., decreased for ibuprofen)
- Altered elimination (e.g., diazepam half clearance almost triples)
- Changed bioavailability (e.g., increased digoxin toxicity) influenced by all of these factors to either reduce or increase bioavailability

Regardless of age-related changes to absorption, distribution, metabolism, and excretion, older people also demonstrate an increased sensitivity to many drugs due to *comorbidity* and polypharmacy. The elderly are at higher risk of an adverse drug effect, have increased severity of effects, are less likely to report adverse effects, and are more likely to be hospitalized or to die due to adverse drug effects.

With increasing age, the amount of saliva produced is significantly reduced, and this can reduce the rate of drug absorption by influencing the gastric pH. Furthermore, older people have reduced gastric acid secretion and reduced acidity (increased pH), which can delay dissolution of oral medications. This is exacerbated by delayed gastric empty due to reduced peristaltic force that reduces the mechanical influences on medication mixing with gastric juices. The surface area for drug absorption is decreased in aging due to intestinal atrophy that, combined with reduced concentration gradient due to poorer blood flow, inhibits passive diffusion of drugs into the bloodstream, further delaying absorption rate. While this does not change the total absorption itself, it does alter the *time to maximum* drug effect.

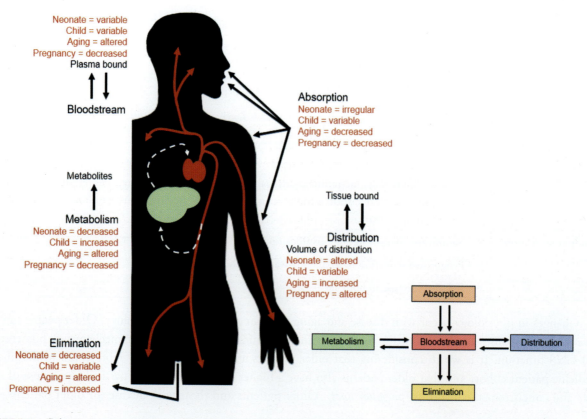

FIGURE 5-1 Schematic representation of the changes to function with age that may affect medications pharmacology.

Drug distribution in the older person can vary due to changes in body composition and critical organ perfusion. The latter will also affect metabolism and elimination with decreased liver and kidney perfusion. The reduction in lean body mass in older people (as much as 19%) will cause an elevation in drug concentrations in muscles for drugs distributed in that manner. The older body also sees an increase of up to 35% in the relative fat composition (adipose tissue) independently of obesity, and despite the increase in fat, older people have a marked decrease in water content of the body. The effects of these changes on drug distribution largely depend on the lipid or water solubility of the drug and its metabolites. Water-soluble drugs show a small *volume of distribution* (V) and increased plasma concentrations with reduced total body water; thus, accommodation needs to be made in reducing loading doses. Conversely, lipid-soluble drugs have a larger volume of distribution and thus a longer half-life. The half-life of water-soluble drugs does not decrease because of the concomitant reduced renal clearance. From the following equation, it is clear that a reduction in volume of distribution in older patients and concomitant reduction in renal clearance will cancel one another out, while the renal reduction potentiates the effects of increased volume of distribution on half-life. A 10% decrease in blood albumin concentration has the effect of increasing the unbound fraction of the drug by a corresponding 10%.

$$T_{1/2} = [0.693 \times V] \div \text{renal clearance}$$

The vast majority of drug metabolism occurs in the liver with minor contributions from the kidneys and lungs. The capacity of the liver to metabolize drugs decreases with age. The 35% to 40% reduction in hepatic perfusion in the elderly has a significant impact on drug delivery to the liver and subsequent rate of metabolism. Liver size can be reduced by 24% to 35% with age. One major influence is the reduced first-pass metabolism of orally absorbed lipid-soluble drugs, which can significantly increase drug bioavailability. Conversely, prodrugs that require metabolism for activation may show decreased or delayed bioavailability. Furthermore, the decreased capacity (up to 60%) of the liver to metabolize drugs for elimination can increase plasma concentrations and prolong biological half-lives of drugs.

For water-soluble drugs, elimination is solely or primarily via renal excretion. In the elderly, the kidneys can show a 20% reduction in size, 30% reduction in glomeruli function, and as much as 50% reduction in normal renal capacity. This functional decline can be further exacerbated by concomitant renal disease. Renal excretion of drugs declines with age, so the elderly should be managed as though they have renal insufficiency. This is particularly important for drugs with a narrow therapeutic index because it increases the likelihood of serious toxicity.

Compliance is simply the extent to which a patient adheres to the instructions provided for a medication. *Concordance* is a variation on this concept that accommodates a negotiation of the instructions between prescriber and patient to develop a medication regime that suits the patient and offers therapeutic benefit. Clearly, the concept of concordance is aimed at addressing perceived issues in compliance. Perhaps the perception that the elderly are less compliant with medications actually relates more to medication errors than deliberate lack of compliance. As few as 18% of the elderly in one study had compliance-related problems with their medication, while as many as 50% of the elderly make errors in their medications. Lack of compliance can result in a reduced therapeutic effect, which may be difficult to differentiate from disease progression. The dose regime may be changed (increased dose) if compliance is not identified as being problematic. Improved compliance after dose adjustment following a period of poor compliance could result in toxicity.

Polypharmacy is very important in the elderly because it relates to the relationship between the greater number of medications taken (typically high in the elderly) and the increased risk of drug interaction, decreased compliance, and increased medication errors. Indeed, medication errors increase 15-fold with an increase in medications from 1 to 4. Polypharmacy is defined by five or more prescription medications, and it has an incidence of 20% to 40% in the over-70 age group. Older patients are frequently prescribed multiple drugs, which make them susceptible to drug-drug interactions. Moreover, older people take more drugs with a narrow therapeutic index, increasing the risk of adverse reactions and drug interactions. Unfortunately, they are also less capable of coping with reaction and interactions due to comorbidity and altered pharmacokinetics.

Insight

With aging comes variations in the absorption, distribution, metabolism, and excretion (ADME) of many drugs. Some drugs, such as digoxin, require caution in older patients because of the potential for toxicity.

Digoxin is an *inotropic* drug that is incompletely absorbed (oral dose) and has a substantial fraction cleared by kidneys with 70% to 85% excreted in urine unchanged. The bioavailability of digoxin varies from 50% to more than 90% of the oral dose, although this increases for gelatin capsules to nearly 100%. It is not uncommon for older patients in medical imaging to be prescribed digoxin.

The half-life of digoxin is 1.5 to 2 days (36–44 h), although this becomes prolonged in renal dysfunction. Digoxin has a volume of distribution of about 7.3 L/kg, but this decreases in renal disease and hypothyroidism (increases in hyperthyroidism). Oral digoxin follows a *two-compartment model* (Fig. 5-2), the first compartment (small volume) being plasma and rapidly equilibrating tissues and the second compartment (large volume) being the more slowly equilibrating tissues. Concentrations in heart, liver, and skeletal muscle tend to be higher than plasma concentrations, while 20% to 30% remains plasma bound. Since cardiac effects are associated with the larger volume, plasma concentrations are not an accurate reflection of pharmacologic effects until there is equilibrium between both compartments (at least 6 h after oral dose). Nonetheless, the distribution half-life of 35 min, *onset of action* (oral) of 30 to 120 min, *time to peak* action of 6 to 8 h (oral) means that pharmacological effects can be seen well before equilibrium. The ideal time to sample is 7 to 14 days after commencement of maintenance regime.

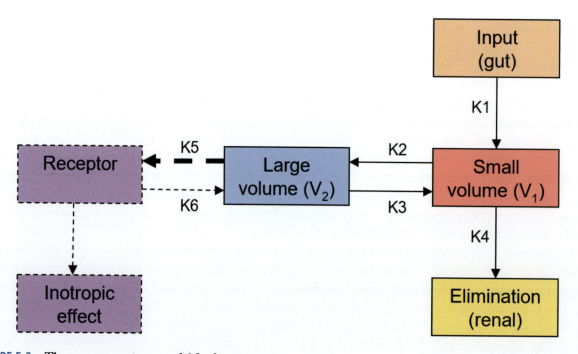

FIGURE 5-2   The two-compartment model for digoxin.

Despite its narrow *therapeutic index* and potential fatal toxicity, particularly in the elderly, digoxin is widely used in the management of congestive heart failure and arrhythmia. Unfortunately, digoxin is associated with a significant increase in hospitalizations and mortality among the elderly. Digoxin toxicity is common in the elderly and relates to a number of factors:

- Reduction in lean body mass
- Decreased GFR
- Decreased muscle mass
- Diuretic-induced potassium loss
- Drug interactions
- Comorbidity

Aging results in prolonged elimination half-life and decreased volume of distribution for digoxin. The most important age-related change is that of deterioration of renal function, and this demands lower dosage to avoid toxicity. Using the two-compartment model, the transfer constant from small to large compartments is increased with aging, elimination is decreased, and both of the compartmental volumes of distribution are reduced. Figure 5-3 provides an overview of the two-compartment model for digoxin in older people, and the two compartments are depicted in Figures 5-4 and 5-5 respectively for digoxin concentration and time curves for normal and older populations.

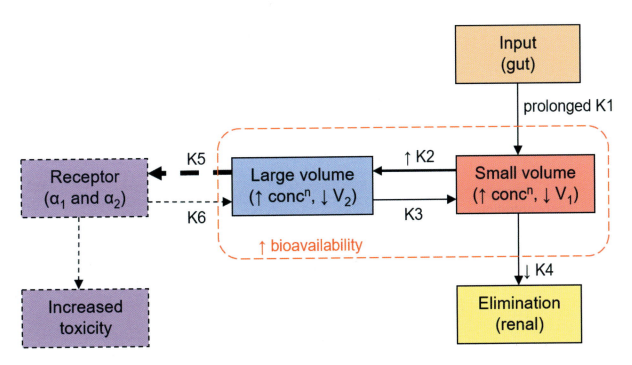

FIGURE 5-3 The two-compartment model for digoxin in the elderly.

64 Pharmacology Primer for Medications

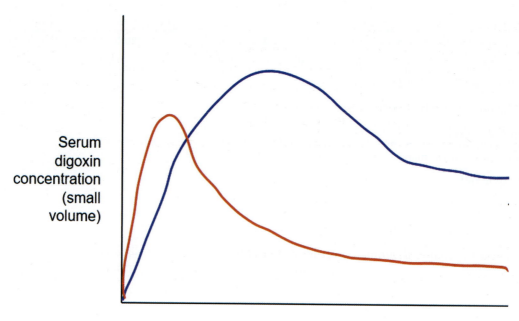

FIGURE 5-4 Digoxin concentration and time curves for normal (red) and elderly (blue) populations for the small volume (plasma). The main features are the delayed time to peak for the elderly population, reflecting delayed absorption. The higher peak for the elderly population reflects the effects on plasma concentration in the reduced volume. The amplitude of the tail in the elderly population reflects the interaction of decreased renal clearance and the large percentage of digoxin that is generally excreted unchanged. The increased area under the curve (AUC) is consistent with increased bioavailability.

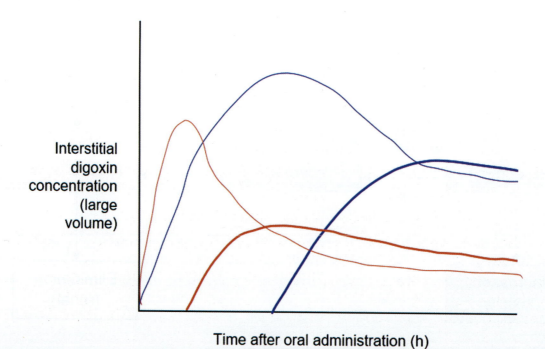

FIGURE 5-5 Digoxin concentration and time curves for normal (red) and elderly (blue) populations for the large volume (interstitial) superimposed for comparison on the small volume (plasma) curves from Figure 5-4 (thin lines). The main features are slightly higher concentrations in the large volume after equilibrium, increased bioavailability in the elderly, and slower clearance in the elderly (slope of line). The increased AUC is consistent with increased bioavailability.

Summary

Age, disease, and pregnancy result in structural and functional changes, and these changes have marked effects on critical organ systems. Altered homeostatic capacity and functional reserve have significant pharmacokinetic implications. Reduced functional reserve increases the vulnerability of older people to disease and drug toxicity. Across the life cycle, there are variations in body composition that, combined with variations in renal function and volume of distribution, alter plasma elimination and bioavailability. An intimate understanding of pharmacology, particularly in the older person, improves the safe use of adjunctive or imaging medications in patients.

References

Armour D, Cairns C. *Medicines in the Elderly*. London, England: Pharmaceutical Press; 2002.

Asperheim K, Favaro J. *Introduction to Pharmacology*. 12th ed. St. Louis, MO: Elsevier; 2012.

Block JH, Beale JM. *Wilson and Gisvold's Textbook of Organic Medicinal and Pharmaceutical Chemistry*. 12th ed. Philadelphia, PA: Lippincott Williams & Wilkins; 2011.

Bryant B, Knights K, Salerno E. *Pharmacology for Health Professionals*. 2nd ed. Sydney, Australia: Mosby Elsevier; 2007.

Currie G. Pharmacology part 1: introduction to pharmacodynamics, *J Nucl Med Technol*. 2018;46:81–86.

Currie G. Pharmacology part 2: introduction to pharmacokinetics. *J Nucl Med Technol*. 2018;46:221–230.

Currie G, Kiat H, Wheat J. Pharmacokinetic considerations for digoxin in older people. *TOCMJ*. 2011;5:130–135.

Cusack BJ. Pharmacokinetics in older persons. *Am J Geriatr Pharmacother*. 2004;2:274–302.

Delafuente JC. Pharmacokinetic and pharmacodynamic alterations in the geriatric patient. *Consult Pharm*. 2008;23:324–334.

El Desoky ES. Pharmacokinetic-pharmacodynamic crisis in the elderly. *Am J Ther*. 2007;14:488–498.

Ewing AB. Altered drug response in the elderly. In: Armour D, Cairns C, eds. *Medicines in the Elderly*. London, England: Pharmaceutical Press; 2002:15–27.

Golan DE, Tashjian AH, Armstrong EJ, Armstrong AW. *Principles of Pharmacology: The Pathophysiologic Basis of Drug Therapy*. 3rd ed. Philadelphia, PA: Lippincott Williams & Wilkins; 2012.

Goodyer LI. Compliance, concordance and polypharmacy in the elderly. In: Armour D, Cairns C, eds. *Medicines in the Elderly*. London, England: Pharmaceutical Press; 2002:371–397.

Greenstein B. *Rapid Revision in Clinical Pharmacology*. New York, NY: Radcliffe Publishing; 2008.

Hacker M, Messer W, Bachmann K. *Pharmacology: Principles and Practice*. London, England: Elsevier; 2009.

Jambhekar SS, Breen PJ. *Basic Pharmacokinetics*. London, England: Pharmaceutical Press; 2009.

Katzung BG, Masters SB, Trevor AJ. *Basic and Clinical Pharmacology*. 12th ed. New York, NY: McGraw Hill; 2012.

Kostrzewski A. Cardiovascular medicines in the elderly. In: Armour D, Cairns C, eds. *Medicines in the Elderly*. London, England: Pharmaceutical Press; 2002.

Mangoni AA, Jackson SHD. Age-related changes in pharmacokinetics and pharmacodynamics: basic principles and practical applications. *Br J Clin Pharmacol*. 2003;57(1):6–14.

McLean AJ, Le Couteur DG. Aging biology and geriatric clinical pharmacology. *Pharmacol Rev*. 2004;56(2):163–184.

Rang H, Dale M, Ritter J, Flower R. *Rang and Dale's Pharmacology*. 6th ed. London, England: Churchill Livingston; 2008.

Waller D, Renwick A, Hillier K. *Medical Pharmacology and Therapeutics*. 2nd ed. London, England: Elsevier; 2006.

CHAPTER 6

Renal Imaging Interventions

Chapter Objectives

Specific learning outcomes (page ix) of this text addressed in this chapter:

- Apply the principles of pharmacology to the safe and effective use of medicines.
- Recognize general, patient-specific, and scenario-specific risks, precautions, and contraindications for use of medicines.
- Apply the pharmacokinetic and pharmacodynamic principles of medications to identify and explain normal and adverse reactions to medications.
- Administer medications safely, effectively, and appropriately according to procedures and within regulatory and statutory parameters.
- Monitor patients for, identify, and manage adverse reactions.

After reading, digesting, reflecting on, and reviewing the content of this chapter, readers should be able to

1. Demonstrate command of key pharmacology terms.
2. Demonstrate enhanced understanding of the principles associated with the pharmacology of renal interventions.
3. Demonstrate critical thinking to effect problem solving related to interventional protocols and procedures.
4. Recognize, explain, and interpret clinical problems and evidence in relation to renal drug use and application.
5. Demonstrate understanding of the mode of action, pharmacokinetics, risks, precautions, contraindications, adverse effects, interactions, and appropriate dosage of key renal medications.
6. Apply knowledge of the general principles and concepts in a translational manner to clinical practice.

Key Terms

adjunctive	bioavailability	drug interaction	interventional	nephrotoxicity
ACE inhibitor	cessation	hypersensitivity	loop diuretic	precaution
adverse reaction	contraindication			

Some of the text, tables, and figures in this chapter were extracted from "Pharmacology Part 3A: Interventional Medications in Renal and Biliary Imaging" by Geoff Currie (*J Nucl Med Technol.* 2018;46:326–334).

Introduction

Patients presenting to the radiology or nuclear medicine department may be taking medication that can interfere with the procedure. Typically, these represent cessation medications, and the period of cessation is largely dependent on the half-life of the medication combined with a clinical decision about the patient's health when that medication is withheld (e.g., other *angiotensin-converting enzyme [ACE] inhibitors* when performing renal scanning in renovascular hypertension). This interference, however, can enhance the procedure by enabling the medical radiation technologist to control the introduction of the medication, deliberately alter physiology, and examine that response (e.g., furosemide diuresis in renography). These types of deliberately administered medications represent interventional medications, which may also be called *imaging medications*. Interventional medications not only enhance the physiological process being evaluated but also can increase the sensitivity and specificity of the procedure. It may also be necessary to administer a medication to alter a patient's condition in some way but without deliberately influencing the physiological response being examined (e.g., sedation of a patient to gain compliance). Drugs used for this purpose are called adjunctive medications and are addressed in Chapter 9.

The scope of practice for medical radiation technologists requires that they display a thorough understanding and working knowledge of indications, contraindications, warnings, precautions, proper use, drug interactions, and adverse reactions for each medication to be used. That understanding and knowledge requires a command of the principles of pharmacology provided in earlier chapters. The content conveyed in the previous chapters should be considered assumed knowledge for this and subsequent chapters. To that end, those foundational principles are not redefined here. The list of interventional and adjunctive medications used in nuclear medicine, radiology, and radiation oncology is long, and an exhaustive examination of all of them is beyond the scope of this text.

Interventional (imaging) medications are medications used to evoke a specific physiological or biochemical response used in conjunction with diagnostic imaging or therapeutic procedures (e.g., captopril). *Adjunctive* medications are medications used to respond to a patient's condition during a procedure (e.g., chloral hydrate). For interventional medications routinely used in renal imaging, this chapter identifies indications for their use; outlines the dosage and administration modes; explains the mode of action and pharmacology; and describes precautions, contraindications, and adverse reactions. Interventional renal scans are among the most commonly performed procedures in general nuclear medicine. Diuretic and ACE inhibition renal imaging (renogram) are the principle interventional applications discussed and are summarized in Table 6-1.

Furosemide (Lasix)

Diuretics generally increase urine volume by inhibiting reabsorption of sodium and chloride in the nephron. There are 3 main classes of diuretics, and the 4th class is added to this discussion because it has an interventional application in brain scanning (Fig. 6-1):

1. *Loop diuretics* (e.g., furosemide)
2. Thiazide diuretics (e.g., hydrochlorothiazide)
3. Potassium-sparing diuretics (e.g., amiloride)
4. Carbonic anhydrase inhibitors (e.g., acetazolamide)

TABLE 6-1 Interventional Medications Used in Renal Scanning*

Drug	Dose	Pharmacokinetics	Mechanism of Action	Contraindications/Cautions	Adverse Effects/Interactions
Furosemide	20–40 mg intravenously in an adult and 1 mg/kg intravenously over 1–2 min for pediatrics	◆ 5 min onset ◆ Peak 15–30 min ◆ Half-life 1.5–2 h ◆ Duration 2–3 h ◆ 99% plasma protein bound	Loop diuretic by inhibiting sodium, potassium, and chloride transport in the ascending portion of loop of Henle.	Contraindicated in anuria, sulfonamide hypersensitivity, and sodium or fluid depletion. Caution in kidney or liver disease, diabetes, gout, lupus, pregnancy, and after urologic procedures.	Tinnitus, allergic reaction, nausea, vomiting, dizziness, blurred vision, headache, hypotension, dehydration. Potential interactions with aspirin, diuretics, digoxin, lithium, antihypertensives, and NSAIDs.
Captopril	25–50 mg tablet orally 60 min before renal scan	◆ 15 min onset ◆ Peak 45–70 min ◆ Half-life 2–3 h ◆ Duration 6–12 h ◆ 30% plasma protein bound	Blocks conversion of angiotensin I to angiotensin II, blocking blood pressure compensation and reducing glomerular filtration.	Contraindicated in angioedema, high renin levels, dehydration, salt depletion, recent dialysis, aortic stenosis, pregnancy, and hypersensitivity. Caution in scleroderma, lupus, depression, diabetes, liver dysfunction, peripheral vascular disease, and dialysis.	Hypotension, dizziness, tachycardia, chest pain, loss of taste, fever, and rash. Can cause a dry cough. Potential interactions with other ACE inhibitors or ARBs, diuretics, hypertensives, NSAIDs, digoxin, and lithium.
Enalapril	Oral dose 20–40 mg 0.04 mg/kg in 10 mL of saline intravenously over 3–5 min to maximum dose of 2.5 mg	◆ 60 min onset ◆ Peak 4–6 h ◆ Half-life 11 hours ◆ Duration 24 h ◆ 50%–60% plasma protein bound If given intravenously, onset is 15 min and peak effect is 1 h.	Same as for captopril except enalapril is ester prodrug converted to enalaprilat in liver after absorption.		

*Duration is the period of significant or measurable effect. Some adverse effects are more likely when used therapeutically than in single interventional doses.

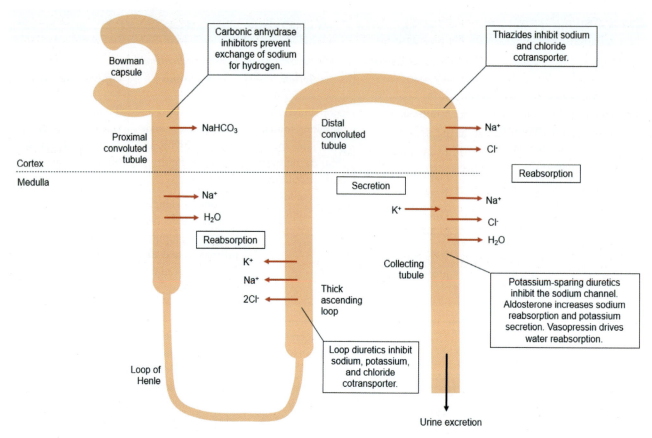

FIGURE 6-1 Schematic representation of the sites of action of different classes of diuretics. Furosemide is a loop diuretic acting on the thick ascending loop of the loop of Henle in the nephron.

Furosemide is a sulfamoylbenzoic acid-based loop diuretic that increases urine volume by inhibiting reabsorption of sodium, potassium, and chloride. While diuresis can occur in proximal and distal tubules in the nephron, it is predominantly situated at the ascending aspect of the loop of Henle; hence the name *loop diuretic*. Loop diuretics are characterized by rapid onset and potent diuretic effects but typically are of a short direction. Furosemide is active inside the lumen of the loop of Henle and therefore relies on adequate glomerular filtration and secretion of furosemide to have its effect. Consequently, furosemide may have a truncated response in renal impairment.

Increasing the flow rate of urine with furosemide allows differentiation of the obstructed kidney (after furosemide clearance half-life >20 min) from the unobstructed kidney (after furosemide clearance half-life <10 min) and the dilated but not obstructed kidney (after furosemide clearance half-life between 10 and 20 min). Furosemide is the diuretic of choice because it has superior peak effects.

There are 2 sodium (Na^+), potassium (K^+), and chloride ($2Cl^-$) cotransporters (*NKCC*): $NKCC_1$ and $NKCC_2$. The former is primarily involved in secretion and the latter primarily in absorption; loop diuretics have an affinity for $NKCC_2$. Transport effectively relies on simultaneous binding to all 3 ion sites, and thus, blockade of just one results in inhibition. Furosemide binds to the chloride-binding site and by doing so inhibits transport of sodium, potassium, and chloride in the loop of Henle (Fig. 6-1). The increased urinary excretion of sodium, potassium, chloride, calcium, and magnesium results in low osmolality, which inhibits the reabsorption of water by the kidney, increasing urine volume. A secondary effect changes the charge difference across the lumen wall, which inhibits calcium and magnesium transport. Furosemide also releases vasodilating prostaglandins, which produce short-duration venodilation.

Furosemide has variable oral bioavailability (10%–100%), while intravenous administration provides 100% bioavailability. It has 95% to 99% plasma protein binding, 50% is excreted unchanged in urine, and the remaining 50% is metabolized in the kidney (conjugated with glucuronic acid in kidney). The elimination half-life is 1.5 to 2 hours, but it can be substantially extended in end-stage renal disease (10 h) and hepatic dysfunction (50–327 min). After intravenous administration, onset of action occurs within 5 minutes with peak activity seen at 15 to 30 minutes and effects of significance lasting 2 to 3 hours.

The clinical role of furosemide tends to be to manage edema in patients with congestive heart failure. It can also be used to treat hypertension. In nuclear medicine, it is used for the evaluation of obstructive uropathy with renography. The standard adult intravenous dose is 20 to 40 mg, and pediatric doses are 0.5 to 1 mg/kg administered intravenously over 1 to 2 minutes. Given the time to peak activity, it can be administered preemptively 15 minutes before the administration of the radiopharmaceutical. More typically, furosemide is administered 15 to 20 minutes after the radiopharmaceutical if radiopharmaceutical retention in the renal pelvis is apparent.

Furosemide is contraindicated in patients with anuresis, those with known hypersensitivity (furosemide specifically or sulfonamides generally), and those significantly dehydrated or with sodium depletion. Furosemide should be administered with caution to prevent injury or suture tearing in patients who have had recent urologic procedures. Patients should be adequately hydrated before administration. It should be used with caution in known kidney or liver disease, pregnancy, diabetes, gout, and lupus. Furosemide is excreted in breast milk.

Adverse reactions to a single dose of furosemide are usually mild and transient and include nausea, vomiting, diarrhea, dizziness, hypotension, headache, tinnitus, rash, electrolyte imbalance, and dehydration. These adverse reactions are more common when furosemide is being used therapeutically. Therapeutic doses of furosemide may also cause vision disturbance, sun sensitivity, hearing impairment, confusion, arrhythmia, limb numbness, tingling and pain, yellow eyes and skin, and abdominal pain. Allergic reactions are possible. Adverse effects on hearing can be minimized with slower injection rates at 4 mg/min.

Furosemide can enhance nephrotoxicity of cephalosporin antibacterials and hearing impairment associated with aminoglycoside antibacterials. It can reduce the effect of antiepileptics such as phenytoin. Cumulative effect with other diuretics can lead to electrolyte imbalance and dehydration. Hypotension can be more severe when used concurrently with ACE inhibitors or angiotensin receptor blockers (ARBs). Furosemide can increase the risk of toxicity of lithium, digoxin, cisplatin and aminoglycosides. Nonsteroidal anti-inflammatory drugs (NSAIDs) decrease diuresis and can exacerbate side effects.

Captopril

The kidneys play an important role in blood pressure regulation through the negative feedback mechanism of the *renin-angiotensin-aldosterone system* (RAAS). A decrease in blood flow through the kidneys (decreased arterial blood pressure) triggers a pressure gradient change between afferent and efferent arterioles in the Bowman capsule. This leads to reduced glomerular filtration and release of renin, which facilitates the production of angiotensin I. As illustrated in Figure 6-2, an ACE converts angiotensin I to angiotensin II, leading to vasoconstriction and increased blood volume, which in turn increases blood pressure. The presence of a hemodynamically significant renal artery stenosis initiates this cascade, resulting in restoration of glomerular filtration (near normal renogram) and hypertension. A 75% stenosis is typically considered necessary for hemodynamic significance, although there is variability in reported cutoffs down to 50% stenosis. Bilateral renal artery stenosis has increased renin production from both kidneys, whereas unilateral disease has increased renin in the diseased kidney and suppressed renin production in the normal kidney.

72 Pharmacology Primer for Medications

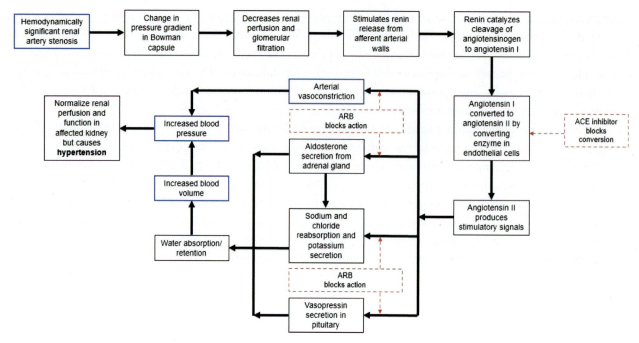

FIGURE 6-2 Flow chart of RAAS response to decreased blood flow (solid lines). Inhibition of this response can be undertaken (dashed lines) by ACE inhibitors acting to prevent conversion of angiotensin I to angiotensin II or by ARBs antagonizing the angiotensin receptor at the numerous sites of action.

Captopril is an ACE inhibitor that competitively blocks the ACE to decrease blood pressure. While captopril is the prototype ACE inhibitor, it differs from most other ACE inhibitors in that it is not an ester prodrug. This property allows more rapid onset of action and shorter duration of effect, making it ideal for an interventional study. Prodrugs such as enalapril have slower onset and longer duration; therefore, therapeutically, they allow a once-per-day dosing regimen.

Captopril blocks the conversion of angiotensin I to angiotensin II. The compensatory vasoconstriction response is thereby inhibited in the efferent arterioles in the kidney, which leads to decreased glomeruli filtration in a kidney with a hemodynamically significant renal artery stenosis. Captopril has an oral bioavailability of 70% to 75%. It has 30% plasma protein binding, 40% to 50% is excreted unchanged in urine, and the remaining 50% to 60% is metabolized in the liver. The elimination half-life is 2 to 3 hours, but this can be increased in renal dysfunction. After oral administration, onset of action occurs within 15 minutes with peak activity seen at 45 to 70 minutes and effects of significance lasting 6 to 12 hours.

Captopril is not the front-line ACE inhibitor but is used for treatment of hypertension in heart failure and post–myocardial infarction. The properties that make it the preferred ACE inhibitor for renal imaging are the same properties that make it inferior to other ACE inhibitors for therapy: onset, half-life, and duration of effect. Captopril is used in conjunction with renal imaging (renogram) for the detection and characterization of the hemodynamic significance of renal artery stenosis in renovascular hypertension. Patients should discontinue ACE inhibitor therapy, including ARBs, prior to the study. The standard dose is 25 mg orally 60 minutes before commencement of the renal scan. However, 50 mg may be required if the requisite change in blood pressure does not occur. Patients should be monitored for 60 minutes after captopril (blood pressure) and kept hydrated (1 L). Improved absorption and bioavailability can be achieved by crushing the tablet prior to administration.

Captopril is contraindicated in patients with known hypersensitivity to captopril, angioedema, high renin levels, dehydration, salt depletion, recent dialysis, or aortic stenosis. Captopril use should be avoided during pregnancy. Captopril should be used with caution in patients with scleroderma, lupus, depression, diabetes, or liver dysfunction. Therapeutically, captopril is not recommended in patients with renovascular disease such as renal artery stenosis, but a single dose for an interventional procedure can be safely undertaken with patient supervision. Captopril is excreted in breast milk but unlikely to be harmful to a nursing infant with relative infant doses on the order of 0.02% of the mother. It should be used with caution in the elderly or those with peripheral vascular disease.

Single doses of captopril for interventional studies may elicit a number of adverse reactions, including hypotension, dizziness, tachycardia, chest pain, loss of taste, fever, and a rash. Longer-term therapy may lead to a dry cough, proteinuria, neutropenia, and thrombocythemia. The intractable dry cough associated with ACE inhibitors is well documented, has implications for therapeutic compliance, and drives some patients toward ARB therapy. The dry cough is thought to be due to incidental inhibition of the enzyme that breaks down bradykinin.

Other ACE inhibitors and ARBs need to be withheld for 3 days prior to the captopril scan or, if the patient is being treated therapeutically with captopril, for 1 day. The patient may experience severe hypotension if captopril is administered concurrently with diuretics or antihypertensive medications. The most serious interaction for ACE inhibitors is hyperkalemia due to the additive effect of potassium retention with diuretics and NSAIDs. Potassium-sparing diuretics and any potassium supplements should be ceased prior to ACE inhibition therapy. Captopril can decrease lithium and digoxin excretion and increase the risk of toxicity for both. Antacids reduce the bioavailability of captopril.

Enalapril

Enalapril is not an ACE inhibitor but rather an ester *prodrug* that is enzymatically converted in the liver to the active metabolite enalaprilat. The principles, mode of action, usual indications, use in nuclear medicine, contraindications, warnings and precautions, adverse reactions, and common interactions are the same as for captopril, discussed previously. Enalapril has an oral bioavailability of 60% and is rapidly *biotransformed* to enalaprilat. Enalaprilat has 50% to 60% plasma protein binding, 90% is excreted in urine, and the remaining 10% is excreted in feces. The elimination half-life is 11 hours but is multiphasic. After oral administration, onset of action occurs within 60 minutes with peak activity seen at 4 to 6 hours and effects of significance lasting 24 hours. The onset and peak times can be reduced to 15 minutes and 60 minutes respectively with intravenous administration.

Enalapril can be administered by oral tablet or intravenous route; however, the benefits of enalapril over captopril (more predictable action) are best demonstrated with an intravenous route. A dose of 0.05 mg/kg diluted in 10 mL of saline is injected intravenously slowly over 5 minutes. If the blood pressure drops more than 30% from baseline, the saline infusion should be increased until blood pressure is back to reference. The renal scan can be commenced at 10 to 15 minutes after enalapril is administered in response to changes in blood pressure. Adverse effects from intravenous enalapril can be reduced using the slow infusion rate (5 min), and this is particularly helpful in reducing the risk of significant hypotension.

Summary

An understanding of basic pharmacology for renal interventional medications allows enhanced practice. Specifically, this deeper understanding of pharmacology, indications, contraindications, warnings, precautions, proper use, drug interactions, and adverse reactions for each medication to be used ensures that nuclear medicine technologists meet the minimum capabilities for their scope of practice. This in turn translates to safer practice and better patient outcomes.

Insight

A *triple whammy* refers to the concurrent use of an ACE inhibitor or an ARB with a diuretic and an NSAID, including the NSAID subclass COX-2 inhibitors, discussed in Chapters 13 and 15. ACE inhibitors or ARBs and diuretics are commonly prescribed together and pose a risk for acute kidney injury. The triple whammy may occur with the addition of a nonprescription NSAID and significantly increases the risk of acute kidney injury. Risk factors for the triple whammy and acute kidney injury include the following:

- Chronic kidney disease
- Liver disease
- Age over 75 years
- Volume depletion
- Ethnicity
- Diabetes
- Heart failure

The triple whammy should be avoided, and careful attention to concurrent medications is critical.

References

Asperheim K, Favaro J. *Introduction to Pharmacology*. 12th ed. St Louis, MO: Elsevier; 2012.

Block JH, Beale JM. *Wilson and Gisvold's Textbook of Organic Medicinal and Pharmaceutical Chemistry*. 12th ed. Philadelphia, PA: Lippincott Williams & Wilkins; 2011.

Bryant B, Knights K, Salerno E. *Pharmacology for Health Professionals*. 2nd ed. Sydney, Australia: Mosby Elsevier; 2007.

Currie G. Pharmacology part 1: introduction to pharmacodynamics. *J Nucl Med Technol*. 2018;46:81–86.

Currie G. Pharmacology part 2: introduction to pharmacokinetics. *J Nucl Med Technol*. 2018;46:221–230.

Currie G. Pharmacology part 3A: interventional medications in renal and biliary imaging. *J Nucl Med Technol*. 2018;46:326–334.

Fine EJ. Interventions in renal scintirenography. *Sem Nucl Med*. 1999;29:128–145.

Golan DE, Tashjian AH, Armstrong EJ, Armstrong AW. *Principles of Pharmacology: The Pathophysiologic Basis of Drug Therapy*. 3rd ed. Philadelphia, PA: Lippincott Williams & Wilkins; 2012.

Hacker M, Messer W, Bachmann K. *Pharmacology: Principles and Practice*. London, England: Elsevier; 2009.

Katzung BG, Masters SB, Trevor AJ. *Basic and Clinical Pharmacology*. 12th ed. New York, NY: McGraw Hill; 2012.

Mettler FA, Guiberteau MJ. *Essentials of Nuclear Medicine Imaging*. 6th ed. Philadelphia, PA: Elsevier/Saunders; 2012.

Park HM, Duncan K. Nonradioactive pharmaceuticals in nuclear medicine. *JNMT*. 1994;22:240–249.

Patrick GL. *An Introduction to Medicinal Chemistry*. 3rd ed. New York, NY: Oxford University Press; 2005.

Rang H, Dale M, Ritter J, Flower R. *Rang and Dale's Pharmacology*. 6th ed. London, England: Churchill Livingston; 2008.

Rossi S (Ed.). *Australian Medicines Handbook 2012*. Adelaide, Australia: Australian Medicines Handbook; 2012:591–598.

Saremi F, Jadvar H, Siegel ME. Pharmacologic interventions in nuclear radiology: indications, imaging protocols, and clinical results. *RadioGraphics*. 2002;22:477–490.

SNMMI-TS Scope of Practice Task Force. Nuclear medicine technologist scope of practice and performance standards. *J Nucl Med Technol*. 2017;45(1):53–64.

Sweetman SC (Ed.). *Martindale: The Complete Drug Reference*. 26th ed. Chicago, IL: Pharmaceutical Press; 2009.

Theobald T. *Sampson's Textbook of Radiopharmacy*. 4th ed. London, England: Pharmaceutical Press; 2011.

Waller D, Renwick A, Hillier K. *Medical Pharmacology and Therapeutics*. 2nd ed. London, England: Elsevier; 2006.

CHAPTER 7

Biliary Imaging Interventions

Chapter Objectives

Specific learning outcomes (page ix) of this text addressed in this chapter:

- Apply the principles of pharmacology to the safe and effective use of medicines.
- Recognize general, patient-specific, and scenario-specific risks, precautions, and contraindications for use of medicines.
- Apply the pharmacokinetic and pharmacodynamic principles of medications to identify and explain normal and adverse reactions to medications.
- Administer medications safely, effectively, and appropriately according to procedures and within regulatory and statutory parameters.
- Monitor patients for, identify, and manage adverse reactions.

After reading, digesting, reflecting on, and reviewing the content of this chapter, readers should be able to

1. Demonstrate command of key pharmacology terms.
2. Demonstrate enhanced understanding of the principles associated with the pharmacology of biliary interventions.
3. Demonstrate critical thinking to effect problem solving related to interventional protocols and procedures.
4. Recognize, explain, and interpret clinical problems and evidence in relation to biliary drug use and application.
5. Demonstrate understanding of the mode of action, pharmacokinetics, risks, precautions, contraindications, adverse effects, interactions, and appropriate dosage of key biliary medications.
6. Apply knowledge of the general principles and concepts in a translational manner to clinical practice.

Key Terms

adjunctive	bioavailability	contraindication	endogenous	opioid agonist
adverse reaction	CCK	drug interaction	hypersensitivity	precaution
augmentation	cessation	ejection fraction	interventional	

Some of the text, tables, and figures in this chapter were extracted from "Pharmacology Part 3A: Interventional Medications in Renal and Biliary Imaging" by Geoff Currie (*J Nucl Med Technol*. 2018;46:326–334).

Introduction

Interventional medications not only enhance the physiological process being evaluated but also can increase the sensitivity and specificity of the procedure. An understanding and working knowledge of the safe use of medicines requires a command of the principles of pharmacology provided in earlier chapters. Interventional hepatobiliary scans are performed frequently in general nuclear medicine. Sincalide stimulation of the gallbladder and morphine augmentation are the principle interventional applications discussed in this chapter and summarized in Table 7-1. The less commonly utilized phenobarbital intervention in the jaundiced neonate is also discussed.

TABLE 7-1	Interventional Medications Used in Biliary Scanning*				
Drug	*Dose*	*Pharmacokinetics*	*Mechanism of Action*	*Contraindications/ Cautions*	*Adverse Effects/ Interactions*
Sincalide	0.02 mcg/kg in 10 mL of saline intravenously over 3–5 min	◆ 5–15 min onset ◆ Peak 40 min ◆ Limited data	Synthetic active portion of CCK stimulates gallbladder contraction and relaxes sphincter of Oddi.	Contraindicated in known hypersensitivity, intestinal obstruction, and pregnancy (spontaneous abortion). Caution with opioids.	Abdominal pain, nausea, dizziness, flushing, urge to defecate, and allergic reaction. No documented interactions.
Morphine	0.04 mg/kg in 10 mL of saline intravenously over 1–2 min (range of 2–4.6 mg). Note this is subanalgesic dose.	◆ 5 min onset ◆ Peak 20 min ◆ Half-life 2 h ◆ Duration 20–50 min ◆ 35% plasma protein bound	Opioid agonist that constricts sphincter of Oddi to increase pressure in common bile duct.	Contraindicated in known hypersensitivity, respiratory depression, and comatose patients. Caution in renal or liver impairment, pregnancy, seizures, head injuries, asthma, hypotension, hypothyroidism, pheochromocytoma, addiction, and dyspnea.	Respiratory depression, hypotension, vomiting, dysphoria, urinary retention, dizziness, sedation, nausea, and constipation. Potential interactions with narcotic analgesics, CNS depressants, benzodiazepines, and monoamine oxidase inhibitors.
Phenobarbital	2.5 mg/kg/ twice daily orally for 5 d prior to study	◆ 30–60 min onset orally ◆ Peak 2–12 h ◆ Half-life 75–120 h ◆ Duration 4 h to 2 d ◆ 45%–60% plasma protein bound	Increases radiotracer uptake and biliary excretion by inducing hepatic enzymes.	Contraindicated in known allergy to phenobarbital and severe respiratory depression. Caution in liver, kidney, or lung dysfunction; the elderly; children; and acute pain.	Sedation, anxiety, respiratory depression, vomiting, dizziness, nausea, headache, and paradoxical excitement. Potential interactions with drugs metabolized by the liver and CNS depressants.

*Duration is the period of significant or measurable effect. Some adverse effects are more likely when used therapeutically than in single interventional doses.

Sincalide

Cholecystokinin (CCK) is an endogenous, 33-amino acid polypeptide hormone secreted in the duodenum in response to a fatty meal. Sincalide (Kinevac) is the *exogenous* active portion (octapeptide) of CCK and is sometimes referred to as CCK-8 to differentiate it from the full polypeptide CCK-33. Sincalide is a synthetic peptide representing the active portion of the endogenous CCK hormone. CCK is released from the duodenal mucosa in response to fat stimuli, which stimulates the contraction of the gallbladder. CCK/sincalide stimulates the dorsal vagus complex, which, through vagal efferents, relaxes the sphincter of Oddi, contracts the gallbladder, and stimulates bile production (Fig. 7-1). The primary mechanism for gallbladder contraction, however, is CCK/sincalide entering the bloodstream to act directly on the gallbladder. Gallbladder contraction occurs when the serum CCK/sincalide levels reach a threshold. Since gallbladder contraction occurs only when serum CCK/sincalide levels reach a threshold, intravenous introduction of CCK-8 is associated with 5 times higher potency. Only limited pharmacokinetic data is available for sincalide. Sincalide administered intravenously has a *bioavailability* of 100%. After intravenous administration, onset of action occurs within 5 to 15 minutes with peak activity seen at 40 minutes. The gallbladder should start emptying within 2 minutes of intravenous administration of sincalide and complete by 11 minutes. A gallbladder ejection fraction of 35% or greater is considered normal.

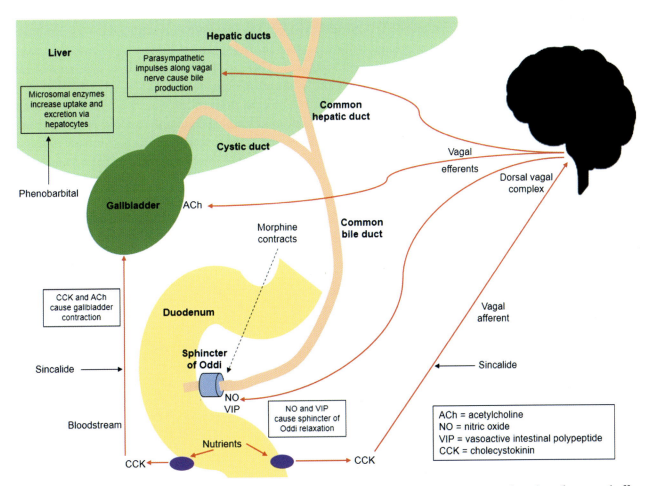

FIGURE 7-1 Schematic representation of the release of CCK to produce gallbladder contraction directly and via vagal afferents. The implications of exogenous sincalide are demonstrated. The relaxation (CCK) and contraction (morphine) effects on the sphincter of Oddi are illustrated. Phenobarbital stimulation of biliary excretion independently of the vagal nerve is also illustrated.

The usual use of sincalide is to contract the gallbladder as an adjunct to cholecystography. It has also been used as a function test of the pancreas in combination with secretin. Endogenous CCK has been used to manage obesity because CCK inhibits gastric motility and increases satiety. Sincalide is used to assess gallbladder function, including calculation of the gallbladder ejection fraction (GBEF), and patency of the biliary system after gallbladder contraction. Sincalide intervention can enhance the specificity of the procedure and shorten the time to reporting the study. The patient should have fasted for a minimum of 4 hours and a maximum of 6 hours to ensure that gallbladder filling of the radiopharmaceutical is not impeded by residual endogenous CCK (45 min half-life) contracting the gallbladder or a full gallbladder due to absence of any endogenous CCK for a long period. The dose of sincalide is 0.02 mcg/kg intravenously over 5 minutes. A larger second dose of 0.04 mcg/kg diluted in 10 mL of saline administered intravenously over 5 minutes may be used if gallbladder contraction is not achieved with the first dose.

There has been some controversy with regard to the correct administration of sincalide: 3- to 5-minute injections or the more physiological 30- to 60-minute infusion. The bulk of the literature is built on the premise that there is variability in the normal value for GBEF among healthy subjects (35%) and, as a result, potential for false positives. The 35% is the value above which we can be reasonably certain (95%) represents absence of gallbladder dysfunction (even if other biliary disease is present). It does not and should not suggest that a value under 35% equates to abnormality or the notion of false positives. A second value that represents the boundary below which there is 95% certainty gallbladder dysfunction is present is required. The literature discrediting the 3- to 5-minute infusion protocol does so on the basis of a single value capturing all, false positives being a poor outcome, overlooking false negatives, and absence of a genuine gold standard. There would be resistance to such a universal change due to the increased demands (time and supervision) of the 60-minute infusion.

Arguments stringently requiring a 60-minute infusion overlook the protocol previously outlined in which a GBEF lower than 35% should consider a second infusion or delayed imaging. Certainly, adverse effects increase with a 3- to 5-minute infusion, but the bulk of the literature remains consistent with the 3- to 5-minute infusion method. Moreover, both FDA and manufacturer (Bracco) describe a rapid injection protocol. Furthermore, the recent literature on which international departments and professional bodies draw insight to inform protocols is quite variable. While key recent literature universally suggests the longer infusion is most appropriate to reduce false positives and unwanted symptoms, there is some debate about whether 30 or 60 minutes should be employed, or indeed whether multiple 10-minute infusions should be used. While physiologically the 60-minute infusion is the best approach, this is not new knowledge. In the 1980s, 60-minute infusions were employed almost universally. But the trade-off between time and the perceived small benefit in reduced variability in the normal GBEF saw the shorter 3- to 5-minute infusion almost universally adopted.

Sincalide is contraindicated in known hypersensitivity or intestinal obstruction. It is contraindicated in pregnancy due to the risk of spontaneous abortion. Sincalide should not be administered after morphine. Adverse reactions are common but transient for sincalide and include abdominal pain and nausea. Less commonly, patients may experience dizziness, flushing, and the urge to defecate. Adverse reactions can be minimized using a diluted dose (10 mL) and slow intravenous infusion (5 min). There are no documented drug interactions as a result of sincalide's short-lived and mild action. Morphine and other opiates should, however, be stopped for 3 half-lives.

Morphine

Morphine is an *opioid agonist* that is mostly selective for μ-opioid receptor (OP_3) but can interact with other opioid receptors (κ and δ) at high doses. As an analgesic, the mechanism of action of opioids is not well understood, but inhibition of substance P release from neurons is a key aspect. Opioid receptors are G protein–coupled transmembrane receptors that can be activated (agonists include morphine), inhibited (antagonists include naloxone), or partially agonized (e.g., buprenorphine).

Morphine increases smooth muscle tone, particularly the sphincters of the gastrointestinal and biliary tracts. Morphine contracts, or constricts, the sphincter of Oddi at the junction of the common bile duct and duodenum (Fig. 7-1), which causes back pressure in the common bile duct. The back pressure in the common bile duct allows a patent cystic duct to fill the gallbladder with bile and radiopharmaceutical. In doing so, it allows differentiation of chronic cholecystitis (incomplete cystic duct obstruction) from acute cholecystitis (complete cystic duct obstruction). It should be noted that for this intervention to be successful, there needs to be adequate clearance of the radiopharmaceutical from the liver after morphine administration. Newer radiopharmaceuticals with rapid clearance may require a second small (top-up) dose of radiopharmaceutical to avoid false-positive studies for acute cholecystitis.

Morphine can be administered via numerous routes, but for hepatobiliary *augmentation*, the dose is administered intravenously. Subanalgesic doses of 0.04 mg/kg intravenously over 3 minutes deliver 100% bioavailability. It has 35% plasma protein binding; 50% is metabolized in the liver (conjugated with glucuronic acid) to morphine-3-glucuronide, which is inactive, and excreted by the kidneys. A further 5% to 15% is metabolized to morphine-6-glucuronide which is more potent than morphine (1–2 h half-life). Ten percent is excreted in the kidneys unchanged, and 10% is excreted as conjugates in bile and feces. The elimination half-life is 2 hours, but morphine-3-glucuronide has an elimination half-life of 2.4 to 6.7 hours. After intravenous administration, onset of action occurs within 5 minutes with peak activity seen at 20 minutes and effects of significance lasting 4 to 5 hours. Morphine crosses the placenta and enters breast milk.

Morphine is primarily a strong opioid analgesic when given in therapeutic doses. Morphine is used for the relief of moderate to severe pain and to relieve anxiety associated with severe pain. It has been used as a hypnotic for insomnia due to pain. Morphine helps to differentiate chronic and acute cholecystitis. Morphine increases the specificity and shortens the duration of the biliary study in these patients (by avoiding delayed imaging). If the gallbladder is not visualized 60 minutes after administration of the biliary radiopharmaceutical, but common bile duct and duodenum are evident, morphine could be considered to avoid delayed imaging. Morphine has no role in the nonvisualized gallbladder in post-cholecystectomy patients. If the duodenum is not visualized, morphine should not be administered. An intravenous administration over 1 to 3 minutes of 0.04 mg/kg of morphine is the standard dose, with imaging continuing for 30 minutes.

While the doses being used in this interventional application are subanalgesic, morphine remains contraindicated in patients with a known allergy to morphine and those with respiratory depression. It should not be used in patients who are comatose. Morphine should be used with caution in patients with seizures, head injuries, asthma, chronic lung disease, hypothyroidism, adrenocortical insufficiency, pheochromocytoma, kidney or liver dysfunction, prostatic hyperplasia, hypotension, shock, inflammatory or obstructive bowel disorders, myasthenia gravis, and pancreatitis. Caution should be employed in cases of opioid addiction. Caution should also be exercised in pregnancy and in mothers who are breast-feeding, as morphine is excreted in breast milk.

While severe adverse reactions are uncommon with subanalgesic doses, a number of adverse reactions can occur, including respiratory depression, dizziness, drowsiness, sedation, nausea, vomiting, constipation, and sweating. With longer-term use, patients may experience dry mouth, facial flushing, headache, vertigo, bradycardia, tachycardia, palpitations, orthostatic hypotension, hypothermia, restlessness, mood changes, decreased libido, hallucinations, and miosis. Large doses of opioids produce respiratory depression and hypotension; circulatory failure and coma are possible. Morphine has a dose-related histamine-releasing effect (unlikely to be of significance in biliary scan doses) that can cause urticaria, pruritus, and hypotension.

Therapeutic doses of narcotic analgesics need to be ceased for 5 half-lives to avoid interference with the biliary scan. While morphine augmentation studies employ subanalgesic doses, consideration should be given to potential interactions with other medications. Morphine interacts with alcohol and other central nervous system (CNS) depressants to enhance respiratory and CNS depression and hypotension. Monoamine oxidase inhibitors can enhance the effects of morphine, and rifampicin can reduce analgesic effects of morphine. There is an additive effect with benzodiazepines, and H_2 antagonists inhibit morphine metabolism. Clomipramine and amitriptyline increase the plasma availability of morphine. Naloxone is a narcotic antagonist and can be used with doses of 0.4 mg intravenously as an adjunctive medication in response to a severe allergic reaction to morphine.

Phenobarbital

Phenobarbital is a long-acting barbiturate *sedative* and *hypnotic* that acts through $GABA_A$ receptor agonism (positive modulation). It also acts as an anticonvulsant. Phenobarbital enhances and accelerates radiopharmaceutical excretion by the biliary system, which allows differentiation of biliary atresia from neonatal hepatitis in the jaundiced neonate. Phenobarbital enhances the entire hepatic transport system independently of vagal induction. Phenobarbital induces microsomal enzymes in the liver, which increases uptake and excretion of a number of compounds, including bilirubin (Fig. 7-1). Consequently, phenobarbital enhances biliary excretion (including biliary radiopharmaceuticals) if the biliary system is patent but not in biliary atresia. Phenobarbital has significant variability with respect to pharmacokinetics. Phenobarbital has an oral bioavailability of 90%. It has 45% to 60% plasma protein binding, 25% is excreted unchanged in urine, and the remainder is only partially metabolized in the liver. The elimination half-life is 75 to 120 hours. After oral administration, onset of action occurs within 30 to 60 minutes with peak activity seen at 2 to 12 hours and effects of significance lasting 4 to 48 hours.

Phenobarbital is used as an antiepileptic to control partial and generalized tonic-clonic seizures. It can also be used in the emergency management of acute seizures. In medical imaging, it is used to differentiate biliary atresia from neonatal hepatitis in the jaundiced neonate and to increase the sensitivity and specificity of the procedure. Phenobarbital is administered orally for 5 days prior to the biliary study at a dose rate of 5 mg/kg/day usually split into 2 doses (i.e., 2.5 mg/kg twice daily for 5 days).

Phenobarbital is contraindicated where there is a known allergy to it and in patients with severe respiratory depression. Caution should be exercised in children and the elderly, acute pain, and depression. Caution is also required for impaired liver, kidney, or lung function. While sedation is the most common adverse reaction, phenobarbital can produce a number of common side effects, including respiratory depression, drowsiness, lethargy, rash, nausea, vomiting, and a paradoxical hyperexcitement in pediatrics. Mood changes and depression can be seen with longer-term use. Nystagmus and ataxia might occur at high doses. Hypersensitivity is uncommon but can occur. By virtue of the role of phenobarbital in activating microsomal enzymes in the liver, it can have a significant negative effect on drugs metabolized in the liver, including analgesics, antibacterials, antiarrhythmics, antidepressants, antiepileptics, antipsychotics, antivirals, beta-blockers, calcium channel blockers, digoxin, ciclosporin, diuretics, theophylline, and some vaccines. Phenobarbital effects can be enhanced by CNS depressants and alcohol.

Summary

An understanding of basic pharmacology for biliary interventional medications allows enhanced practice. Specifically, this deeper understanding of pharmacology, indications, contraindications, warnings, precautions, proper use, drug interactions, and adverse reactions for each medication to be used ensures that medical radiation technologists meet the minimum capabilities for their scope of practice. This in turn translates to safer practice and better patient outcomes.

References

Block JH, Beale JM. *Wilson and Gisvold's Textbook of Organic Medicinal and Pharmaceutical Chemistry*. 12th ed. Philadelphia, PA: Lippincott Williams & Wilkins; 2011.

Bryant B, Knights K, Salerno E. *Pharmacology for Health Professionals*. 2nd ed. Sydney, Australia: Mosby Elsevier; 2007.

Currie G. Pharmacology part 2: introduction to pharmacokinetics. *J Nucl Med Technol.* 2018;46:221–230.

Currie G. Pharmacology part 3A: interventional medications in renal and biliary imaging, *J Nucl Med Technol.* 2018;46:326–334.

Golan DE, Tashjian AH, Armstrong EJ, Armstrong AW. *Principles of Pharmacology: The Pathophysiologic Basis of Drug Therapy.* 3rd ed. Philadelphia, PA: Lippincott Williams & Wilkins; 2012.

Hacker M, Messer W, Bachmann K. *Pharmacology: Principles and Practice.* London, England: Elsevier; 2009.

Katzung BG, Masters SB, Trevor AJ. *Basic and Clinical Pharmacology.* 12th ed. New York, NY: McGraw Hill; 2012.

Krishnamurthy S, Krishnamurthy GT. Cholecystokinin and morphine pharmacological intervention during 99mTc-HIDA cholescintigraphy: a rational approach. *Sem Nucl Med.* 1996;26:16–24.

Mettler FA, Guiberteau MJ. *Essentials of Nuclear Medicine Imaging.* 6th ed. Philadelphia, PA: Elsevier/Saunders; 2012.

Park HM, Duncan K. Nonradioactive pharmaceuticals in nuclear medicine. *JNMT.* 1994;22:240–249.

Rang H, Dale M, Ritter J, Flower R. *Rang and Dale's Pharmacology.* 6th ed. London, England: Churchill Livingston; 2008.

Rossi S (Ed.). *Australian Medicines Handbook 2012.* Adelaide, Australia: Australian Medicines Handbook; 2012: 591–598.

Saremi F, Jadvar H, Siegel ME. Pharmacologic interventions in nuclear radiology: indications, imaging protocols, and clinical results. *RadioGraphics.* 2002;22:477–490.

SNMMI-TS Scope of Practice Task Force. Nuclear medicine technologist scope of practice and performance standards. *J Nucl Med Technol.* 2017;45(1):53–64.

Sweetman SC (Ed.). *Martindale: The Complete Drug Reference.* 26th ed. Chicago, IL: Pharmaceutical Press; 2009.

Theobald T. *Sampson's Textbook of Radiopharmacy.* 4th ed. London, England: Pharmaceutical Press; 2011.

Tulchinsky M, Colletti PM, Allen TW. Hepatobiliary scintigraphy in acute cholecystitis. *Sem Nucl Med.* 2012;42:84–100.

Waller D, Renwick A, Hillier K. *Medical Pharmacology and Therapeutics.* 2nd ed. London, England: Elsevier; 2006.

Ziessman HA. Sincalide cholescintigraphy—32 years late: evidence-based data on its clinical utility and infusion methodology. *Sem Nucl Med.* 2012:42:79–83.

CHAPTER 8

Cardiac Imaging Interventions

Chapter Objectives

Specific learning outcomes (page ix) of this text addressed in this chapter:

- Apply the principles of pharmacology to the safe and effective use of medicines.
- Recognize general, patient-specific, and scenario-specific risks, precautions, and contraindications for use of medicines.
- Apply the pharmacokinetic and pharmacodynamic principles of medications to identify and explain normal and adverse reactions to medications.
- Administer medications safely, effectively, and appropriately according to procedures and within regulatory and statutory parameters.
- Monitor patients for, identify, and manage adverse reactions.

After reading, digesting, reflecting on, and reviewing the content of this chapter, readers should be able to

1. Demonstrate command of key pharmacology terms.
2. Demonstrate enhanced understanding of the principles associated with the pharmacology of cardiac interventions, adjunctive medications, and cessation drugs.
3. Demonstrate critical thinking to effect problem solving related to interventional protocols and procedures.
4. Recognize, explain, and interpret clinical problems and evidence in relation to cardiac drug use and application.
5. Demonstrate understanding of the mode of action, pharmacokinetics, risks, precautions, contraindications, adverse effects, interactions, and appropriate dosage of key cardiac medications.
6. Apply knowledge of the general principles and concepts in a translational manner to clinical practice.

Key Terms

afterload	cardiac glycoside	drug interaction	interventional	preload
beta blocker	cessation	endogenous	methylation	purine nucleoside
bioavailability	chronotropic	flow reserve	paradoxical	receptor
bronchodilation	collateral supply	inhibition	phosphodiesterase	sympathomimetic
bronchospasm	dromotrophic	inotropic	precaution	vasodilator

Some of the text, tables, and figures in this chapter were extracted from "Pharmacology Part 4: Nuclear Cardiology" by Geoff Currie (*J Nucl Med Technol.* 2019;47:97–110).

Introduction

Interventional (imaging) medications are medications used to evoke a specific physiological or biochemical response used in conjunction with diagnostic imaging or therapeutic procedures (e.g., adenosine and dobutamine). In cardiology, imaging is commonly undertaken following pharmacological stress testing in nuclear medicine and radiology (myocardial perfusion single-photon emission computerized tomography [SPECT], positron emission tomography [PET], stress echocardiography, cardiac computerized tomography [CT], and cardiac magnetic resonance imaging [MRI]). Adjunctive medications are medications used to respond to a patient's condition during a procedure (e.g., salbutamol and aminophylline). Given that patients present for evaluation of serious cardiac conditions and may become stressed because of the exercise or medications used during the evaluation, it is not uncommon to require adjunctive medication in response to a patient's change in status while in the imaging department. Patients who present for imaging also are likely to be taking medication that can interfere with the procedure, particularly with the stress test component of the procedure. These represent cessation medications, and the period of cessation is largely dependent on the half-life of the medication. An understanding of indications, contraindications, warnings, precautions, proper use, drug interactions, and adverse reactions for each medication is outlined in this chapter.

Pharmacological Stress Testing

Stress testing in imaging aims to create a disparity in blood flow between normal and stenosed arteries. This can be achieved either by increasing the myocardial oxygen demand or by *vasodilation* of coronary arteries (Fig. 8-1). Generally, exercise is considered the preferred method of cardiac stress testing, but pharmacologic stress testing can overcome a number of limitations to exercise and the associated imaging procedure. There are essentially two approaches to pharmacological stress testing: vasodilators and positive *inotropic* agents. Vasodilators such as adenosine and dipyridamole have a direct and potent impact on *coronary flow reserve* to accentuate the blood flow differences between normal and diseased vessels (Fig. 8-2). Positive inotropic agents, such as dobutamine, increase cardiac workload, potentially inducing myocardial ischemia (Fig. 8-3). Both dipyridamole and dobutamine have been used for performing stress tests in medical imaging. Vasodilatory and positive inotropic-based interventional agents are discussed in this chapter and summarized in Table 8-1.

Adenosine

Adenosine is a potent *vasodilator* endogenous adenine *purine* nucleoside that is a class V antidysrhythmic drug due to its effect on the atrioventricular (AV) node. Adenosine is a natural regulator of blood flow and coronary demand, acting directly on adenosine cell surface receptors (Fig. 8-2). Adenosine also modulates sympathetic neurotransmission. There are four main adenosine receptor subtypes:

1. A_1, blocks AV conduction, reduces force of cardiac contraction (negative inotropic and chronotropic action), triggers decreased glomerular filtration rate, cardiac depression, renal vasoconstriction, decreased central nervous system (CNS) activity, and bronchoconstriction.
2. A_{2A}, triggers anti-inflammatory response, vasodilation, decreased blood pressure, decreased CNS activity, inhibition of platelet aggregation, and bronchodilation.
3. A_{2B}, stimulates phospholipase activity, release of mast cell mediators, and actions on colon and bladder (contributes to bronchoconstriction).
4. A_3, stimulates phospholipase activity and release of mast cell mediators (contributes to bronchoconstriction).

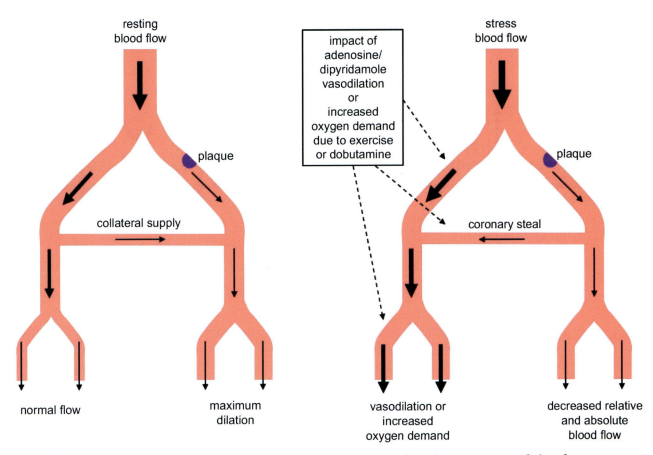

FIGURE 8-1 Schematic representation of the general principle of pharmacological stress in myocardial perfusion imaging. Ischemic myocardium may maintain resting blood supply with collateral vessels and resting vasodilation. Under pharmacologic vasodilation or increased oxygen demand (exercise or inotropic), the blood flow between normal and stenosed vessels will exaggerate the blood flow difference and expose coronary flow reserve (the difference between maximum and resting flow rates). The variation in coronary flow reserve between normal and stenosed vessels may be further influenced by coronary steal.

Endogenous adenosine is produced in vascular smooth muscle cells and leaves the cell. In the extracellular space, endogenous and exogenous adenosine can couple with the 4 types of adenosine receptors. Receptors A_1 and A_3 couple with an adenylate cyclase inhibitory G protein. Receptors A_{2A} and A_{2B} couple with an adenylate cyclase–stimulating G protein. Receptor A_{2A} specifically produces coronary and peripheral vasodilation by reducing intracellular calcium. Receptor A_{2A} stimulates adenylate cyclase activity, which enhances the production of cyclic adenosine monophosphate (cAMP) to produce vasodilation and arterial smooth muscle relaxation. As a result, normal arteries dilate, while atherosclerotic arteries do not. The resulting exaggeration in the difference between the blood flow in normal coronary arteries and the blood flow in atherosclerotic coronary arteries causes differential perfusion patterns. Adenosine is rapidly transported inside the cell (erythrocytes and vascular endothelial cells) where it is rapidly metabolized to inosine via adenosine deaminase or to adenosine monophosphate (AMP) via adenosine kinase–mediated phosphorylation. This rapid transport and metabolism results in the very short half-life of less than 10 seconds. Adenosine is also metabolized by xanthine oxidase in the intracellular space of endothelial, smooth muscle, and red blood cells.

86   Pharmacology Primer for Medications

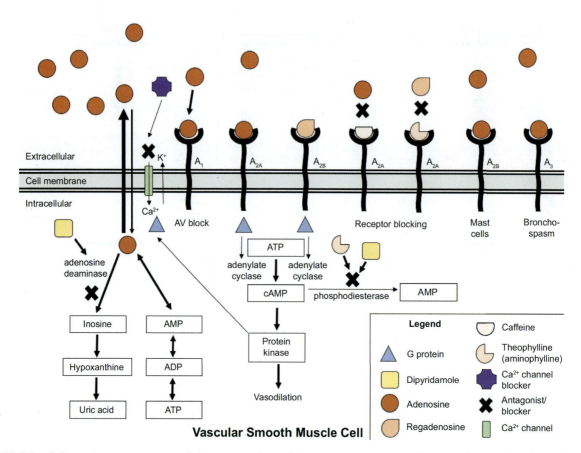

FIGURE 8-2 Schematic representation of the action of vasodilating agents in a vascular smooth muscle cell. Endogenous adenosine is produced in vascular smooth muscle cells and leaves the cell. In the extracellular space, endogenous and exogenous adenosine can couple with the 4 types of adenosine receptors. Receptor A_1 couples with an adenylate cyclase–inhibitory G protein to produce AV block and some bronchoconstriction. Receptor A_3 couples with an adenylate cyclase–inhibitory G protein to produce bronchoconstriction. Receptor A_{2B} couples with an adenylate cyclase–stimulating G protein to produce mast cell degranulation, peripheral vasodilation, and antiplatelet activity. Receptor A_{2a} couples with an adenylate cyclase–stimulating G protein to convert adenosine triphosphate (ATP) to cAMP and produce coronary and peripheral vasodilation. Regadenoson is selective for receptor A_{2a} to produce vasodilation. Caffeine has greater selectivity for receptors A_1 and A_{2a} to antagonize those actions. Theophylline (aminophylline and tea) has 3 to 5 times higher potency than caffeine in antagonizing receptors A_1 and A_{2A}, while theobromine (typical of chocolate) has lower potency than caffeine. Dipyridamole antagonizes adenosine deaminase, which reduces adenosine metabolism and thus increases availability of adenosine in the extracellular space. Dipyridamole is also a phosphodiesterase inhibitor and so blocks conversion of cAMP to AMP, further increasing vasodilation. Calcium channel blockers act to antagonize the voltage-dependent calcium channel to block vasodilation.

The *chronotropic, dromotropic,* and *inotropic* actions associated with the receptor A_1 allow adenosine to be used for managing sinoatrial (SA) node activity, AV node conductivity, and ventricular automaticity. The main indication of adenosine is to restore sinus rhythm in paroxysmal supraventricular tachycardia. Adenosine is used as a vasodilatory agent for the performance of cardiac stress testing for those unable to exercise adequately (e.g., vascular disease, respiratory disease, musculoskeletal limitations, calcium channel blockers, beta-blockers, poor motivation) and in cardiac PET. Adenosine increases coronary blood flow 4 to 5 times normal in normal blood vessels and to a lesser extent in stenosed vessels. This exaggeration in blood flow differences between normal and stenosed vessels is the basis for detecting hemodynamically significant disease. The dose is administered intravenously as 140 mcg/kg/min for 6 minutes or, alternatively, as incremental doses each minute of 50 mcg/kg/min, then 75 mcg/kg/min, then 100 mcg/kg/min, and then 140 mcg/kg/min for 4 minutes for a 7 minute protocol (Fig. 8-4). The radiopharmaceutical is injected intravenously 3 minutes after commencement of the adenosine infusion.

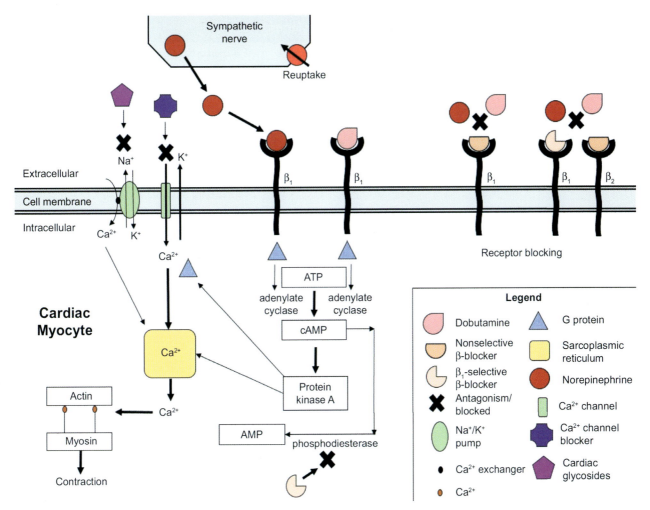

FIGURE 8-3 Schematic representation of the action of inotropic and chronotropic agents in a cardiac myocyte. Endogenous norepinephrine is released from the sympathetic nerve. Note that in a reuptake mechanism failure (e.g., heart failure), excess norepinephrine is available for β1 activation. In the extracellular space, endogenous norepinephrine and exogenous dobutamine can couple with β1-receptors. Receptor β1 couples with an adenylate cyclase–stimulating G protein to drive increased intracellular calcium, which facilitates formation of actin-myosin cross-bridges and produces an increased force and rate of contraction. This response can be antagonized by a β-blocker either nonselective (e.g., propranolol) or selective for β1 (e.g., atenolol). Calcium channel blockers act to antagonize the voltage-dependent calcium channel to block the inotropic and chronotropic contraction response. Likewise, cardiac glycosides such as digoxin antagonize the sodium-potassium pump to increase intracellular calcium via the calcium exchanger, increasing the force of contraction.

Patients with sick sinus syndrome, second- or third-degree AV block, or patients with asthma and a history of bronchospasm represent contraindications for adenosine use. Adenosine is relatively contraindicated in known hypersensitivity, unstable angina, oral dipyridamole use, and hypotension. Adenosine should be used with caution in patients on medications that suppress sinoatrial (SA) or AV nodes (additive or synergistic effects may result). Adenosine itself is not selective for particular receptor subtypes. Consequently, a number of unwanted effects accompany adenosine stress. These are generally resolved rapidly by cessation of the infusion, since adenosine has a duration of action less than 1 minute, and it has a very short biological half-life (<10 sec).

TABLE 8-1 Interventional Medications Used for Cardiac Stress Testing*

Drug	Dose	Pharmacokinetics	Mechanism of Action	Contraindications/Cautions	Adverse Effects/Interactions
Adenosine	50 mcg/kg/min intravenously, increasing to 140 mcg/kg/min maintained for 4 min with radiopharmaceutical administered at 1 min. Alternative approach: 140 mcg/kg/min for 6 min with radiopharmaceutical administered at 3 min	◆ Rapid onset ◆ Peak <1 min ◆ Half-life <10 sec ◆ Duration <1 min constant infusion ◆ No plasma protein bound	Vasodilation through activation of adenosine receptor A_{2a}.	Contraindicated in AV block, severe bronchospasm or asthma, known hypersensitivity. Use with caution in hypotension, unstable angina, oral dipyridamole therapy, medications that suppress SA or AV nodes. Long-standing methylxanthines need cessation for 5 half-lives.	Adverse reactions include chest, neck, jaw, or arm pain; headache; flushing; dyspnea; ECG changes. Bronchospasm is possible, especially in people with asthma. Adverse reactions reversed with cessation of infusion. Interactions include caffeine/xanthine drugs or foods.
Dipyridamole	0.56 mg/kg intravenously in 20–40 mL of saline over 4 min with radiopharmaceutical administered at the end of 4 min infusion	◆ 1–2 min onset ◆ Peak 4 min ◆ Half-life 10–12 h ◆ Duration can be prolonged without reversal ◆ 90%–99% plasma protein bound	Inhibits cellular uptake of adenosine to increase availability of endogenous adenosine. Vasodilation through activation of adenosine receptor A_{2a}.	Same as for adenosine.	Same as for adenosine except adverse reactions reversed with aminophylline.
Regadenoson	0.4 mg in 5 mL intravenous bolus followed by 5 mL saline flush and immediate administration of the radiopharmaceutical	◆ 0.5–2.3 min onset ◆ Duration 2.3 min ◆ Half-life is triphasic with 2–4, 30, and 120 min respectively ◆ 20%–30% plasma protein bound	Vasodilation through selective activation of adenosine receptor A_{2a}.	Same as for adenosine except potentially more flexible in mild to moderate airways disease.	Same as for adenosine except less bronchoconstriction but has risk of seizures.

TABLE 8-1	Interventional Medications Used for Cardiac Stress Testing*				
Drug	*Dose*	*Pharmacokinetics*	*Mechanism of Action*	*Contraindications/ Cautions*	*Adverse Effects/Interactions*
Dobutamine	15 mcg/kg/min intravenously, increasing to 20 mcg/kg/min, 30 mcg/kg/min, and 40 mcg/kg/min every 3 min	◆ 1–2 min onset ◆ Duration 10 min ◆ Half-life 2–3 min ◆ 40% plasma protein bound	Synthetic catecholamine β_2-adrenoreceptor agonist that produces increased rate and force of contraction.	Contraindicated in hypertrophic cardiomyopathy, uncontrolled hypertension, unstable angina, atrial fibrillation, β-blocker use, known hypersensitivity. Use with caution in myocardial infarction and cardiogenic shock. β-Blockers need cessation for 5 half-lives.	Adverse reactions include angina, palpitations, headache, nausea, tachycardia. Adverse reactions reversed with cessation of infusion or β-blockers. Interactions include blood pressure medications, β-blockers, tricyclic antidepressants, MAOIs, CNS stimulants, potassium-depleting drugs.

*Duration is the period of significant or measurable effect. Some adverse effects are more likely when used therapeutically than in single interventional doses.

Commonly seen adverse reactions include chest pain, pain in the throat/jaw and arm, headache, flushing, and dyspnea. Electrocardiogram (ECG) changes and AV block are also occasionally noted. Some patients experience lightheadedness, gastrointestinal discomfort, paresthesia, and hypotension. It is worth noting that 10.6% of patients experience these adverse effects several hours after cessation of the infusion despite the very short half-life. Despite being an antiarrhythmic medication, adenosine can potentiate arrhythmia. Bronchospasm, particularly in people with asthma, is a significant potential adverse reaction. Caffeine and similar xanthine products potentiate adenosine. Adenosine effects are potentiated by dipyridamole.

Dipyridamole

Dipyridamole is an indirect potent vasodilator pyridopyrimidine compound with adenosine reuptake inhibition and *phosphodiesterase inhibition* producing vasodilatory and antiplatelet activity. Dipyridamole is a pyramidopyrimidine compound with both vasodilatory and antithrombotic effects. Adenosine deaminase is an enzyme that catalyzes the deamination of adenosine to inosine (Fig. 8-2). Dipyridamole inhibits adenosine deaminase, which is an enzyme involved in cellular uptake of adenosine. By blocking cellular uptake in myocardial, endothelial, and blood cells, dipyridamole increases extracellular interstitial adenosine. Consequently, the increased adenosine has increased reactivity with adenosine receptors that regulate coronary blood flow, which leads to vasodilation. In blood cells, inhibition of phosphodiesterase increases cAMP, which reduces activation of cell aggregation. Dipyridamole is incompletely absorbed from the gut, has 90% to 99% plasma protein binding, and has a 10- to 12-hour half-life. It is metabolized in the liver and eliminated mostly in bile with a small fraction via urine.

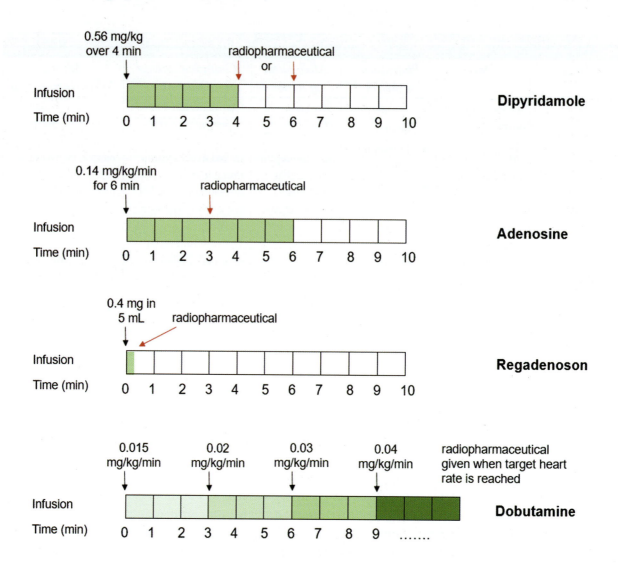

FIGURE 8-4 Comparison of the infusion techniques for the main pharmacological stress agents.

Dipyridamole is used as an antiplatelet medication for thromboembolism prophylaxis, especially after stroke or valve replacement (usually in oral dose form). Dipyridamole is used as an indirect vasodilatory agent for the performance of cardiac stress testing for those unable to exercise adequately (e.g., vascular disease, respiratory disease, musculoskeletal limitations, calcium channel blockers, beta-blockers, poor motivation). Dipyridamole is also used for exercise radionuclide ventriculography (technetium-99 [^{99m}Tc]-labeled red blood cells). A dose of 0.56 mg/kg of dipyridamole diluted in 20 to 40 mg of saline is infused intravenously over 4 minutes. The maximum vasodilatation occurs at 4 minutes after the end of the infusion, so the radiopharmaceutical is administered at 3 to 5 minutes postinfusion (Fig. 8-4).

Patients with sick sinus syndrome, second- or third-degree AV block, or patients with asthma and history of bronchospasm represent contraindications for adenosine use. Hypersensitivity to dipyridamole or aminophylline are also relative contraindications. Since adenosine shunts endocardial blood flow to the epicardium, there may be a reduction in collateral blood supply or induction of ischemia. Severe ischemic symptoms may occur. Orthostatic hypotension may also occur. Severe hepatic dysfunction needs to be managed with caution because of liver metabolism. Caution should also be exercised in known hypotension, aortic stenosis, heart failure, recent myocardial infarction, coagulation disorders, and angina. Careful consideration should be exercised in patients not abstaining from xanthine medications and products due to potential false negative.

Forty-seven percent of patients report adverse reactions, of which 0.26% are severe. Significant adverse reactions can be treated with intravenous aminophylline or nitroglycerine for chest pain (discussed later in this chapter). Frequent adverse reactions include chest pain, headache, and dizziness. Less commonly, patients experience nausea, flushing, tachycardia, dyspnea, hypotension, and ECG changes. Patients with severe coronary artery disease (CAD) or conduction abnormalities are at greater risk of adverse effects. Dipyridamole can potentiate the effects of anticoagulants and potentially inhibit fludarabine uptake, reducing efficacy. Interestingly, alcohol (ethanol) consumption has also been reported to increase adenosine levels by decreasing adenosine reuptake. Thus, alcohol consumption might potentiate the effects of dipyridamole and decrease antagonism by xanthines (reduce the half-life of caffeine).

Regadenoson

Regadenoson is a potent adenosine derivative vasodilator with selectivity for receptor A_{2A}. Regadenoson is an adenosine derivative that is a selective A_{2A} agonist and extends several potential advantages over adenosine (Fig. 8-2):

- It is given as an intravenous bolus at a fixed dose, which "uncomplicates" the infusion process.
- It produces less undesirable side effects (e.g., AV block and bronchospasm) due to the A_{2A} selectivity.
- It could be used in patients with mild to moderate reactive airways disease.

Most clinical evaluations tend to focus on it being "not inferior" to adenosine rather than on any specific tangible benefits over adenosine. Regadenoson is given by intravenous bolus injection with onset of action (increased coronary blood flow) occurring at 0.5 to 2.3 minutes after administration, with 2.3 minutes being the recognized duration of action. Approximately 20% to 30% of Regadenoson is plasma protein bound, and unlike adenosine, it is not rapidly metabolized. Regadenoson undergoes triphasic elimination with half-lives of 2 to 4 minutes, 30 minutes, and 2 hours respectively.

Regadenoson was developed specifically for stress testing, providing vasodilatory pharmacological stress with specific application in patients with mild to moderate airways disease. The standard dose is 0.4 mg in 5 mL by intravenous bolus injection followed by a 5 mL bolus saline flush, after which the radiopharmaceutical dose is injected (Fig. 8-4). Contraindications are the same as for adenosine with some flexibility in mild to moderate airways disease.

Regadenoson has a 13-fold lower affinity for A_1 receptors than A_{2A} but is 10 times more potent than adenosine. Despite the selective A_{2A} agonism designed to eliminate bronchoconstriction, there is a surprisingly high incidence of dyspnea reported. The most common adverse reactions include dyspnea, headache, nausea, abdominal discomfort, and ventricular conduction abnormalities, all occurring more frequently than with adenosine. Less frequently than with adenosine, flushing, chest pain, angina, and AV block can occur. The use of Regadenoson has an increased risk of seizures not evident with adenosine. Interactions are as per adenosine.

Dobutamine

Dobutamine is a sympathomimetic beta-1 (β_1)-agonist with positive inotropic (increased contractility) and chronotropic (increased heart rate) effects. Adrenergic β-receptors are important to understand in cardiac pharmacology and are discussed further under the section "Beta-blockers." There are three subtypes of β-adrenergic receptors designed to respond to catecholamines:

- β_1-receptors are found in the heart and kidneys with responsibility for increasing the rate and force of cardiac contraction and renin secretion respectively.
- β_2-receptors are found in the lungs, liver, and skeletal muscle, causing, when activated by an agonist, vasodilation, bronchodilation, glycogenolysis, and glucagon release.
- β_3-receptors are found in adipose tissue with responsibility for lipolysis.

Dobutamine is a powerful positive inotropic and chronotropic sympathomimetic drug with a primary mechanism of action through direct stimulation of β_1-receptors of the sympathetic nervous system. Dobutamine also demonstrates weak β_2-agonist activity (vasodilation) and α_1-agonist activity (increases intracellular calcium concentrations). In the extracellular space, endogenous norepinephrine and exogenous dobutamine can couple with β_1-receptors (Fig. 8-3). Receptor β_1 couples with an adenylate cyclase–stimulating G protein to drive increased intracellular calcium, which facilitates formation of actin-myosin cross-bridges and produces an increased force and rate of contraction. Arbutamine has been used as an alternative to dobutamine with similar inotropic and chronotropic actions but less peripheral vasodilation. Dobutamine is inactive orally. The onset of action is 1 to 2 minutes after intravenous injection, and the duration of action is 10 minutes. The half-life after intravenous injection is just 2 to 3 minutes. Dobutamine is rapidly metabolized in the liver and conjugates with glucuronic acid before being excreted mainly in urine with a small fraction in feces.

Dobutamine is used to treat acute heart failure and septic shock by increasing cardiac output. The primary advantage of dobutamine in stress testing is the minimal β_2 activity, which significantly reduces the risks in those with respiratory compromise. The absence of bronchospasm makes dobutamine the pharmacological stress agent of choice (over dipyridamole, adenosine, and regadenoson) for patients with asthma or obstructive airways disease. From a practical standpoint, dobutamine can be employed in patients who have consumed caffeine, and it is ideal in patients who are limited physically from undertaking exercise stress. Dobutamine is administered as an incremental dose of 15 mcg/kg/min up to 40 mcg/kg/min every 3 minutes (Fig. 8-4). The radiopharmaceutical is administered when the target heart rate is reached.

Hypersensitivity to dobutamine, hypertrophic cardiomyopathy, noncessation of β-blockers, uncontrolled hypertension, unstable angina, atrial fibrillation, aortic stenosis, ventricular arrhythmias, and pheochromocytomas are the main contraindications. Caution should be exercised when using dobutamine in patients with acute myocardial infarction and cardiogenic shock. It is possible that dobutamine can interfere with the uptake of the radiopharmaceutical in myocardial perfusion imaging; therefore, vasodilators are preferred.

A wide range of adverse effects are possible with sympathomimetics, and this reflects sympathetic nervous system stimulation. Dose-related increases in heart rate and blood pressure, angina, and palpitation can occur. There is a greater risk of arrhythmia and decreased blood pressure. Angina, palpitations, headache, nausea, and tachycardia are seen in 31% to 70% of patients. While a short half-life allows adverse reaction resolution with infusion cessation, a fast-acting β-blocker (e.g., esmolol) may be used to reverse dobutamine. Dobutamine will interact with medications that affect blood pressure and with β-blockers. Severe interactions to be avoided can occur with monoamine oxidase inhibitors (MAOIs), tricyclic antidepressants, CNS stimulants, and drugs that deplete potassium (e.g., diuretics, corticosteroids, aminophylline).

Adjunctive Medications

Adjunctive medications are medications that may be used to directly respond to the patient's status during a nuclear medicine procedure. The crash cart/emergency trolley is discussed in Chapter 12, so the discussion in this chapter is limited to the reversal of pharmacologic interventions and the use of salbutamol and nitroglycerin to manage acute adverse reactions. These adjunctive medications are discussed next and summarized in Table 8-2.

TABLE 8-2 Adjunctive medications commonly used in nuclear cardiology. Some adverse effects are more likely when used therapeutically than in single adjunctive doses.

Drug/Indication/Dose	Pharmacokinetics/Mechanism of Action	Contraindications/Cautions	Adverse Effects/Interactions
Aminophylline Reverse dipyridamole 125–250 mg by slow intravenous	◆ Rapid onset and peak ◆ Half-life 8 h ◆ 50%–70% plasma protein bound Antagonizes all adenosine receptors	No absolute contraindication, but caution in patients with porphyria, hyperthyroidism, hypertension, arrhythmia, heart failure, and liver dysfunction.	Adverse effects include CNS stimulation, gut disturbances, headache, and palpitations. Interactions include xanthine products and medications, medications altering liver metabolism, acyclovir, allopurinol, some antiarrhythmics, antidepressants, cimetidine, disulfiram, fluvoxamine, interferon-α, macrolide antibacterials and quinolones, oral contraceptives, thiabendazole, viloxazine, phenytoin and antiepileptics, phenobarbitone, ritonavir, rifampicin, sulfinpyrazone, lithium, macrolides, pancuronium, and phenytoin.
Nitroglycerin Relieve acute angina 300–600 mcg sublingual tablet or 1–2 sprays of 400 mcg each onto or under the tongue or 2–3 mg buccal tablet	◆ 1–3 min onset ◆ Half-life 2–3 min ◆ Duration 30–60 min Facilitates nitric oxide metabolism, which causes vasodilation and reduced preload and afterload	Contraindicated in hypotension, hypovolemia, and increased intracranial pressure. Contraindicated with the use of phenytoin, alteplase, levofloxacin, and sildenafil. Caution in renal and liver dysfunction and hypothyroidism.	Adverse reactions include flushing, dizziness, tachycardia, and headache. Interaction include alcohol, antihypertensives and vasodilators.
Salbutamol Relieve dyspnea and bronchospasm 1–2 inhalations of 100 mcg each with a third inhalation if necessary 1 min after the second	◆ 5 min onset ◆ Peak 60 min ◆ Half-life 4–6 h ◆ Duration 3–6 h Direct-acting $β_2$-agonist to dilate bronchi	Contraindicated in hypotension. Caution in hyperthyroidism, myocardial insufficiency, hypertension, arrhythmia, and diabetes mellitus.	Adverse reactions include tremor, palpitations, tachycardia, anxiety, headaches, peripheral vasodilation, muscle cramps, hyperglycemia, and hypersensitivity. Interactions with other $β_2$-agonists, corticosteroids, diuretics, xanthines, β-blockers, and antidepressants.

Aminophylline

Aminophylline is a *methylxanthine* that is described as a xanthine-based antiasthma class medication. Aminophylline itself is a *prodrug* that, after administration, rapidly releases theophylline as its active bronchodilating constituent. Aminophylline is also a phosphodiesterase inhibitor; antagonizes CNS adenosine receptors, causing stimulation; and has diuretic action stronger than caffeine. While theophylline antagonizes all adenosine receptors, it has a greater effect on A_2 receptors. Antagonism of A_1 receptors reduces bronchoconstriction, increases CNS activity, and increases cardiac contraction force, while antagonism of A_{2A} receptors blocks vasodilation, blocks antiplatelet activity, and increases CNS activity (Fig. 8-2). Theophylline also inhibits phosphodiesterase, causing an increase in cAMP, which in turn leads to smooth muscle relaxation and stimulation of cardiac muscles. Inhibition of phosphodiesterase, in theory at least, results in bronchodilation and increased cardiac contraction rate and force, but these effects generally require therapeutic doses.

Aminophylline is the prodrug ester derivative of theophylline. Aminophylline (or theophylline in vivo) has higher affinity for adenosine receptors than does adenosine itself and thus provides effective blockade. Aminophylline does not reduce the amount of either dipyridamole or adenosine but simply displaces them due to preferential binding. Theophylline gut absorption is unpredictable and can cause gastric irritation. Consequently, theophylline is given as the more soluble aminophylline, which is rapidly hydrolyzed into theophylline and ethylenediamine at a ratio of 2:1 and a half-life of several minutes. Theophylline is 50% to 70% plasma protein bound and is metabolized in the liver; it is excreted in urine, and 10% of the urine excretion is unchanged. Theophylline and caffeine are metabolized in the liver by CYP450 with elimination half-lives of 8 and 4 to 6 hours respectively. The half-lives do, however, vary significantly among individuals. In particular, nicotine smoking decreases the half-life by 50%, oral contraceptive use doubles the half-life, the last trimester of pregnancy substantially increases the half-life (15 h), liver disease increases the half-life, alcohol consumption decreases the half-life, and age increases half-life.

As an antiasthmatic medication, aminophylline is not the first-line therapy but rather is reserved for unresponsive, life-threatening acute asthma. It can be used as a general bronchodilator in asthma and chronic obstructive airways disease management. Theophylline competitively antagonizes adenosine at all adenosine receptor subtypes to reverse the effects of dipyridamole infusion. There is no need to reverse adenosine infusion because of the short half-life of less than 10 seconds; however, the prolonged activity of dipyridamole in increasing availability of extracellular adenosine requires antagonism. The standard reversal dose is 125 to 250 mg of aminophylline by slow intravenous infusion to avoid adverse CNS and cardiovascular stimulant effects. There are several approaches, including reversal only when patient symptoms warrant and aminophylline reversal in all patients immediately following the stress test. An alternative approach adopted in some clinical sites is to use aminophylline reversal only in severe symptoms or if mild symptoms are not resolved by a strong cup of coffee.

There are no specific contraindications, but caution should be exercised in patients already taking xanthine medications, peptic ulcer disease (oral dose), porphyria, hyperthyroidism, hypertension, cardiac arrhythmia, heart failure, liver dysfunction, and epilepsy. Hypersensitivity to the ethylenediamine component of aminophylline is possible. Tolerance can occur. Dose dependent adverse effects include CNS stimulation, gut disturbances (even when aminophylline is administered intravenously), nausea, vomiting, diarrhea, abdominal pain, headache, insomnia, anxiety, irritability, tremor, and palpitations. Overdosage can cause excessive diuresis, dehydration, tachycardia, hypotension, and metabolic acidosis. Overdosage can be treated with activated charcoal to increase elimination and decrease absorption of oral doses or β-blockers.

Theophylline can interact with other medications that can enhance or reduce liver metabolism. Xanthine effects are additive with aminophylline. The effects of aminophylline can be potentiated by $β_1$-agonists and diuretics. Clearance of aminophylline can be reduced by acyclovir, allopurinol, some antiarrhythmics, antidepressants, cimetidine, disulfiram, fluvoxamine, interferon-α, macrolide antibacterials and quinolones, oral contraceptives, thiabendazole, and viloxazine. Clearance can be increased by phenytoin and antiepileptics, phenobarbitone, ritonavir, rifampicin, and sulfinpyrazone. Theophylline can reduce the concentrations of lithium, macrolides, pancuronium, and phenytoin.

Nitroglycerin (Glyceryl Trinitrate)

Essentially, nitroglycerin is a nitrovasodilator/organic nitrate that enhances oxygen delivery and reduces oxygen demand. Nitrates and nitrogen compounds enter the endothelial cell and are converted from arginine to nitric oxide (and citrulline), which in turn stimulates guanylate cyclase metabolism in smooth muscle cells (Fig. 8-5). The resultant cyclic guanosine monophosphate (cGMP) activates a protein kinase, causing protein phosphorylation. Vasodilation is associated with the reduction in calcium concentration and dephosphorylation of myosin. Nitroglycerin results in pooling of blood in veins, and by reducing the amount of blood returned to the heart, it decreases preload (left ventricular end diastolic volume) and decreases myocardial oxygen demand.

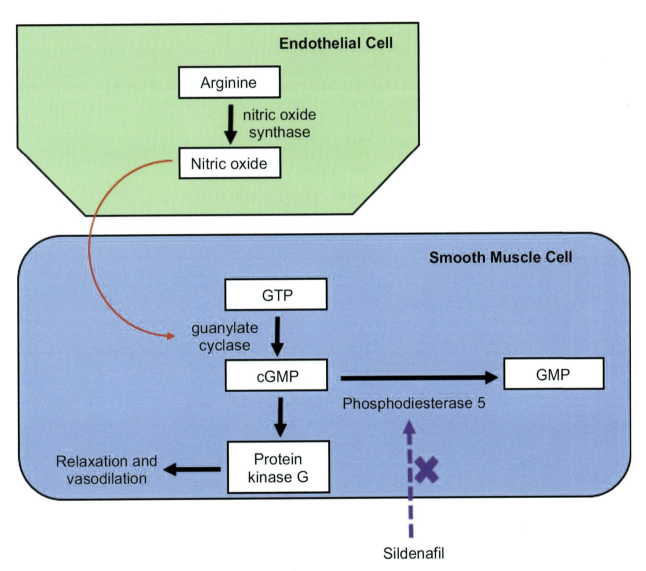

FIGURE 8-5 Schematic representation of the production of nitric oxide in endothelial cells with subsequent activation of guanylate cyclase in smooth muscle cells. This facilitates the conversion of guanine triphosphate (GTP) to cGMP, activating protein kinase G, which leads to smooth muscle relaxation and vasodilation. It is worth noting that cGMP is converted to GMP by phosphodiesterase-5. Thus, the use of phosphodiesterase inhibitors such as sildenafil block this conversion, potentiating the effects of cGMP. It is essential, therefore, to be aware of potential sildenafil use in patients who may receive cardiac medications and, in particular, nitroglycerin.

At low doses, nitroglycerin produces venodilation and reduced preload. Higher doses produce arterial dilation, which reduces afterload (resistance against contraction). Reducing both preload and afterload effectively reduces the primary determinants of myocardial oxygen demand. Nitroglycerin also causes dilation of coronary (and collateral) vessels to more efficiently distribute blood and oxygen to ischemic tissues. Two important relationships need to be outlined for nitroglycerin: First, nitric oxide reacts with metals, thiols, and oxygen and as such can modify proteins, lipids, and DNA. Second, phosphodiesterase-5 inhibitors used for erectile dysfunction, such as sildenafil (Viagra), function by potentiating the effects of nitric oxide in the corpora cavernosa.

Nitroglycerin is rapidly absorbed from oral mucosa, but bioavailability is reduced by extensive first-pass metabolism in the liver. Other routes of administration see rapid activation by liver metabolism. Effects are therapeutic immediately after intravenous administration, after 1 to 3 minutes after sublingual or buccal administration, and 30 to 60 min after transdermal or ointment application. Duration of effect varies from 3 to 5 minutes for intravenous, 30 to 60 minutes for sublingual to 3 to 5 hours for buccal; and 24 hours for transdermal. Nitroglycerin is metabolized in the liver and eliminated via the kidneys with a plasma half-life of 2 to 3 minutes.

Nitroglycerin is the initial therapy for treating ischemia and angina pectoris. It has also been used for treatment of heart failure and myocardial infarction. It is used to treat acute angina in response to stress testing and is generally administered in the form of sublingual spray or buccal tablets for rapid onset and relief of symptoms. For application in nuclear medicine in response to acute angina,

- One 300 to 600 mcg sublingual tablet is placed under the tongue.
- One or two sprays of 400 mcg each are directed onto or under the tongue.
- One 2 to 3 mg buccal tablet is placed between the upper lip and gum.
- Sublingual tablet or spray doses can be repeated if necessary, but failure to respond to repeated doses requires medical intervention.

Nitroglycerin is contraindicated with phenytoin, alteplase, and levofloxacin. Concurrent use with phosphodiesterase-5 inhibitors such as sildenafil is also contraindicated. Nitrates are contraindicated in cardiomyopathy, hypotension, hypovolemia, aortic or mitral stenosis, severe anemia, and increased intracranial pressure. Caution should be exercised in renal and liver dysfunction and in hypothyroidism. Sublingual and buccal preparations can reduce effectiveness associated with changes to oral moisture. Tolerance can develop.

Flushing, dizziness, tachycardia, and headache are common adverse reactions. Larger doses can lead to vomiting, restlessness, vision disturbances, hypotension, and syncope. On rare occasions, it may lead to cyanosis, respiratory dysfunction, and bradycardia. Alcohol, antihypertensives, and other vasodilators that enhance hypotension are the main interactions.

Salbutamol

Direct-acting sympathomimetic β_2-agonists, such as salbutamol, dilate the bronchi by direct action (Fig. 8-6). Salbutamol mimics the effects of endogenous norepinephrine by coupling with bronchial smooth muscle cell surface β_2-receptors. Receptor β_2 couples with a G protein, stimulating adenylate cyclase to decrease intracellular calcium. This leads to calcium efflux from the cell and uptake in the sarcoplasmic reticulum, stripping calcium from actin-myosin bridges to produce smooth muscle relaxation and bronchodilation. Short-acting salbutamol is given by inhalation for direct action and symptom relief. Salmeterol is a longer-acting β_2-agonist used regularly as a symptom preventer.

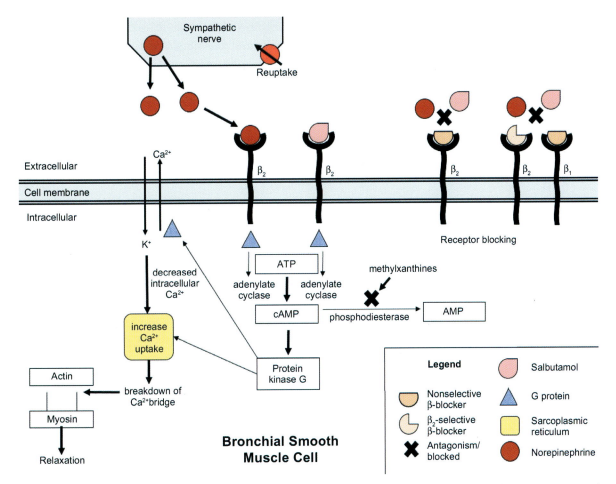

FIGURE 8-6 Schematic representation of the action of β-agonism in a bronchial smooth muscle. Endogenous norepinephrine is released from the sympathetic nerve. In the extracellular space, endogenous norepinephrine and exogenous salbutamol can couple with β₂-receptors. Receptor β₂ couples with an adenylate cyclase–stimulating G protein to produce decreased intracellular calcium through calcium efflux and uptake in the sarcoplasmic reticulum, leading to a reduction in actin-myosin bridge formation and thereby producing smooth muscle relaxation and bronchodilation. Inhibition of phosphodiesterase conversion of cAMP to AMP by methylxanthines (e.g., caffeine, theobromine, theophylline) further decreases intracellular calcium. This response can be antagonized by a β-blocker either nonselective (e.g., labetalol) or selective for β₂ (e.g., butoxamine).

After inhalation, 10% to 20% of the dose reaches the lower airways for direct action on smooth muscle. The direct action and rapid onset combined with the half-life makes salbutamol a short-acting bronchodilator suitable as a symptom reliever. It is not metabolized in the lung but does undergo first-pass metabolism in the liver. Of the remainder not inhaled, that component swallowed will be readily absorbed from the gut. Salbutamol and its metabolites are rapidly excreted in urine with a small amount of fecal elimination. Plasma half-life is 4 to 6 hours. Onset of action is rapid following inhalation (<5 min), with peak effect at 1 hour and duration of action lasting 3 to 6 hours. If given orally, onset of action is 30 min, peak is 2 to 3 hours, and duration is 6 hours.

High intravenous doses have been used to delay labor. Salbutamol is a bronchodilator for reversible airways obstruction (e.g., asthma and chronic obstructive airways disease). In nuclear medicine and radiology, patients having reversible respiratory difficulties during or after stress testing, including exercise, may have symptom relief with salbutamol. For relief of acute bronchospasm, 1 to 2 inhalations of 100 mcg each is administered, with a third inhalation if necessary 1 minute after the second. This same dose can be given prophylactically before stress testing.

Hypotension is the main contraindication. Hyperthyroidism, myocardial insufficiency, hypertension, arrhythmia, and diabetes mellitus are the main precautions. Plasma potassium levels should be monitored in severe asthma to minimize synergistic effects of medications causing hypokalemia. Adverse effects are reduced through inhalation and selectivity for $β_2$. Tremor, palpitations, tachycardia, anxiety, headaches, peripheral vasodilation, muscle cramps, and hyperglycemia are the main adverse reactions. Hypersensitivity has occurred; it may manifest as paradoxical bronchospasm, angioedema, urticaria, and hypotension. An increased risk of hypokalemia is associated with concurrent use with other $β_2$-agonists, corticosteroids, diuretics, and xanthines. Concurrent use with other sympathomimetics may cause sympathetic excitation, while β-blockers antagonize effects. Antidepressant medications may potentiate cardiovascular effects (e.g., tachycardia).

Cessation Medications

There are a number of medications a patient may be taking that can interfere with nuclear cardiology studies, directly or through interference with the stress component of the study. A blanket cessation rule may be in place to uncomplicate patient preparation, but 3 considerations need to be mentioned: (1) The imaging procedure may be attempting to assess patient status on the medication. (2) Withholding the medication may compromise the patient, including the patient's ability to have the procedure. (3) Not all cessation medications apply to each stress testing approach. How long medications are withheld should be determined by their half-life; typically, 5 half-lives is adequate. Medications that are generally ceased for stress testing are discussed here and summarized in Table 8-3.

TABLE 8-3 Cessation Medications Commonly Used in Nuclear Cardiology Should Be Stopped for 5 Half-lives of the Medication

Drug	*Cessation Window*	*Comment*
Nitrates	12–24 h for exercise, vasodilator, and dobutamine stress testing	24 h of cessation should be used for long-acting nitrates. 1 h cessation could be used for short-acting nitrates delivered in sublingual forms. For patches, cessation commences at the time the patch is removed.
β-Blockers	48 h for exercise and dobutamine stress testing	24 h is sufficient for those with shorter half-lives, but more than 48 h may be required for longer half-lives. Refer to specific half-life if β-blocker is used for potential variations.
Calcium channel antagonists	48 h for exercise, vasodilator and dobutamine stress testing	24 h is sufficient for those with shorter half-lives, but more than 48 h may be required for longer half-lives. Refer to specific half-life if calcium channel blocker is used for potential variations.
Methylxanthine food and drinks including caffeine	12–24 h for vasodilator stress testing	There is unlikely to be a marginal benefit beyond 24 h cessation. However, 6 h could be sufficient for those with mild consumption. Caffeine and theophylline products (coffee, tea, etc.) are of importance, while theobromine (chocolate) is less likely to have benefits from cessation.
Methylxanthine medications	1–5 d for vasodilator stress testing depending on formulation	Refer to the specific half-life of the medication to determine appropriate cessation period. Most medications are theophylline based or contain caffeine; thus, 24 h is adequate for most (unless in a controlled-release form).
Dipyridamole	12–24 h for vasodilator stress testing	The half clearance time for dipyridamole should allow a cessation period of 12 h to be used if urgent.
Digoxin	2 wk for exercise and dobutamine stress testing	Longer should be considered in known renal dysfunction.

Xanthines

Xanthines are purines found throughout the body and structurally resemble adenine and guanine. The basic xanthine structure is therefore similar to the adenine portion of adenosine, and this similarity allows antagonism of adenosine. Methylation (CH_3) of the xanthine produces a number of methylxanthines, including caffeine, theobromine, and theophylline. Caffeine is typically found in coffee, tea, guarana, and yerba mate; theobromine in chocolate and yerba mate; and theophylline mostly in tea (and aminophylline).

While theophylline antagonizes all adenosine receptors (Fig. 8-2), it has a greater effect on A_2-receptors. Caffeine tends to be more selective for A_1 and A_{2A}, and theobromine has higher activity for A_1. Generally speaking, a single cup of strong coffee provides sufficient caffeine to block less than 20% of A_1 and A_{2A} receptors. To achieve 50% antagonism would require 5 times higher plasma concentrations, and 80% antagonism would need 25 times higher plasma concentrations. Methylxanthines also inhibit phosphodiesterase, causing an increase in cAMP, which in turn leads to smooth muscle relaxation (Fig. 8-6) and stimulation of cardiac muscles (Fig. 8-3). While this potentially results in bronchodilation and increased cardiac contraction rate and force, therapeutic-range doses might be required.

Structurally, xanthine is a weak antagonist, and the simple addition of a methyl (CH_3) group in theobromine increases receptor affinity by a factor of 40. A further methyl group (theophylline and caffeine) provides affinity 80 times that of xanthine. Adenosine has significantly lower affinity than theophylline, allowing theophylline to displace adenosine at receptors. The NH_3 and CH_3 groups on various xanthines also change their potency. While caffeine has high affinity, it has poor potency; theobromine has low affinity and low potency; and theophylline has high affinity and high potency. This raises the question whether chocolate (theobromine) should be ceased prior to a myocardial perfusion stress test.

Beta-Blockers

As previously outlined, there are three subtypes of β-adrenergic receptors. The two of interest are

- $β_1$-receptors, found in the heart and kidneys, with responsibility for increasing the rate and force of cardiac contraction and renin secretion respectively.
- $β_2$-receptors, found in the lungs, liver, and skeletal muscle, causing vasodilation, bronchodilation, glycogenolysis, and glucagon release.

Antagonists of the β-adrenergic receptors are referred to as β-blockers and function by competitive blockade of the actions of catecholamines (Figs. 8-3 and 8-5). β-Blockers can be selective for either $β_1$ (atenolol, bisoprolol, esmolol, and metoprolol) or $β_2$ (butoxamine); however, it is common for β-blockers to be nonselective (propranolol, sotalol, oxprenolol, and pindolol) or nonselective for α- and β-receptors (labetalol and carvedilol), although they do not generally act on $β_3$. A clinically important role of β-blockers is to limit the response to exercise or other excitatory stimuli. Thus, at exercise or excitation, $β_1$-blockers (or cardioselective blockers) work to reduce heart rate, cardiac output, and arterial pressure. At high doses, selective $β_1$-blockers can also inhibit the action of $β_2$-receptors. This is particularly important in nuclear cardiology because β-blockers limit maximal response to exercise; thus, pharmacologic vasodilation stress is required for patients on a β-blocker whose medication cannot be withheld for the purpose of stress testing. Furthermore, β-blockers in those with asthma can inhibit bronchodilation. Dobutamine stress, as a β-agonist, is unsuitable in patients on β-blockers for obvious reasons. Furthermore, β-blockers limit vasodilation of skeletal muscles and can potentially reduce exercise capacity. As a selective $β_2$-blocker, butoxamine would not require cessation prior to an exercise or dobutamine stress test.

Using the 5 half-life rule of thumb for cessation of medications prior to exercise or dobutamine stress testing, the following cessation times apply:

- Atenolol for 30 to 35 hours (half-life 6–7 h, 50% bioavailability, 85%–100% renal elimination)
- Bisoprolol for 50 to 60 hours (half-life 10–12 h, 80% bioavailability, 50% renal elimination/50% hepatic elimination)

- Metoprolol for 15 to 25 hours (half-life 3–5 h, 40% bioavailability, 90% hepatic elimination)
- Propranolol for 15 to 30 hours (half-life 3–6 h, 25% bioavailability, 99% hepatic elimination)
- Sotalol for 35 to 90 hours (half-life 7–18 h, 100% bioavailability, 90% renal elimination)
- Oxprenolol for 5 to 15 hours (half-life 1–3 h, 24%–60% bioavailability, 95% hepatic elimination)
- Pindolol for 15 to 20 hours (half-life 3–4 h, 75% bioavailability, 50% renal elimination/50% hepatic elimination)
- Labetalol for 30 to 40 hours (half-life 6–8 h, 20% bioavailability, 95% hepatic elimination)
- Carvedilol for 30 to 50 hours (half-life 6–10 h, 25% bioavailability, 75% hepatic elimination)

Calcium Channel Blockers

Calcium channel blockers stop the influx of calcium through the calcium channel of cell membranes in both cardiac myocytes and smooth muscle cells. Calcium channel blockers decrease the intracellular calcium concentration, reducing the release of calcium from the sarcoplasmic reticulum and thus blunting the calcium-driven excitation-contraction coupling of actin-myosin cross-bridges. Consequently, calcium channel blockers reduce cardiac contraction force (negative inotrope), which makes them incompatible with effective exercise or pharmacological stress testing (Figs. 8-2 and 8-3). Calcium channel blockers can be used to treat angina, tachyarrhythmia, and hypertension.

Calcium channel blockers are metabolized in the liver (CYP3A4) to metabolites that tend to have their own activity. Given the CYP3A4 metabolism, a wide variety of drug interactions can occur, and this varies from one medication to another; however, generally, calcium channel blockers interact with β-blockers, carbamazepine, cyclosporin, digoxin, and inhibitors of CYP3A4 (e.g., grapefruit juice).

Using the 5 half-life rule of thumb for cessation of medications prior to exercise or pharmacological stress testing, the following cessation times apply:

- Amlodipine for 175–225 hours (half-life 35–45 h, 65% bioavailability)
- Diltiazem for 20 hours (half-life 4 h, 40%–50% bioavailability)
- Felodipine for 75–100 hours (half-life 15–20 h, 15%–20% bioavailability)
- Nifedipine for 10 hours (half-life 2 h, 50% bioavailability)
- Verapamil for 20 hours (half-life 4 h, 20% bioavailability)

Nitrates

Organic nitrates, such as glyceryl trinitrate, were discussed in detail earlier and outlined in Figure 8-6. As a cessation medication, the aforementioned vasodilatory effects in reducing both cardiac preload and cardiac afterload can potentially interfere with the effectiveness of exercise and vasodilatory and dobutamine stress testing. Unlike adenosine and dipyridamole, importantly, nitrates dilate collateral blood supply.

When considering the period of cessation prior to a myocardial perfusion stress test, consideration must be given to both the medication half-life and the dose form. The relatively rapid action of sublingual and buccal dose forms can reduce the cessation period compared to controlled-release dose forms (tablet or patches). More important is the elimination half-life. Short-duration nitrates such as glyceryl trinitrate, with a plasma half-life of 2 to 3 minutes, taken in the hours immediately preceding the stress test are unlikely to be prohibitive of performing the stress test, especially if delivered via sublingual or buccal routes. Conversely, longer-acting nitrates such as isosorbide mononitrate, with its 5-hour plasma half-life, regardless of the route of administration, require cessation for 24 hours. Cessation commencement is when the last dose was administered or when the patch was removed.

Digoxin

Digoxin is a cardiac glycoside that originates from the foxglove plant (digitalis). Digoxin is used to treat heart failure and cardiac arrythmias. The action of digoxin is associated with the inhibition of the sodium-potassium pump (Fig. 8-3). Inhibition of the sodium-potassium pump increases intracellular sodium, and this inhibits the efflux of calcium, increasing uptake of calcium in the sarcoplasmic reticulum. In turn, this provides more calcium ions for release to form actin-myosin bridges, which produce the excitation-contraction coupling and an increased cardiac contraction force (inotrope). It should be noted that the increased contraction force and cardiac output are achieved without increased oxygen demand. Digoxin produces a paradoxical negative chronotropic action (decreased rate of contraction) and slows AV conduction velocity (negative dromotropic). This is achieved by increasing resting membrane potentials, leading to decreasing the sensitivity of the SA and AV nodes to sympathetic and catecholamine stimuli. The plasma half-life of digoxin is 20 to 50 hours, which increases to 3 to 5 days in renal dysfunction. Digoxin is primarily eliminated unchanged by the kidneys (80%), with the remainder being eliminated by the biliary system without liver metabolism. Clearly, these actions interfere with exercise or dobutamine stress testing and require cessation for 2 weeks, longer in patients with renal dysfunction.

Digoxin has a narrow therapeutic index and extensive list of drug interactions, perhaps the most important of which are those that increase digoxin serum levels (increased absorption or delayed elimination) and risk toxicity (e.g., amiodarone, calcium channel blockers, quinine, and spironolactone). Digoxin is also associated with significant adverse effects, including nausea, vomiting, diarrhea, anorexia, visual disturbances, confusion, agitation, sleep disturbances, and less commonly, arrhythmias. Caution should be exercised when used with patients who have renal or thyroid dysfunction, electrolyte imbalances, and acute myocardial infarction. It is contraindicated in patients with heart block, ventricular arrhythmia, obstructive cardiomyopathy, cor pulmonale, constrictive pericarditis, and known hypersensitivity to digoxin.

Insight

Caffeine is almost completely absorbed (99%) in the gastrointestinal tract within 45 minutes of consumption; however, plasma concentrations resulting from the same caffeine ingestion can vary among individuals by as much as sixteen-fold. Caffeine is metabolized in the liver by CYP450, with an elimination half-life of 4 to 6 hours, but this can increase with oral contraception use, pregnancy, and liver disease, or it can decrease with nicotine and alcohol use. The major metabolites of caffeine include paraxanthine, which approximates caffeine in potency, theobromine (low potency), and theophylline (3–5 times more potent).

Managing methylxanthine cessation, therefore, requires an understanding of the affinity and potency and the sources of caffeine:

- 150 mL of coffee contains 40 to 180 mg of caffeine.
- 150 mL of decaffeinated coffee contains 2 to 8 mg of caffeine.
- 150 mL of tea, including iced tea, contains 24 to 50 mg of caffeine.
- 150 mL of cocoa contains only 2 to 7 mg of caffeine.
- 28 g of milk chocolate contains 1 to 15 mg of caffeine.
- 28 g of dark chocolate contains 5 to 36 mg of caffeine.
- 180 mL of soft drink contains 15 to 24 mg of caffeine.
- 180 mL of energy drink, such as Red Bull, contains 80 mg of caffeine.

Caffeine (100 mg or more) is also contained in some medications, including but not limited to migraine medications, pain relievers, diuretics, cold remedies, menstrual products, weight control medications, and stimulants.

A single cup of coffee produces serum caffeine levels of 0.004 mM, blocking 18% of adenosine receptors, while toxicity occurs at 0.25 mM (90% blockade). In the unlikely scenario of caffeine toxicity in a stress test patient, 6 half-lives (30 h) would return serum caffeine levels to the equivalent of 1 cup of coffee. Also unlikely is 50% receptor blockade (0.02 mM), but this would require only 2 half-lives (10 h) to return to the equivalent of a single cup. Thus, the first 12 hours of caffeine abstinence provides a tangible benefit to patient preparation (dipyridamole and adenosine stress patients), while the marginal benefit beyond 24 hours is very small. A more intuitive approach might lead to greater compliance with both patient preparation and scanning.

References

Al Jaroudi W, Iskandrian AE. Regadenoson: a new myocardial stress agent. *J Am Coll Cardiol*. 2009;54:1123–1130.

Asperheim K, Favaro J. *Introduction to Pharmacology*. 12th ed. St Louis, MO: Elsevier; 2012.

Bengalorkar GM, Bhuvana K, Sarala N, Kumar TN. Regadenoson. *J Postgrad Med*. 2012;58:140–146.

Block JH, Beale JM. *Wilson and Gisvold's Textbook of Organic Medicinal and Pharmaceutical Chemistry*. 12th ed. Philadelphia, PA: Lippincott Williams & Wilkins; 2011.

Bruns RF, Daly JW, Snyder SH. Adenosine receptor binding: structure activity analysis generates extremely potent xanthine antagonists. *Proc Natl Acad Sci*. 1983;80:2077–2080.

Bryant B, Knights K, Salerno E. *Pharmacology for Health Professionals*. 2nd ed. Sydney, Australia: Mosby Elsevier; 2007.

Buhr C, Gössl M, Erbel R, Eggebrecht H. Regadenoson in the detection of coronary artery disease. *Vasc Health Risk Manag*. 2008;4:337–340.

Currie G. Pharmacology part 1: introduction to pharmacodynamics, *J Nucl Med Technol*. 2018;46:81–86.

Currie G. Pharmacology part 2: introduction to pharmacokinetics. *J Nucl Med Technol*. 2018;46:221–230.

Currie G. Pharmacology part 4: nuclear cardiology, *J Nucl Med Technol*. 2019;47:97–110.

Currie G, Wheat J, Wang L, Kiat H. Pharmacology in nuclear cardiology. *Nucl Med Commun*. 2011; 32:617–627.

Currie G, Kiat H, Wheat J. Pharmacokinetic considerations for digoxin in older people. *TOCMJ*. 2011;5:130–135.

Druz RS. Current advances in vasodilator pharmacological stress perfusion imaging. *Semin Nucl Med*. 2009;39:204–209.

Gao Z, Li Z, Baker SP. Novel short-acting A2A adenosine receptor agonists for coronary vasodilation: inverse relationship between affinity and duration of action of A2A agonists. *J Pharmacol Exp Ther*. 2001;298:209–218.

Golan DE, Tashjian AH, Armstrong EJ, Armstrong AW. *Principles of Pharmacology: The Pathophysiologic Basis of Drug Therapy*. 3rd ed. Philadelphia, PA: Lippincott Williams & Wilkins; 2012.

Greenstein B. *Rapid Revision in Clinical Pharmacology*. New York, NY: Radcliffe Publishing; 2008.

Hacker M, Messer W, Bachmann K. *Pharmacology: Principles and Practice*. London, England: Elsevier; 2009.

Jambhekar SS, Breen PJ. *Basic Pharmacokinetics*. London, England: Pharmaceutical Press; 2009.

Katzung BG, Masters SB, Trevor AJ. *Basic and Clinical Pharmacology*. 12th ed. New York, NY: McGraw Hill; 2012.

Mettler FA, Guiberteau MJ. *Essentials of Nuclear Medicine Imaging*. 6th ed. Philadelphia, PA: Elsevier/Saunders; 2012.

Park HM, Duncan K. Nonradioactive pharmaceuticals in nuclear medicine. *JNMT*. 1994;22:240–249.

Patrick GL. *An Introduction to Medicinal Chemistry*. 3rd ed. New York, NY: Oxford University Press; 2005.

Rang H, Dale M, Ritter J, Flower R. *Rang and Dale's Pharmacology*. 6th ed. London, England: Churchill Livingston; 2008.

Rossi S (Ed.). *Australian Medicines Handbook 2012*. Adelaide, Australia: Australian Medicines Handbook; 2012: 591–598.

Saremi F, Jadvar H, Siegel ME. Pharmacologic interventions in nuclear radiology: indications, imaging protocols, and clinical results. *RadioGraphics*. 2002;22:477–490.

Sweetman SC (Ed.). *Martindale: The Complete Drug Reference*. 26th ed. Chicago, IL: Pharmaceutical Press; 2009.

Theobald T. *Sampson's Textbook of Radiopharmacy*. 4th ed. London, England: Pharmaceutical Press; 2011.

Travin MI, Wexler JP. Pharmacological stress testing. *Semin Nucl Med*. 1999;29:298–318.

Waller D, Renwick A, Hillier K. *Medical Pharmacology and Therapeutics*. 2nd ed. London, England: Elsevier; 2006.

Zaret BL, Beller GA. *Clinical Nuclear Cardiology: State of the Art and Future Directions*. 3rd ed. Philadelphia, PA: Elsevier Mosby; 2005.

CHAPTER 9

Other Imaging Interventions

Chapter Objectives

Specific learning outcomes (page ix) of this text addressed in this chapter:

- Apply the principles of pharmacology to the safe and effective use of medicines.
- Recognize general, patient-specific, and scenario-specific risks, precautions, and contraindications for use of medicines.
- Apply the pharmacokinetic and pharmacodynamic principles of medications to identify and explain normal and adverse reactions to medications.
- Administer medications safely, effectively, and appropriately according to procedures and within regulatory and statutory parameters.
- Monitor patients for, identify, and manage adverse reactions.

After reading, digesting, reflecting on, and reviewing the content of this chapter, readers should be able to

1. Demonstrate command of key pharmacology terms.
2. Demonstrate enhanced understanding of the principles associated with the pharmacology of outlined interventions, adjunctive medications, and cessation drugs.
3. Demonstrate critical thinking to effect problem solving related to interventional protocols and procedures.
4. Recognize, explain, and interpret clinical problems and evidence in relation to drug use and application.
5. Demonstrate understanding of the mode of action, pharmacokinetics, risks, precautions, contraindications, adverse effects, interactions, and appropriate dosage of key medications.
6. Apply knowledge of the general principles and concepts in a translational manner to clinical practice.

Key Terms

adverse reaction	drug interaction	histamine	nephrotoxicity	proton pump
bioavailability	endogenous	hypersensitivity	paradoxical	sedative
cessation	flow reserve	hypnotic	precaution	receptor
contraindication	inhibition	mast cell		

Some of the text, tables, and figures in this chapter were extracted from "Pharmacology Part 3B: General Nuclear Medicine: Other Interventions and Adjunctive Medications" by Geoff Currie (*J Nucl Med Technol.* 2019;47:3–12).

Introduction

The list of medications used as either interventional or adjunctive medications is long, and an exhaustive examination of all medications used in medical radiation science is beyond the scope of this chapter. Medications commonly used adjunctively and, less commonly, interventionally in medical radiation science are outlined in detail. These medications are summarized in Tables 9-1 and 9-2.

Less Common Interventional Studies

A number of interventional procedures in general nuclear medicine are performed relatively infrequently. Acetazolamide evaluation of cerebral flow reserve and the use of H_2 histamine antagonists or proton pump inhibitors to enhance detection of Meckel's diverticulum are discussed in this section and summarized in Table 9-1. Glucagon and pentagastrin are excluded, as these previously used approaches in Meckel's diverticulum detection have been largely replaced by H_2 histamine and proton pump inhibitors. Rarely utilized interventions for diabetic gastroparesis assessment also are excluded (metoclopramide and erythromycin).

Acetazolamide

Acetazolamide is a sulfonamide carbonic anhydrase inhibitor. Regional cerebral blood flow and cerebral flow reserve can be assessed by perfusion imaging at rest and after vasodilation. Decreased flow reserve will not demonstrate the same increased flow in response to vasodilation as areas with normal vascular supply. The predominant site for carbonic anhydrase is in the proximal tubule of the kidney (Fig. 9-1), where it facilitates carbon dioxide hydration and carbonic acid dehydration reactions. This reaction controls bicarbonate reabsorption in the kidney. By inhibiting carbonic anhydrase, acetazolamide effectively causes sodium bicarbonate diuresis and an overall reduction of total body stores of bicarbonate. Urinary alkalinization is linked to metabolic acidosis, which results from the profound inhibition and blockade of bicarbonate reabsorption in the proximal tubule. Rapid and potent cerebral vasodilation follows acetazolamide injection due to the decrease in pH resulting from cerebral carbonic acidosis after inhibition of carbon dioxide clearance. The increased cerebral perfusion is due to intra- and extracellular acidosis (Fig. 9-2). Cerebral flow response is not immediate, with a slow increase over a period of 15 to 25 minutes before returning to normal. This increases cerebral blood volume by 9% and cerebral blood flow by 50% in normal vascular territories. While normal vessels readily dilate, diseased vessels do not, which allows the interventional study (compared to baseline) to exaggerate the blood flow difference between regions with normal and diseased vasculature. Acetazolamide has an intravenous bioavailability of 100%. It has 70% to 90% plasma protein binding, and 90% is excreted unchanged in urine. The elimination half-life is 3 to 6 hours. After intravenous administration, onset of action occurs within 30 minutes with peak activity seen by 2 hours and duration of effect of 12 hours from a single dose.

A number of other indications documented are in the literature, including the following:

- Weak diuretic
- Can be used in the acute management of glaucoma by minimizing the intraocular pressure
- Second- or third-line therapy in epilepsy, particularly in absence seizures, tonic-clonic seizures, and myoclonic seizures
- Preferred agent for prophylaxis of altitude sickness syndrome
- Has also been used for the treatment of macular edema, Meniere disease, and neuromuscular disorders and to decrease intracranial pressure in idiopathic intracranial hypertension
- Decreased nephrotoxicity in patients taking methotrexate

TABLE 9-1	Less Commonly Used Interventional Medications*				
Drug	Dose	Pharmacokinetics	Mechanism of Action	Contraindications/ Cautions	Adverse Effects/ Interactions
Acetazolamide	1 g diluted in sterile water intravenously over 2 min	◆ 30 min slow onset ◆ Peak 2 h ◆ Duration 12 h ◆ Half-life 3–6 h ◆ 70%–90% plasma protein bound	Carbonic anhydrase inhibitor causing sodium bicarbonate dieresis and vasodilation in the brain in response to cerebral carbonic acidosis (carbon dioxide clearance inhibition).	Contraindicated in sodium or potassium depletion, hyperchloremic acidosis, Addison disease, closed-angle glaucoma, and severe renal or liver dysfunction. Caution in acute stroke, kidney or liver disease, diabetes, gout, lupus, hypotension, and pregnancy.	Tingling sensation, flushing, dizziness, blurred vision, confusion, nausea, headache, tinnitus, and allergic reaction. Potential interactions with aspirin, lithium, cyclosporin, amphetamines, other diuretics, antihypertensives, salicylates, hypoglycemics, phenytoin, sodium bicarbonate, anticoagulants, and cardiac glycosides.
Cimetidine	300 mg orally, 4 times over 24 h for an adult and 20 mg/kg in 20 mL of saline intravenously over 20 min in pediatrics	◆ 30–60 min onset ◆ Peak 1 h ◆ Half-life 2 h ◆ Duration 4–6 h ◆ 20% plasma protein bound	H_2 histamine receptor blocker that reduces gastric acid secretion and volume. It impedes ^{99m}Tc-pertechnetate secretion.	Contraindicated in known hypersensitivity. Caution in renal or cardiovascular dysfunction.	Headache, dizziness, diarrhea, muscle pain, confusion, and bradycardia. Potential interactions with medications metabolized in the liver. It can also alter bioavailability of drugs reliant on stomach pH for absorption.
Ranitidine	300 mg orally for adults and 1 mg/kg intravenously over 20 min for pediatrics	◆ 60 min onset ◆ Peak 2–3 h ◆ Half-life 2–3 h ◆ Duration 4–13 h ◆ 15% plasma protein bound			
Omeprazole	40 mg orally morning before and morning of the scan	◆ 60 min onset ◆ Peak 2 h ◆ Half-life 0.5 h ◆ Duration 3–5 d ◆ 95% plasma protein bound	Proton pump inhibitor (irreversible) that suppresses stomach acid secretion and impedes ^{99m}Tc-pertechnetate secretion.	Contraindicated in known hypersensitivity. Caution in liver dysfunction. Ranitidine is preferred in pediatrics.	Infrequent but include headache, dizziness, abdominal pain, diarrhea, nausea, vomiting, and rash. Potential interactions with diazepam, phenytoin, warfarin, and medications reliant on gastric acidity for absorption.

*Duration is the period of significant or measurable effect. Some adverse effects are more likely when used therapeutically than in single interventional doses.

TABLE 9-2 Common Adjunctive Medications in General Nuclear Medicine*

Drug	Dose	Pharmacokinetics	Mechanism of Action	Contraindications/ Cautions	Adverse Effects/Interactions
Chloral hydrate	30–50 mg/kg to a maximum of 1 g	◆ Good gut absorption, rapid metabolism ◆ Onset 30–60 min ◆ Elimination half-life 7–11 h and effects of significance 4–8 h	Prodrug converted to trichloroethanol that modulates GABA to cause CNS depression.	Contraindicated in significant liver, kidney, or cardiac dysfunction. Caution in respiratory insufficiency and known hypersensitivity.	Nausea, vomiting, diarrhea, dizziness, ataxia, drowsiness, headache, confusion, and paradoxical excitement. Potential interactions with ethanol, warfarin, and CNS depressants.
Diazepam (benzodiazepam)	1–10 mg orally individualized on basis of age and liver/kidney function	◆ Onset 15–45 min ◆ Peak 30–90 min ◆ Half-life 46 h ◆ Duration can be prolonged ◆ 100% bioavailability orally ◆ 98%–99% plasma protein bound ◆ Biphasic elimination with rapid component followed by slower 1–2 d half-life	Inhibition through modulation of GABA and neuronal inhibition.	Contraindicated in COPD, severe liver or lung disease, sleep apnea, and hypersensitivity. Caution in CNS depression, dependence, glaucoma, liver or kidney dysfunction, depression, pregnancy, and lactation.	Drowsiness, sedation, muscle weakness, ataxia, vertigo, headache, confusion, and paradoxical excitement all with increased risk in elderly. Potential interactions with CNS depressants, including antihistamines and drugs metabolized by the liver.
Bisacodyl	5–15 mg single oral dose	◆ Minimal absorption after oral administration ◆ Onset 6–8 h	Stimulant laxative increases stool water retention and peristalsis.	Contraindicated in bowel obstruction. Caution in liver impairment.	Gastric irritation, cramping, and fluid or electrolyte imbalance. Potential interactions with medications that change gastric acidity.
Heparin	10–15 units per milliliters of blood being labeled in vitro	◆ Highly plasma protein bound with variable elimination based on dose (slow for low doses) ◆ Rapid onset with effects lasting 3–6 h	Combines with antithrombin III to inactivate numerous clotting factors.	Contraindicated in known sensitivity, acute bacterial endocarditis, high bleeding risk. Caution in those using anticoagulants and in asthma, liver dysfunction, and animal protein allergy.	Bleeding, hemorrhage, and hypersensitivity. Potential interaction with anticoagulants (including NSAIDs and aspirin).

*Duration is the period of significant or measurable effect. Some adverse effects are more likely when used therapeutically than in single adjunctive doses.

Chapter 9 | Other Imaging Interventions 109

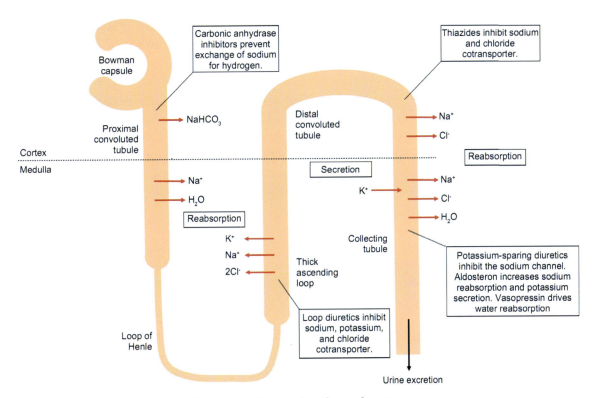

FIGURE 9-1 Schematic representation of the action of acetazolamide as a diuretic.

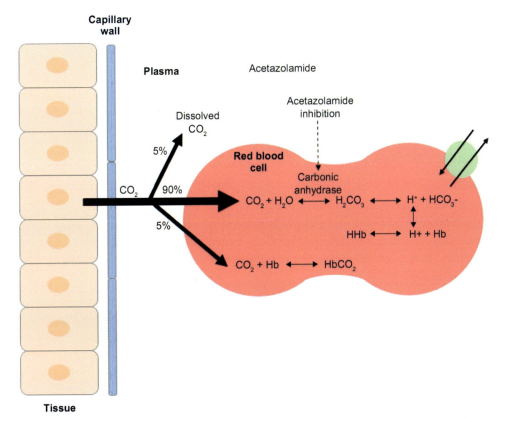

FIGURE 9-2 Schematic representation of the impact of acetazolamide in inhibiting carbonic anhydrase, increasing serum carbon dioxide, which leads to increased cerebral perfusion.

In medical imaging, the clinical use is to increase cerebral blood flow to perform a stress test on the brain and assess cerebral flow reserve in patients with transient ischemic attacks, stroke, carotid artery stenosis, and other vascular disorders and for differentiating vascular dementia from other causes of dementia. The standard dose is 1 g acetazolamide diluted in 10 mL of sterile water, which is then administered by slow intravenous (over 2 min). Typically, this administration is done 25 to 30 minutes before the radiopharmaceutical administration.

Acetazolamide is contraindicated in cases of sodium or potassium depletion, hyperchloremic acidosis, Addison disease, adrenal insufficiency, and marked hepatic or renal impairment. It is also contraindicated in hepatic cirrhosis because of the risk of hepatic encephalopathy. It should not be used in patients who have chronic closed-angle glaucoma. Caution should be applied with acetazolamide use in known kidney or liver disease, diabetes, gout, lupus, hypotension, and pregnancy. Care should be taken where there is a known sulfonamide allergy. Acetazolamide can cause hyperglycemia in people with diabetes. Severe electrolyte imbalance can occur due to diuresis, severe renal disease may lead to nephrotoxicity, and caution should be exercised in patients with increased cerebral pressure. Acetazolamide is excreted in breast milk but need not be ceased even for therapeutic doses (as opposed to single interventional administrations).

For acetazolamide, any adverse reactions tend to be mild and transient, but they can include tingling sensations (extremities and mouth particularly), blurred vision, headache, dizziness, and confusion. Some patients experience flushing, nausea, tinnitus, and changes in taste. The diuretic effect can lead to urinary urgency. These adverse reactions can be minimized using the slow intravenous infusion (over 2 min). Longer-term use (therapeutic doses) can also lead to sun sensitivity, loss of appetite, increased body hair, hearing loss, tachycardia/arrhythmia, bleeding, bruising, hematuria, and mood changes.

Acetazolamide has a number of important interactions that need consideration: First, it makes the urine alkaline and therefore decreases excretion of urine, which may enhance the effects of renally excreted or metabolized drugs (e.g., amphetamines, cyclosporine). Second, if used in conjunction with aspirin and other salicylates, acetazolamide can cause acidosis and central nervous system (CNS) toxicity. Third, if the patient is taking other antiepileptic drugs, the effects can be cumulative. Finally, alkalization of the urine increases the solubility of methotrexate in the urine. Consequently, excretion of methotrexate is enhanced, and this can be used to decrease nephrotoxicity in those patients. There are a number of other reported interactions between acetazolamide and other medications potentially causing toxicity, including but not limited to carbamazepine, lithium, mexiletine, methadone, phenobarbital, phenytoin, and quinidine.

Cimetidine

The gastric mucosa concentrates ^{99m}Tc-pertechnetate, including in Meckel's diverticula. Cimetidine is an H$_2$ histamine receptor antagonist that reduces gastric acidity. The detection of a Meckel's diverticulum can be enhanced by either increasing the uptake at the site or reducing migration of activity away from the site. While the ^{99m}Tc-pertechnetate accumulation is not affected, the change in gastric acidity in response to cimetidine reduces the secretions into the gastric lumen, concentrating the radiopharmaceutical. This effect also applies to Meckel's diverticula, enhancing visualization.

Histamine is released from mast cells and stimulates H$_2$ receptors in the gastric parietal cells to increase gastric acid secretion. Cimetidine is an H$_2$ histamine antagonist that inhibits histamine stimulation of receptors (Fig. 9-3) and thus reduces both the volume and the concentration of hydrochloric acid in the stomach by as much as 50% to 70%. Cimetidine has an oral bioavailability of 60% to 70%. It has 20% plasma protein binding and is partially (25%) metabolized in the liver, with 50% of the oral dose excreted unchanged in urine. The elimination half-life is 2 hours, but this can be increased in renal dysfunction. After oral administration, onset of action occurs within 30 to 60 minutes, with peak activity seen at 60 minutes if taken on an empty stomach and 120 minutes with food, and effects of significance last 4 to 6 hours. While cimetidine crosses the placenta and is excreted in breast milk, it is safe to use in both situations.

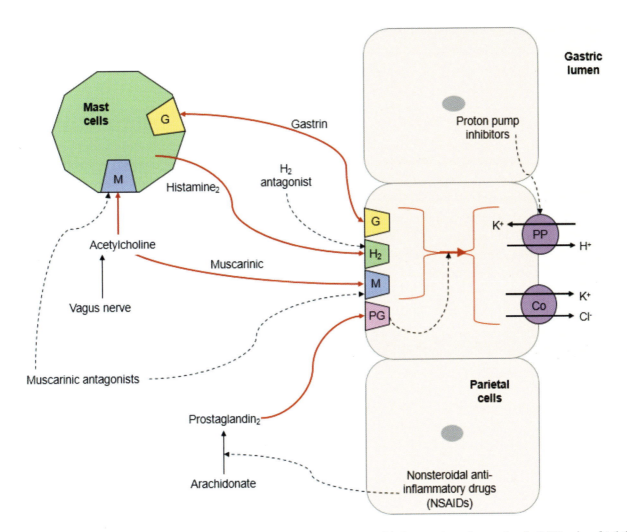

FIGURE 9-3 Schematic representation of the action of receptors responsible for gastric acid secretion (solid lines) and inhibitors of gastric acid secretion (dashed lines).

Cimetidine is used to treat peptic ulcer disease, gastroesophageal reflux, dyspepsia, and stress ulcers by reducing gastric acid secretion. It has also been used for people at risk of aspiration during childbirth or general anesthesia. In medical imaging, it enhances radiopharmaceutical accumulation and visualization in Meckel's diverticulum, improving the sensitivity of the test. The cimetidine can be administered orally as an 800 to 1,600 mg single dose 24 hours prior to the Meckel's diverticulum study. Alternatively, 300 mg orally, 4 times during the 24 hours prior to the study, can be used. Oral administration is not always practical because of compliance associated with the regime, so a single dose intravenously of 300 mg in 100 mL of 5% dextrose for adults over 20 minutes (or 20 mg/kg in pediatrics) 1 hour before the study can be used. The intravenous dose can be diluted in 20 mL of normal saline and administered over 2 minutes, but this can increase the adverse reaction rate.

Known hypersensitivity to the medication is a contraindication for use. Renal impairment should be managed by a reduced dose, and slow intravenous administration should be used in preference to rapid bolus administration for patients with cardiovascular impairment. Cimetidine is well tolerated and has a good safety profile. Nonetheless, patients may experience dizziness, confusion, headache, diarrhea, or bradycardia. Adverse reactions tend to self-resolve but can be limited by extending the intravenous administration over a longer period of time (e.g., up to 20 min). Cimetidine has a weak antiandrogenic effect, and gynecomastia, decreased libido, and impotence have also been shown to occasionally occur in men, but these conditions are usually reversible. Cimetidine and other H_2

antagonists can reduce the absorption of drugs reliant on gastric acidity, including dasatinib, ketoconazole, and itraconazole. Cimetidine decreases hepatic metabolism of warfarin, phenytoin, propranolol, nifedipine, chlordiazepoxide, diazepam, tricyclic antidepressants, lidocaine, theophylline, and metronidazole, which increases serum levels of these medications.

Ranitidine

Ranitidine is an H_2 histamine antagonist that reduces gastric acidity in the same way as cimetidine. Ranitidine and cimetidine share the same drug class, general information, mode of action (Fig. 9-3), clinical use, use in nuclear medicine, contraindications, and precautions. Adverse reactions and common interactions have similarities but also some important differences that should be highlighted. Ranitidine has an oral bioavailability of 50%. It has 15% plasma protein binding and is partially (4%–6%) metabolized in the liver, with 30% of the oral dose excreted unchanged in urine. The elimination half-life is 2 to 3 hours, but this can be increased in renal dysfunction. After oral administration, onset of action occurs within 60 minutes, with peak activity seen at 2 to 3 hours (independent of fasting) and effects of significance lasting 4 to 13 hours. Ranitidine crosses the placenta and is excreted in breast milk but is safe to use in both situations.

Ranitidine is administered orally as a 300 mg dose to adults or as 1 mg/kg to a maximum dose of 50 mg intravenously over 20 minutes in pediatrics. The imaging procedure commences 1 hour after ranitidine administration. The adverse reactions are the same for ranitidine as for cimetidine except ranitidine does not have the androgenic effects associated with cimetidine. Unlike cimetidine, ranitidine does not affect CYP450 and therefore has little effect on the metabolism of other medications in the liver. As with other H_2 antagonists, ranitidine alters absorption of medications reliant on gastric acidity for absorption, as outlined for cimetidine.

Omeprazole

The detection of a Meckel's diverticulum can be enhanced by either increasing the uptake at the site or reducing migration of activity away from the site. Proton pump inhibitors decrease gastric acidity, which increases the availability of radiopharmaceutical (^{99m}Tc-pertechnetate) for accumulation in the Meckel's diverticulum. Omeprazole is a proton pump inhibitor that inhibits the secretion of gastric acid by inhibiting the proton pump. The proton pump is the enzyme system of hydrogen potassium adenosine triphosphatase (H+/K+ ATPase) in the gastric parietal cell (Fig. 9-3). In essence, when sufficient omeprazole accumulates or binds to the proton pump, the final step in acid production is inhibited, which suppresses acid secretion. The action is irreversible inhibition, which is reflected in the long duration of effect relative to the elimination half-life.

Omeprazole is rapidly but variably absorbed after oral administration with an oral bioavailability of 30% to 40%. It has 95% plasma protein binding and is extensively metabolized in the liver, with 80% of metabolites excreted in urine and the remaining 20% by feces. The elimination half-life is 0.5 hours, but this can be increased in renal dysfunction. After oral administration, onset of action occurs within 60 minutes, with peak activity seen at 120 minutes and effects of significance lasting 3 to 5 days. Omeprazole has increased bioavailability in the elderly and with liver dysfunction.

Omeprazole is used for the treatment of peptic ulcer, NSAID-induced ulceration, esophageal erosion due to acid reflux, and Zollinger-Ellison syndrome. It is generally used in conditions in which gastric acid inhibition may relieve symptoms, including aspiration, dyspepsia, gastroesophageal reflux disease, and peptic ulcer. Proton pump inhibitors have also been used to reduce gastric acidity in the management of *Helicobacter pylori*. In nuclear medicine, it is used to enhance radiopharmaceutical accumulation in Meckel's diverticulum by inhibiting the excretion from parietal cells (not affecting initial uptake). Omeprazole comes as a capsule formulation, which should be taken orally whole; the capsule should not be crushed, chewed, opened. Therapeutically, omeprazole is administered as a single 20 to 40 mg dose daily for 4 to 8 weeks. For Meckel's diverticulum preparation and in consideration of pharmacokinetic information, omeprazole should be administered as a 40 mg dose on the morning preceding the scan and again on the day of the scan.

Omeprazole use is contraindicated in known sensitivity. The main precaution for omeprazole use is in patients with liver dysfunction. There is a potential risk of drug accumulation (due to high degree of liver metabolism); however, this is unlikely to present issues for isolated use as an interventional medication for Meckel's diverticulum imaging. Omeprazole is well tolerated, and adverse reactions are minor. The risk of adverse reaction is further reduced with an isolated interventional dose. Nonetheless, the possibility of a number of adverse reactions should be considered, including abdominal pain, dizziness, headache, nausea, vomiting, diarrhea, flatulence, and rash. Omeprazole is metabolized by CYP2C19 and CYP3A4 and so can alter metabolism of many other medications. Of note is the potential of omeprazole to increase plasma concentrations of diazepam, phenytoin, and warfarin. Omeprazole can also decrease absorption of medications reliant on stomach acidity, including atazanavir, dasatinib, ketoconazole, and itraconazole.

Adjunctive Medications Common in General Nuclear Medicine

A number of adjunctive medications are employed in medical radiation science, with the most common being associated with sedation, anxiolytics, laxatives, and anticoagulation. Specific medications used for these purposes vary among clinical centers. Consequently, a prototype approach is adopted to medication selection to allow general understanding that can be translated for more specific application where alternative medications are used. For example, diazepam is the prototype anxiolytic medication and is widely used clinically and therapeutically; however, some clinical departments may utilize alternative benzodiazepams (e.g., temazepam) or other drug classes (e.g., barbiturates). As outlined in Table 9-2, this discussion focuses on diazepam as an anxiolytic, chloral hydrate for sedation, bisacodyl as a laxative, and heparin for anticoagulation.

Chloral Hydrate

Chloral hydrate is a simple chemical structure that is structurally similar to ethanol and chloroform. A combination of chloral hydrate with alcohol produces the potentially toxic additive effects known as "knockout drops" or a "Mickey Finn." Chloral hydrate is a prodrug that is converted to trichloroethanol. It is a powerful hypnotic with CNS depressant properties that has been used for pediatric sedation in nuclear medicine, but its mode of action remains uncertain. It is thought to act by modulating the inhibitory properties of gamma-aminobutyric acid (GABA) in neurotransmission. Chloral hydrate is absorbed well from the gut and is rapidly metabolized to trichloroethanol in the liver. The elimination half-life is 7 to 11 hours. After oral administration, onset of action (sedation) occurs within 30 to 60 minutes, and effects of significance last 4 to 8 hours.

Chloral hydrate is used as a sedative-hypnotic and as premedication for medical procedures. Chloral hydrate is used for the sedation of pediatric patients for imaging procedures. The prescribed pediatric dose is 30 to 50 mg/kg to a maximum of 1 g as an oral liquid given 45 to 60 minutes prior to the procedure. Doses of 100 mg/kg up to 2 g can be used in pediatrics with respiratory monitoring.

Chloral hydrate is contraindicated with significant liver, kidney, or cardiac dysfunction. Chloral hydrate should be used with caution in respiratory insufficiency. Hypersensitivity reactions can occur, as can paradoxical excitement. The effects can last more than 24 hours, so driving or using machinery should be avoided. Chloral hydrate is excreted in breast milk and can cause infant sedation.

There are a number of common adverse reactions to chloral hydrate, including nausea, vomiting, diarrhea, dizziness, ataxia, drowsiness, lightheadedness, headache, hallucination, confusion, and paradoxical excitement. Hypersensitivity can lead to rash. Gastric irritation, abdominal distention, and flatulence have also been reported.

It is possible with overdose to cause respiratory and cardiac depression. Alcohol is the main interaction because trichloroethanol competes with ethanol for metabolism. There is a potential additive effect associated with concurrent use of other CNS depressants. Chloral hydrate is known to alter the effects of warfarin.

Diazepam

Benzodiazepams are widely used hypnotics and anxiolytics due to their superior safety profile, which includes fewer dose-related effects, lower fatality from toxicity and overdose, lower abuse potential, less adverse effects, and less serious drug interactions. Diazepam is the prototype diazepam, with newer variations (e.g., lorazepam) having shorter durations of effect and thus further improved safety profiles. Diazepam is a CNS depressant that has specific functions to reduce anxiety. Diazepam acts on the GABA receptor. GABA is an endogenous inhibitory neurotransmitter that causes increased chloride permeability, hyperpolarization, and decreased excitability of the neuron. Diazepam is not a GABA agonist, but rather it modulates the binding of GABA to the $GABA_A$ receptor, further inhibiting the neuron.

Diazepam is a long-acting benzodiazepam with metabolites that have their own activity (e.g., temazepam). It has an oral bioavailability of almost 100%, being easily and completely absorbed after oral administration. It has 98% to 99% plasma protein binding and is extensively metabolized in the liver with excretion in urine in the form of conjugated or free metabolites. The elimination half-life is biphasic with a rapid elimination phase followed by a second phase with a half-life of 1 to 2 days. After oral administration, onset of action occurs within 15 to 45 minutes, depending on the presence or absence of food, with peak activity seen at 30 to 90 minutes and effects of significance being prolonged by the 2- to 5-day half-life of active metabolites. Diazepam crosses the placenta and is excreted in breast milk, which means, as outlined shortly, that it should be used with caution in these situations.

Diazepam is used for short-term management of anxiety, muscle spasm, premedication for sedation, and as an adjunctive medication for managing seizures in the acute setting. In radiology and nuclear medicine, it is used to minimize anxiety in claustrophobic patients, especially those undergoing single-photon emission computed tomography (SPECT), positron emission tomography (PET), and magnetic resonance imaging (MRI). Diazepam can be administered intravenously, intramuscularly, rectally, and orally; however, for ease of use as an anxiolytic in nuclear medicine, the oral route is typically employed. Doses should be individualized on the basis of age, liver and kidney function, and purpose, with typical doses ranging from 1 to 10 mg. If diazepam is being used for sedation, 10 to 20 mg intravenously over 2 to 4 minutes is used in adults.

Diazepam is contraindicated in patients with chronic obstructive pulmonary disease (COPD), other severe respiratory disease, severe liver disease, sleep apnea, glaucoma, myasthenia gravis, patients for whom dependence has developed, and patients with hypersensitivity. Diazepam use should be avoided for those already with CNS depression. Diazepam should be used for only short periods, and withdrawal can be protracted. It should be used with caution in glaucoma, liver and kidney dysfunction, depression, psychosis, the elderly and very young, during pregnancy, and while lactating.

Adverse reactions have an increased risk of occurrence in the elderly. The most common adverse reactions to diazepam are drowsiness, sedation, muscle weakness, and ataxia. Less frequently, patients may experience vertigo, headache, and confusion; and with ongoing use, patients may experience depression, dysarthria, changes in libido, tremor, visual disturbances, urinary issues, gastrointestinal disturbances, and amnesia. Paradoxical excitement is possible. Additive effects may be seen with other CNS depressants, including alcohol, sedating antihistamines, opioids, sedatives, and antidepressants. Many drugs metabolized in the liver, including H_2 antagonists, can inhibit diazepam metabolism and thus prolong its effect.

Bisacodyl

There are a number of classifications for laxatives that might be employed for interventional purposes (refer also to Chapter 15):

- Fecal softeners use wetting agents to mix water and fatty substances with the feces (e.g., docusate) but have a 1- to 3-day onset of action.
- Bulk-forming agents cause water absorption, bowel distention, and reflex bowel activity (e.g., psyllium), with a lag in onset of 12 hours to 3 days.
- Osmotics increase the volume of liquid in the bowel lumen (e.g., lactulose), with onset of 1 to 3 hours.
- Lubricants coat the surface of the feces to aid passage (e.g., liquid paraffin), with onset of 6 to 8 hours.
- Stimulants increase peristalsis via innervation (e.g., bisacodyl), with onset of 6 to 12 hours. This category includes sodium picosulfate, typically used for bowel preparation for medical procedures.
- Combination therapy can also be used (e.g., softener and stimulant).

Bisacodyl is a stimulant laxative that increases water retention in the stool and stimulates peristalsis in the bowel. As such, it is effective for clearing the bowel of fecal content but should not be used regularly for constipation. Bisacodyl has minimal absorption. The small amount that may be absorbed after oral administration has 99% plasma protein binding, is metabolized in the liver, and is eliminated via the kidneys. After oral administration, onset of action occurs within 6 to 8 hours.

The usual use is for preparation for medical procedures and for treatment of severe constipation. In medical imaging, it is used to differentiate intraluminal bowel activity from pathological accumulation by stimulating fecal progression and passage in studies where colonic activity can obscure pathology (e.g., gallium-67 [^{67}Ga] citrate studies for non-Hodgkins lymphoma or abdominal infection, and ^{123}I-metaiodobenzylguanidine [mIBG] abdominal imaging). The oral dose of enteric-coated tablets should not be taken within 1 hour of ingestion of milk or antacids. The tablet should not be crushed or chewed to avoid gastric irritation and abdominal cramping. The oral dose is typically 5 to 15 mg as a single daily dose for constipation and up to 30 mg for bowel cleansing ahead of procedures.

Bisacodyl should not be used when the bowel is obstructed. Caution should be exercised in patients with liver impairment because of liver metabolism of the small fraction absorbed. There are few major adverse reactions other than the expected local reactions that include gastric irritation and cramping. Fluid and electrolyte depletion is possible. Possible interactions with medications that change gastric acidity (e.g., H_2 antagonists, proton pump inhibitors) may alter the effects of bisacodyl.

Heparin

There are 5 main categories of anticoagulant medications:

- Vitamin K antagonists (e.g., warfarin)
- Antithrombin III–dependent anticoagulants (e.g., fondaparinux)
- Direct thrombin inhibitors (e.g., lepirudin)
- Direct factor X inhibitors (e.g., rivaroxaban)
- Heparin and low-molecular-weight heparins

Heparin is a substance composed of repeating units of a disaccharide attached to a central protein, and as a result, this unfractionated form has a variety of molecular weights. Heparin is formed in mast cells of the lung, liver, and intestinal mucosa. Heparin used for human injection tends to be derived from either porcine mucosa or bovine lung. This is an important consideration for patients with cultural beliefs that may prohibit the use of products originating from these animals. Fractionated heparins are the low-molecular-weight heparins separated for more predictable use (actions and adverse reactions).

Heparin combines with antithrombin III, which is a naturally occurring clotting factor found in plasma. The heparin–antithrombin III complex has numerous actions:

- It inactivates thrombin factor IIa (most pronounced effect) and factors IXa, Xa, XIa, and XIIa.
- Inactivation of thrombin prevents fibrin formation and activation of factors V and VIII.
- Inactivation of factor Xa prevents conversion of prothrombin to thrombin, which prevents the formation of fibrin from fibrinogen.

Heparin is useful in preventing clot formation and growth and in vivo venous thrombosis, but it does not break down existing clots.

Heparin is inactive orally and has an intravenous bioavailability that is somewhat erratic. It is highly plasma protein binding, and only a small fraction is excreted unchanged in urine. The elimination is dose dependent with a rapid saturation process at higher doses and slower renal elimination at lower doses. The elimination half-life, therefore, averages 1.5 hours but ranges from 30 minutes for low doses and up to 6 hours for higher doses. After intravenous administration, onset of action occurs rapidly, with effects of significance lasting less than 3 to 6 hours. Heparin does not cross the placenta.

Heparin is used to prevent and treat (without actually breaking them down) venous thromboembolism and to prevent blood clots during surgery (prophylactically). It is used intravenously in preference to oral warfarin because onset of action is immediate and it can be reversed, if necessary, with protamine sulfate. Heparin is used to prevent blood clotting during blood labeling procedures or to maintain intravenous lines. The specific dose of heparin used will depend on the technique and local protocol. For example, some sites may use pre-heparinized blood tubes, while others may add a small volume of heparin to a syringe containing blood. Caution should be exercised when considering the order of adding heparin, as it can label to the radionuclide. A typical dose for blood labeling is 10 to 15 units per milliliter of blood.

Heparin is contraindicated in patients with heparin hypersensitivity, acute bacterial endocarditis, and bleeding risk (e.g., recent surgery or childbirth, peptic ulcer, severe liver disease, severe hypertension, hemophilia, cerebral aneurysm, or hemorrhage). Heparin should be used with caution when patients are concurrently using dextran, dipyridamole, or thrombolytics. It should also be used with caution in patients with asthma, allergy to animal proteins, and liver dysfunction.

Bleeding and hemorrhage are the most common adverse reactions to heparin. Hypersensitivity reactions can occur. A number of important interactions can occur with heparin, including an increased risk of bleeding when used with other anticoagulants (e.g., aspirin and NSAIDs), and this risk of hemorrhage is particularly concerning when used with thrombolytics, dextran, and dipyridamole.

Insight

From "Pediatric Brown Adipose Tissue (BAT) on FDG PET: Diazepam Intervention" by J. Cousins, M. Czachowski, A. Muthukrishnan, and G. Currie (*J Nucl Med Technol.* 2017;45(2):82–86).

Brown adipose tissue (BAT) is responsible for nonshivering thermogenesis, which produces heat in the BAT cells to maintain body temperature. BAT is highly vascular and mitochondria-rich compared to white adipose tissue. BAT is metabolically stimulated by the sympathetic nervous system, which is why both MIBG and sestamibi have been used to document distribution of BAT. BAT utilizes glucose as a source of adenosine triphosphate to generate heat, providing a pathway by which ^{18}F-fluorodeoxyglucose (FDG) can localize within BAT. BAT, or brown fat, has been widely reported to have an impact on the efficacy of ^{18}F-FDG PET in oncology. BAT remains a confounder on ^{18}F-FDG PET studies in oncology with the potential for both false-positive and false-negative results.

There are a number of important predisposing factors for BAT on ^{18}F-FDG PET; in particular, age and gender. BAT plays an important role in children to maintain core body temperature; consequently, one might expect to see greater incidence of BAT on pediatric ^{18}F-FDG PET scans. A number of reports indicate that BAT is more common in females. BAT is also, understandably, more common in colder temperatures (e.g., winter versus summer).

Given the role of BAT in managing core body temperature, warming patients has been used to reduce BAT on ^{18}F-FDG PET. While warming provides a noninvasive, inexpensive, and universal approach to BAT reduction, there are a number of failings that see it ineffective as a standalone solution. First, the approach assumes core body temperature and BAT activation are managed with a short-term strategy. Sympathetic activation associated with ambient thermal conditions reflects a wider window of days rather than the period immediately adjacent ^{18}F-FDG injection. Second, the higher degree of BAT activation in pediatrics may limit the success of warming strategies, leading to potential false-positive and false-negative findings.

A number of pharmaceutical approaches have been used to minimize BAT on ^{18}F-FDG PET. Propranolol (a nonselective β-blocker) has been the most widely reported pharmacologic approach to BAT reduction in ^{18}F-FDG PET. The propranolol blocks epinephrine and norepinephrine on β-receptors and thus prevents the stimulation of BAT to produce heat. Importantly, anxiety and stress have been reported to both increase muscle uptake of ^{18}F-FDG and activate BAT, which suggests a role for diazepam. Diazepam has been used to reduce muscle accumulation of ^{18}F-FDG in anxious patients, but as a lipid-soluble drug stored in adipose tissue, diazepam success will be dose dependent and subject to associated pharmacokinetic influences.

In a retrospective analysis of 139 cases for patients ages 9 to 21 years, 71 consecutive patients had a warm blanket protocol, and 68 consecutive patients had a warm blanket plus diazepam (0.27 mg/Kg to a maximum of 10 mg). There was a statistically significant decrease in the presence of BAT for those patients administered diazepam (16.2%) compared to those without diazepam administered (33.8%) (P = 0.0167).

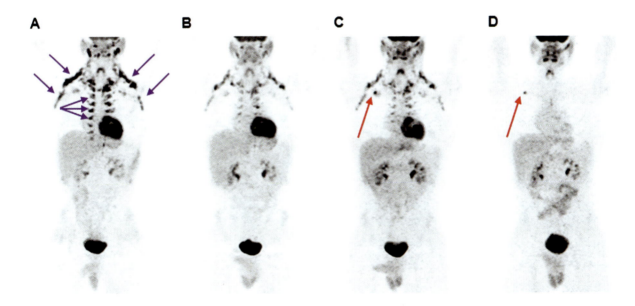

FIGURE 9-4 (A) Baseline ^{18}F-FDG PET study with warm blankets and extensive BAT (purple arrows). (B) The 3-month follow-up ^{18}F-FDG PET with warm blankets demonstrated no change. (C) The 6-month follow-up ^{18}F-FDG PET study with warm blankets demonstrated prospectively no significant change. Nonetheless, retrospectively, there appears to be increased focal accumulation in the right upper chest (red arrows). (D) At the 9-month follow-up, ^{18}F-FDG PET study following warm blankets and diazepam intervention, suppression of BAT, and clear demarcation of focal disease in the upper right chest was demonstrated.

This impact is highlighted in a number of cases. Here, a 17-year-old male presented with non-Hodgkin lymphoma for evaluation (Fig. 9-4). The patient underwent a series of four ^{18}F-FDG PET scans over a period of 9 months. The first 3 PET studies used warm blankets, and the fourth used a combination of warm blankets and 10 mg diazepam. As demonstrated in Figure 9-4, marked accumulation in the neck, supraclavicular, mediastinum, and paravertebral regions are suggestive of extensive BAT accumulation of ^{18}F-FDG. At 9 months, the study demonstrates suppression of BAT accumulation, washout of cardiac accumulation, and a focal area of ^{18}F-FDG accumulation in the right upper chest representing new disease. On baseline and 3-month scans, this region is associated with mild and more diffuse accumulation of ^{18}F-FDG likely to be BAT. On the 6-month study, however, the previous activity has superimposed focal accumulation of ^{18}F-FDG representing new disease that is noted only retrospectively once BAT suppression has been achieved with diazepam. The case provides an interesting paradox. While BAT accumulation of ^{18}F-FDG was reduced with warming and diazepam, cardiac accumulation of ^{18}F-FDG also was reduced. This finding might be expected to have a negative impact on cardiac ^{18}F-FDG PET imaging. It has been reported previously with patient warming reducing both BAT and cardiac ^{18}F-FDG accumulation. Cardiac glucose metabolism depends on numerous factors, but increased sympathetic activity drives increased metabolic demand for glucose, and cooler ambient conditions may be associated with increased cardiac sympathetic activity.

References

Agrawal A, Nair N, Baghel NS. A novel approach for reduction of brown fat uptake on FDG PET. *BJR*. 2009;82:626–631.

Asperheim K, Favaro J. *Introduction to Pharmacology*. 12th ed. St Louis, MO: Elsevier; 2012.

Block JH, Beale JM. *Wilson and Gisvold's Textbook of Organic Medicinal and Pharmaceutical Chemistry*. 12th ed. Philadelphia, PA: Lippincott Williams & Wilkins; 2011.

Bryant B, Knights K, Salerno E. *Pharmacology for Health Professionals*. 2nd ed. Sydney, Australia: Mosby Elsevier; 2007.

Currie G. Pharmacology part 1: introduction to pharmacodynamics, *J Nucl Med Technol*. 2018;46:81–86.

Currie G. Pharmacology part 2: introduction to pharmacokinetics. *J Nucl Med Technol*. 2018;46:221–230.

Cypess AM, Lehman S, Williams G, et al. Identification and importance of brown adipose tissue in adult humans. *NEJM*. 2009;360:1509–1517.

Golan DE, Tashjian AH, Armstrong EJ, Armstrong AW. *Principles of Pharmacology: The Pathophysiologic Basis of Drug Therapy*. 3rd ed. Philadelphia, PA: Lippincott Williams & Wilkins; 2012.

Greenstein B. *Rapid Revision in Clinical Pharmacology*. New York, NY: Radcliffe Publishing; 2008.

Hacker M, Messer W, Bachmann K. *Pharmacology: Principles and Practice*. London, England: Elsevier; 2009.

Hany TF, Gharehpapagh E, Kamel EM, Buck A, Himms-Hagen J, von Schulthess GK. Brown adipose tissue: a factor to consider in symmetrical tracer uptake in the neck and upper chest region. *Eur J Nucl Med*. 2002;29:1393–1398.

Jambhekar SS, Breen PJ. *Basic Pharmacokinetics*. London, England: Pharmaceutical Press; 2009.

Katzung BG, Masters SB, Trevor AJ. *Basic and Clinical Pharmacology*. 12th ed. New York, NY: McGraw Hill; 2012.

Kiss B, Dallinger S, Findl O, Rainer G, Eichler H, Schmetterer B. Acetazolamide-induced cerebral and ocular vasodilation in humans is independent of nitric oxide. *Am J Physiolo Regul Integr Comp Physiol*. 1999;276:R1661–R1667.

Leung DK, Heertum RL. Interventional nuclear brain imaging. *Semin Nucl Med*. 2009;39:195–203.

Mettler FA, Guiberteau MJ. *Essentials of Nuclear Medicine Imaging*. 6th ed. Philadelphia, PA: Elsevier/Saunders; 2012.

O'Loughlin S, Currie G, Trifonovic M, Kiat H. Impact of ambient temperature on cardiac accumulation of FDG. *J Nucl Med Technol*. 2014;42:186–193.

Park HM, Duncan K. Nonradioactive pharmaceuticals in nuclear medicine. *JNMT*. 1994;22:240–249.

Parysow O, Mollerach AM, Jager V, Silvina R, Roman JS, Gerbaudo VH. Low-dose oral propranolol could reduce brown adipose tissue F-18 FDG uptake in patients undergoing PET scans. *Clin Nucl Med*. 2007;32:351–357.

Patrick GL. *An Introduction to Medicinal Chemistry*. 3rd ed. New York, NY: Oxford University Press; 2005.

Rang H, Dale M, Ritter J, Flower R. *Rang and Dale's Pharmacology*. 6th ed. London, England: Churchill Livingston; 2008.

Rossi S (Ed.). *Australian Medicines Handbook 2012*. Adelaide, Australia: Australian Medicines Handbook; 2012: 591–598.

Saremi F, Jadvar H, Siegel ME. Pharmacologic interventions in nuclear radiology: indications, imaging protocols, and clinical results. *RadioGraphics*. 2002;22:477–490.

Skillen A, Currie G, Wheat J. Thermal control of brown adipose tissue in ^{18}F-FDG PET. *J Nucl Med Technol*. 2012;40:99–103.

Soderlund V, Larsson SA, Jacobsson H. Reduction of FDG uptake in brown adipose tissue in clinical patients by a single dose of propranolol. *Eur J Nucl Med Mol Imaging*. 2007;34:1018–1022.

Sweetman SC (Ed.). *Martindale: The Complete Drug Reference*. 26th ed. Chicago, IL: Pharmaceutical Press; 2009.

Tatsumi M, Engles JM, Ishimori T, Nicely O, Cohade C, Wahl RL. Intense ^{18}F-FDG uptake in brown fat can be reduced pharmacologically. *J Nucl Med*. 2004;45:1189–1193.

Theobald T. *Sampson's Textbook of Radiopharmacy*. 4th ed. London, England: Pharmaceutical Press; 2011.

Truong MT, Erasmus JJ, Munden RF, et al. Focal FDG uptake in mediastinal brown fat mimicking malignancy: a potential pitfall resolved on PET/CT. *AJR*. 2004;183:1127–1132.

Vorstrup S, Henriksen L, Paulsen OB. Effect of acetazolamide on cerebral blood flow and cerebral metabolic rate for oxygen. *J Clin Invest*. 1984;74:1634–1639.

Vorstrup S, Brun B, Lassen NA. Evaluation of the cerebral vasodilatory capacity by the acetazolamide test before EC-IC bypass surgery in patients with occlusion of the internal carotid artery. *Stroke*. 1986;17:1291–1298.

Waller D, Renwick A, Hillier K. *Medical Pharmacology and Therapeutics*. 2nd ed. London, England: Elsevier; 2006.

Yudd AP, Van Heertum RL, Masdeu JC. Interventions and functional brain imaging. *Semin Nucl Med*. 1991;21:153–158.

CHAPTER 10

Iodinated CT Contrast

Chapter Objectives

Specific learning outcomes (page ix) of this text addressed in this chapter:

- Apply the principles of pharmacology to the safe and effective use of medicines.
- Recognize general, patient-specific, and scenario-specific risks, precautions, and contraindications for use of medicines.
- Apply the pharmacokinetic and pharmacodynamic principles of medications to identify and explain normal and adverse reactions to medications.
- Administer medications safely, effectively, and appropriately according to procedures and within regulatory and statutory parameters.
- Monitor patients for, identify, and manage adverse reactions.

After reading, digesting, reflecting on, and reviewing the content of this chapter, readers should be able to

1. Demonstrate command of key pharmacology terms.
2. Demonstrate enhanced understanding of the principles associated with the pharmacology of computed tomography (CT) contrast.
3. Demonstrate critical thinking to effect problem solving related to CT contrast protocols and procedures.
4. Recognize, explain, and interpret clinical problems and evidence in relation to CT contrast use and application.
5. Demonstrate understanding of the mode of action, pharmacokinetics, risks, precautions, contraindications, adverse effects, interactions, and appropriate dosage of CT contrast.
6. Apply knowledge of the general principles and concepts in a translational manner to clinical practice.

Key Terms

anaphylactic	extravasation	hypersensitivity	nephrotoxicity	resistance
anaphylactoid	flow friction	hypertonic	nonionic	saturated
biphasic	inorganic	hypotonic	oligomerization	tolerability
chemotoxic	iodinated	isotonic	osmolality	tonicity
dimer	ionic	monomer	prophylactic	tri-iodinated
dissociate	ionicity	nephropathy	radio-opacification	viscosity

Some of the text, tables, and figures in this chapter were extracted from "Pharmacology Part 5: CT and MRI Contrast" by Geoff Currie (*J. Nucl Med Technol.* 2019;47:189–202).

Introduction

In imaging, a contrast agent is any agent that is administered to the patient in order to improve the visualization of an organ, tissue, or pathology. Generally, contrast agents are positive (increase opacity), but some negative contrast agents (decrease opacity; e.g., air, gases) exist. In the context of this chapter, the positive contrast agents associated with iodinated contrast agents in computed tomography (CT) are outlined. It should be noted, however, that iodinated contrast agents are used outside of CT.

While contrast agents have become safer and better tolerated in recent decades, adverse reactions still occur to varying degrees. Consequently, it is essential that those administering contrast or monitoring patients after contrast administration are familiar with the pharmacology and adverse reactions associated with those contrast agents. Foundations of pharmacology and pharmacokinetics outlined in previous chapters are considered assumed knowledge. This insight and understanding facilitate early detection of adverse reactions and inform a response with the most appropriate management.

CT Contrast

Ideally, a contrast agent for CT would be able to provide opacification of blood vessels, organs, and tissues without altering physiology or producing toxicity. The iodine molecule can absorb x-rays to provide contrast and has been the basis of intravenous contrast since 1929. The development of organic iodinated compounds emerged because the inorganic sodium iodide was too toxic for regular or routine use. Today, CT contrast is based on the structure that emerged in the 1950s: tri-iodinated derivatives of benzoic acid that were ionic and high osmolality. Current agents are either monomers or dimers (one or two benzene rings), ionic or nonionic, high or low osmolality, or isotonic, and they vary in viscosity. It is important to note that almost all current CT contrast agents are iodine based. The emergence of nonionic CT contrast created the misnomer that they were noniodinated; nonionic does not mean that the contrast agent contains no iodine. More than 50 million CT studies are performed in the United States each year, an estimated 50% (25 million) of which include intravenous contrast. Worldwide, an estimated 75 million intravenous CT contrast doses are administered annually.

Properties of CT Contrast

A number of key properties of iodinated contrast agents influence their behavior, efficiency, and adverse reaction risk profile. There is an interplay among these properties that optimizes the degree of radio-opacification and the tolerability and toxicity of iodinated contrast agents (Table 10-1):

- *Iodine concentration* is the amount of iodine per unit volume of the contrast solution administered (expressed as milligrams per milliliter [mg/mL]).
- *Osmolality* is a measure of the number of active particles when the contrast agent is dissolved in 1 kg of water, expressed as milliosmoles per kilogram (mOsm/kg).
- *Viscosity* is internal or flow friction, resistance, or thickness of the fluid.
- *Ionicity* is the tendency for the contrast agent to separate into charged species (ions) when dissolved in solution.
- *Oligomerization* refers to the chemical structure being either a monomer or dimer.
- The dose delivered to the patient can vary in both relative (mg/kg) and absolute (mg I) terms but also in the time course over which it is administered.

TABLE 10-1 Optimizing the Key Properties of Intravenous CT Contrast*			
Contrast	Iodine Concentration mg/mL	Osmolality mOsm/kg Water	Viscosity mPa/s (37°C)
Ionic monomer (HOCM)	Up to 400	1,400–2,100	
Ionic dimer (HOCM)	320	600	
Nonionic monomer (LOCM)	Up to 350	600–800	
Nonionic dimer (IOCM)	320	290	
Human serum	3.2–4	290	1.5–2.0
Ionic monomers			
Amidotrizoic acid (Urografin)	146	1,690	8.5
Amidotrizoate-meg (Angiografin)		1,530	
Ioxitalaminic acid (Telebrix)	350	2,130	7.5
Nonionic monomers			
Iohexol (Omnipaque)	240, 300, 350	500, 690, 880	3.3, 6.1, 10.6
Iopamidol (Isovue)	200, 300, 370	413, 616, 796	2.0, 4.7, 8.6
Ioxilan (Oxilan)	350	695	4.6
Iopromide (Ultravist)	370	780	9.5
Ioversol (Optiray)	320	702	5.8
Iomeprol (Iomeron)	350	618	7.5
Iobitridol (Xenetix)	350	915	10.0
Ionic dimers			
Ioxaglate (Hexabrix)	320	580	7.5
Nonionic dimers			
Iodixanol (Visipaque)	320	290	11.4
Iotrolan (Isovist)	300	320	8.1

Abbreviations: HOCM, high osmolality contrast media; IOCM, iso-osmolar contrast media (IOCM); LOCM, low osmolality contrast media.

*Optimization of these properties has resulted in an evolution to contrasts that are easier to use and have low intravenous toxicity and fewer adverse effects (frequency and severity).

Iodine concentration among iodinated CT contrast agents ranges from 11% to 46%, with higher iodine concentrations providing both better radio-opacification but higher risk of adverse reaction. Today, most current-generation CT contrast agents are nonionic; however, they often vary significantly in terms of iodine content. The dimer configuration is designed to reduce the risk of adverse reaction and toxicity without compromising radio-opacification. Typically, the iodine concentration of common iodinated contrast agents is on the order of 300 mg/mL, but they can range from 200 mg/mL to 400 mg/mL (Table 10-1). Indeed, the same contrast agent maybe be marketed and branded with varying iodine concentrations (e.g., Omnipaque 240, Omnipaque 300, and Omnipaque 370). Increasing iodine concentration increases viscosity.

Osmolality introduces the concept of *tonicity*—hypertonic or isotonic, for example. Tonicity relates to the impact of the osmolality of a solution on the surrounding cells. Isotonic solutions (like most radiopharmaceuticals) have an osmolality that equals blood (290 mOsm/kg water) and thus have no impact on surrounding cells. Hypertonic solutions have a higher osmolality than blood, which results in water being drawn out of blood cells. Iodinated contrast agents in CT can have an osmolality 7 times that of blood. Hypotonic solutions have a lower osmolality than blood, which results in water being taken into blood cells. Iodinated contrast agents are classified as high osmolality contrast media (HOCM), low osmolality contrast media (LOCM), or iso-osmolar contrast media (IOCM) (Table 10-1). There are no hypotonic iodinated contrast agents. Both HOCM and LOCM are hypertonic, but to varying degrees. Older iodinated contrast agents are typically HOCM (1,300–2,140 mOsm/kg water), and newer contrast agents, developed in the 1980s and later, are typically LOCM (600–850 mOsm/kg water). As outlined shortly in relation to adverse reactions, osmolality contributes to the incidence of non-anaphylactoid adverse reactions mediated by endothelial damage, movement of fluid among compartments, and cell deformation. IOCM iodinated contrast agents are a more recent development, with osmolality that equals that of blood. Given the aim of iodinated CT contrast agents is to have sufficient iodine concentration for radio-opacification, the ratio of iodine atoms to particles in solution is important; HOCM is 0.5, LOCM is 3.0, and IOCM is 6.0. Adverse effects attributable to osmolality include pain, flushing, nausea, vomiting, and dehydration. Contrast osmolality higher than blood (HOCM and LOCM) results in movement of water from interstitial spaces into the vascular compartment, which causes increased blood viscosity, endothelial damage, hypervolemia, vasodilation, edema with neurotoxicity, decreased myocardial contractility, and toxicity.

The *viscosity* of iodinated CT contrast agents is the flow friction, resistance, or thickness of the contrast media. Iodinated contrast is significantly more viscous than radiopharmaceuticals, which has an impact on intravenous injectability, flow rate, and gauge of cannula required. Viscosity can be reduced by injecting the contrast at body temperature (37°C) rather than room temperature, and it is worth noting that viscosity of iodinated contrast media at 20°C is approximately twice that of the same agent at 37°C. Viscosity is influenced by the molecular structure and composition of the contrast agent, with inclusion of sodium decreasing viscosity but increasing endothelial irritation compared to meglumine. LOCM has higher viscosity than HOCM, and viscosity increases with iodine content (Table 10-1). Viscosity plays an important role in renal tolerance, contributing significantly to the risk of contrast-induced nephrotoxicity. High-viscosity intravenous iodinated contrast agents require longer infusion times, while low viscosity allows the use of a rapid bolus, a key factor in optimizing the contrast agent for imaging protocol. High-viscosity intravenous contrast agents also exert an influence on the local circulation. Water is used as the reference standard for viscosity at 1 centipoise (cps); plasma is 1.5 to 2 cps; and iodinated CT contrast agents range from 2.0 cps for low iodine concentration, nonionic, and monomer-based contrast up to 11.4 cps.

Contrast agents used intravenously in CT are tri-iodinated derivatives of benzoic acid (Fig. 10-1). A monomer is a simple molecule or base unit that can undergo polymerization. In the case of iodinated contrast agents, it is a 2,4,6-tri-iodinated benzene ring (Fig. 10-1). A dimer is two bonded monomer units following polymerization to form a two-unit oligomer. Monomers have higher osmolality than dimers, with dimers typically being LOCM or IOCM (Table 10-1). Covalently bonded iodine atoms associated with CT contrast agents are within the range of x-ray wavelengths and so can produce attenuation. This attenuation is enhanced by the close proximity of the tri-iodinated configuration. Importantly, the benzine ring structure reduces the risk of toxicity.

Ionic iodinated CT contrast agents dissociate into ion pairs, while nonionic do not (Fig. 10-1). Nonionic does not mean noniodinated, nor does it mean LOCM even though most nonionic contrast is LOCM. Fully saturated tri-iodinated benzoic acid derivative monomer CT contrast agents dissociate into ions in solution, the anion containing the iodine atoms and the cation containing sodium and/or meglumine. These are typically hypertonic (osmolality 5 times that of blood) and alter the plasma tonicity. Consequently, adverse reactions are common. The dimer form (2 tri-iodinated benzoic acid rings) allows high iodine content but low osmolality because a single cation is still all that is required. Only the anion is radio-opaque because it carries the iodine atoms, but the cation is needed for the solution to be formed.

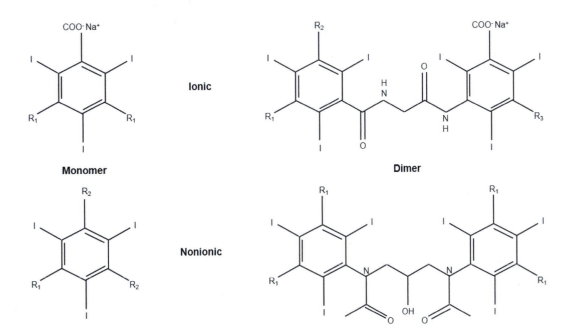

FIGURE 10-1 The chemical structure of iodinated CT contrast agents is based on the 2,4,6-tri-iodinated benzene ring and provides the four major classifications of iodinated CT contrast agents: ionic monomer (top left), ionic dimer (top right), nonionic monomer (bottom left), and nonionic dimer (bottom right). For ionic contrast media, the carboxyl group (COOH) ionizes (COO$^-$) with sodium or meglumine to form anion and cation pairs. Side chains (R) vary but tend to be longer for nonionic contrast.

Nonionic monomer CT contrast agents have a longer side chain than ionic monomers (Fig. 10-1), which increases the molecular weight, decreases the osmolality, but does not change the iodine concentration. The nonionic dimer structures tend to be isotonic. Low osmolality agents are less toxic and have fewer adverse reactions. The four major classifications of iodinated CT contrast agents are ionic monomer, ionic dimer, nonionic monomer, and nonionic dimer (Fig. 10-1).

Individual doses for patients should be tailored in consideration of the properties outlined previously and the following:

- Iodine concentration
- Volume of dose
- Patient height, weight, age, and gender
- Venous accessibility
- Renal function
- Pharmacokinetic model (discussed below)
- Injection rate
- Target organ
- Target enhancement
- CT scanner and imaging protocol

Mechanism of Action

While a discussion of the physical principles of x-ray production in CT is beyond the scope of this chapter, it is important to briefly revise key principles that contribute to the effectiveness of iodinated CT contrast media. An incident x-ray can undergo photoelectric absorption following interaction with an inner shell electron of an atom in the attenuating medium when the x-ray energy is fractionally in excess of the binding energy of the electron. The subsequent ejection and replacement of the electron from an outer shell results in production of a characteristic x-ray.

The photoelectric interaction does not occur when the incident x-ray energy is less than the binding energy of the electron. If, however, the incident energy is equal to the binding energy, the photoelectric effect becomes possible and a disproportionate increase in attenuation occurs. Beyond the binding energy equivalent for the incident x-ray, the probability of photoelectric interaction decreases. The K-edge refers to the abrupt increase in attenuation when the energy of the incident x-ray approximates the K-shell binding energy, which is measured in kiloelectron volts (keV) (Fig. 10-2).

The human body is largely composed of low atomic mass elements with corresponding low K-shell binding energies. Higher atomic masses associated with, among many elements, iodine, gadolinium, and lead have high K-shell binding energies producing characteristic x-rays with relatively high energies. This principle allows higher atomic mass elements to be utilized for contrast media or detector material.

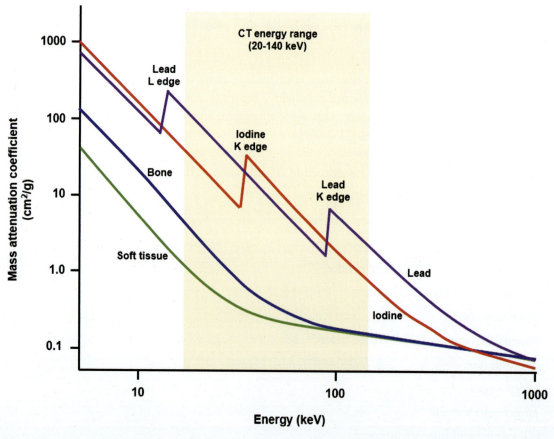

FIGURE 10-2 Schematic representation on log-log scales of the mass attenuation coefficient against x-ray energy. The iodine K-edge at 33 keV demonstrates an abrupt increase in attenuation producing equivalent attenuation greater than lead and several orders of magnitude greater than bone and soft tissue. It should also be noted that within the range of 30 to 100 keV, attenuation coefficients for biological tissues remain fairly uniform, while the contrast agent (iodine) varies substantially.

Since the photoelectric effect has a higher probability of occurring between low-energy x-rays and high atomic mass elements, it provides excellent properties as a CT contrast agent. Iodine, for example, has approximately 350 times higher attenuation than soft tissue at the same energy. This property can be exploited in CT contrast imaging. The K-shell binding energy for x-rays is 33.2 keV for iodine, but rather than attempting imaging with a monochromatic beam at that energy, kilovolt peak (60–80 kVp) can be optimized to produce a good proportion of x-rays in the 33 to 40 keV range. In this energy range, attenuation is greater for iodine than it is for lead (Fig. 10-2).

Pharmacokinetics

Iodinated CT contrast agents are best described using a two-compartment model (Fig. 10-3). Iodinated contrast agents demonstrate rapid peak plasma concentration at 2 minutes after intravenous. A biphasic plasma profile represents rapid diffusion of the contrast from the plasma compartment into the interstitial compartment and then slow urinary clearance. The peak plasma concentration at 2 minutes after intravenous shortens to 1 minute with higher doses. Only 1% to 3% of iodinated contrast agents are plasma protein binding. As contrast diffuses into the extravascular space, water is drawn from extravascular space into the intravascular space due to osmolality. Tight junctions prevent movement of contrast into extravascular spaces in the brain, testes, and neural tissues.

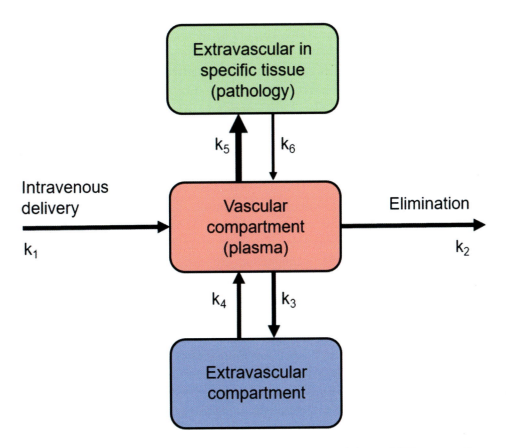

FIGURE 10-3 Modified two-compartment model for iodinated CT contrast or gadolinium MRI contrast administered intravenously. The second extravascular compartment represents pathological tissue that may enhance with contrast administration and therefore be differentiated by surrounding normal tissue by a greater rate constant (k_5 over k_3 or k_4 over k_6). Refer to Chapter 3 for more detailed interpretation of compartment models and rate constants.

The biphasic half-lives vary from one agent to the next but tend to be approximately 7 minutes (range of 2–30 min) and 1.6 hours (range 1–2 h), but these half-lives universally increase with increasing contrast dose. In renal dysfunction, elimination half-life can increase to 40 hours or longer. The intravenous CT contrast agents do not undergo metabolism and are almost exclusively excreted by glomeruli filtration in urine unchanged in a similar fashion to inulin. The proportion of the contrast dose in urine is variable among agents, but in normal patients, it is in the range of 12% at 10 minutes, 50% at 1 hour, 83% at 3 hours, and virtually 100% at 24 hours.

Calcium or magnesium has been added to newer contrast agents to reduce toxicity. All ionic contrast media bind in vivo to calcium and magnesium. If given orally, CT contrast agents are absorbed from the intestine, glucuroconjugated, strongly plasma protein bound, and then rapidly concentrated and eliminated in the biliary system.

Adverse Reactions

Adverse effects are common and classified in several overlapping ways: by type of reaction, by severity of reaction, or by mechanism of reaction (Fig. 10-4). Based on a classification of the type of adverse reaction, contrast agents in CT can produce general reactions or organ-specific reactions. Organ specific reactions include toxicity associated with renal, cardiovascular, pulmonary or neurological systems. General reactions can be acute or delayed, with the latter tending to be skin reactions. Acute general reactions can be mild and self-limiting in nature or moderate to severe, requiring intervention. The incidence of adverse reactions to intravenous iodinated contrast is higher for ionic than for nonionic contrast (Table 10-2). The most common adverse reactions to CT iodinated contrast are hives (52.5%) and nausea (17.6%). Prior adverse reactions to CT contrast are a significant predictor of a subsequent reaction. There is a prevalence of 17% to 35% for adverse reactions to ionic contrast in those with previous reactions and 5% for nonionic contrast. Other predictors or risk factors for developing an adverse reaction to iodinated intravenous contrast include a history of asthma, history of allergies, heart disease, dehydration, sickle cell disease, polycythemia, myeloma, and underlying renal disease. Risks of adverse reactions are also higher in infants and the elderly, during periods of anxiety, and with the use of medications such as beta (β)-blockers, nonsteroidal anti-inflammatories (NSAIDs), and interleukin-2.

Fatal adverse reactions can occur but rarely (1 in 170,000 cases), but with 25 million CT contrast studies annually in the United States, that equates to 150 deaths in the annually. The risk of a fatal adverse effect increases for women, the elderly, Anglo-Saxon, and those with comorbidity. This has been referred to as the four Ws: women, wrinkled, white, and weakened. Generally, the cause of death in fatal CT contrast reactions are associated with renal failure (58%), anaphylaxis/allergy (19%), cardiopulmonary arrest (10%), respiratory failure (8%), and stroke/cerebral hypoxia (4%).

Delayed general adverse reactions occur 1 hour to 1 week after the intravenous contrast injection. Delayed reactions tend to be skin reactions and are more likely for dimeric isomolar agents or in young adults, women, and those with a history of allergy.

Describing adverse reactions to contrast by the mechanism creates three classifications: *anaphylactoid*, chemotoxic (organ specific), and vasovagal. Anaphylactic reactions are associated with an allergen-immunoglobulin G (IgE)–mediated release of chemical mediators such as histamine from mast cells. Anaphylactoid reactions like those of iodinated contrast agents are similar to anaphylactic reactions in terms of activation of mast cells, but they are not initiated by the allergen-IgE complex. This is important to understand because it means that an anaphylactoid CT contrast reaction can occur with the first administration (no sensitization), reaction severity is not dose related (test doses are unhelpful), and a previous history of contrast reaction increases the risk of a subsequent reaction but does not mean it will occur. Non-anaphylactoid reactions are dose dependent. Nonetheless, patients with asthma, food or medication allergies, mastocytosis, and prior contrast reactions are at highest risk of an anaphylactoid reaction.

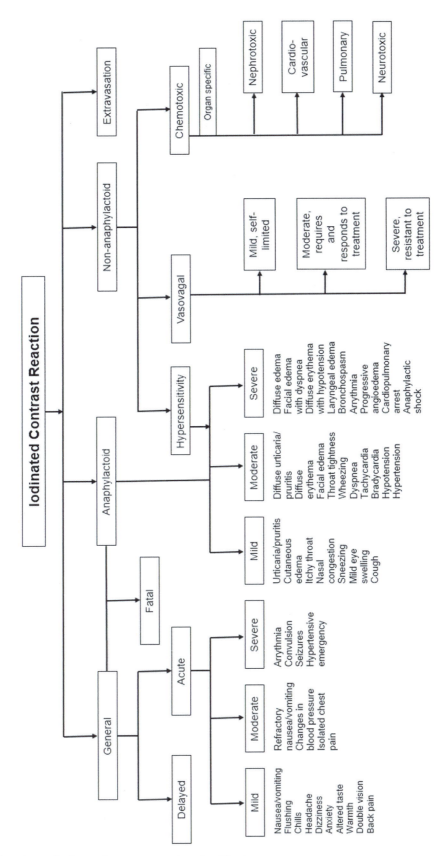

FIGURE 10-4 Flow chart of iodinated contrast reaction classification.

TABLE 10-2	Incidence Rates (%) of Adverse Reactions to Iodinated Intravenous Contrast Agents			
Reaction Type	*Ionic*	*Nonionic*	*Ionic HOCM*	*Nonionic LOCM/IOCM*
Mild	15%	3%		
Moderate	1–2%	0.2%–0.4%		
Severe	0.2%	0.04%	0.22%	0.04%
Fatal	0.0006%	0.0006%		
Overall			13%	3%
Delayed	2%–4% for nonionic dimer	0.5%–1% for ionic and nonionic monomers	12.5% for CT with intravenous contrast	10% for CT without intravenous contrast
Extravasation	0.04%–0.2% for mechanical power injectors			
Contrast-induced nephropathy	1%–3% in normal renal function	12%–27% in renal impairment	50% in diabetic nephropathy	

Chemotoxic adverse reactions are associated with the ionicity, iodine concentration, viscosity, osmolality, injection rate, and dose of the contrast agent, all contributing to alterations to homeostasis. Contrast-induced nephrotoxicity suffers a lack of uniform definition around the degree of resulting renal dysfunction, but incidence does vary with baseline renal function status. There is a 1% to 3% risk of developing nephrotoxicity in patients with normal baseline renal function, 12% to 27% in those with preexisting renal dysfunction, and 50% in those with diabetic nephropathy. Preventative strategies include 6 to 12 hours of prehydration followed by 4 to 12 hours of posthydration, and the use of nonionic contrast at the minimum dose. N-acetylcysteine, at 600 mg twice daily for 48 hours prior to the study, has also been used prophylactically. Sodium bicarbonate infusion starting 1 hour before contrast administration and continued until 6 hours after contrast administration has also been used.

Screening patients on the basis of health history and renal function is perhaps the best strategy for minimizing acute contrast-induced nephrotoxicity. Estimated glomerular filtration rate (GFR) from serum creatinine levels has been used effectively to predict risk. A GFR greater than 60 mL/min/1.73 m^2 is associated with negligible risk of contrast-induced nephrotoxicity. Conversely, a GFR of 30 to 60 mL/min/1.73 m^2 is associated with a moderate risk of contrast-induced nephrotoxicity and a GFR of less than 30 mL/min/1.73 m^2 is associated with a high risk (relatively contraindicated) of contrast-induced nephrotoxicity. Serum creatinine levels should be assessed prior to CT contrast administration in patients with a history of renal disease, a family history of renal disease, diabetes, myeloma, or collagen vascular disease or if they are on medications such as metformin, NSAIDs, and aminoglycosides. Creatinine assessment is also recommended in patients with a history of renal transplant, renal tumor, or renal surgery; in patients with end-stage liver disease; and in patients with severe congestive heart failure.

The molecular weight of iodinated contrast agents allows ready filtration in the glomeruli. The virtual 100% elimination of iodinated contrast agents via the glomeruli creates potential for nephrotoxicity. Iodinated contrast nephrotoxicity is generally associated with a number of mechanisms (Fig. 10-5). First, hypertonic solutions in the renal tubules reduce water reabsorption, which leads to tubular swelling, increased intrarenal pressure, and a decrease in both renal blood flow and GFR. Concurrently, increased viscosity increases tubular pressure. Second, tubular cell damage results with a decrease in clearance of para-aminohippurate and an increase in excretion of enzymes in the proximal tubules. Medullary hypoxia resulting from vasoconstriction and decreased blood flow also contribute to tubular cell damage. Tubular cell damage both reduces GFR and increases oxidative stress. Third, cytotoxicity causes endothelial damage resulting in vasoconstriction and decreased GFR, and it increases oxidative stress. Vasoconstriction can be exacerbated in diabetes and vasoconstrictive drugs.

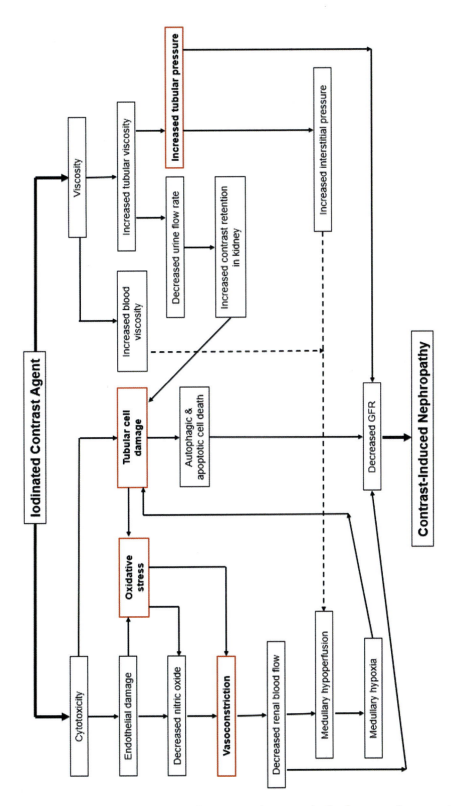

FIGURE 10-5 Flow chart outlining the interplay among factors contributing to the development of contrast-induced nephrotoxicity. As outlined by bold boxes, vasoconstriction, oxidative stress, tubular cell damage, and increased tubular pressure are the key drivers associated with cytotoxicity and viscosity as mediators.

Cardiovascular toxicity results in increased incidence or severity of cardiovascular adverse reactions to iodinated contrast agents. Underlying heart disease increases the risk of cardiovascular toxicity. Neurotoxicity associated with iodinated contrast agents results from an alteration in the blood-brain barrier due to the hypertonicity. Clearly, LOCM and IOCM agents reduce this risk. Headache, confusion, seizures, altered consciousness, visual disturbances, and dizziness are the most common signs of neurotoxicity.

Vasovagal reactions manifest as bradycardia and hypotension because the involuntary reflex slows heart rate and dilates blood vessels in the legs. Vasovagal reactions are not necessarily attributed to the contrast agent itself but to a sympathetic nervous system response to fear or pain. Clearly, anxiety can exacerbate this reaction. With more blood in the legs and less in the brain, patients may get lightheaded and faint. Elevating the patient's legs in combination with 6 to 10 L/min of oxygen is generally adequate treatment.

Life-threatening reactions usually occur in first 20 minutes after intravenous contrast. Of severe or fatal adverse reactions to iodinated CT contrast agents, 94% to 100% occur within 20 minutes of contrast administration.

Management of Adverse Reactions

Prevention is better than cure. Prophylactic medications to reduce but not necessarily eliminate risk include 32 mg of methylprednisolone orally 12 hours and 2 hours prior to contrast administration (Lasser protocol) and 50 mg of diphenhydramine orally 1 hour before contrast administration plus 50 mg of prednisone orally 13 hours, 7 hours, and 1 hour before contrast administration (Greenberger protocol). The Lasser protocol reduces adverse reactions from 9% to 6.4% for ionic contrast, while the Greenberger protocol has been reported to decrease the incidence of adverse reaction to ionic contrast from 9% to 7%. Antihistamines are often used prophylactically in high-risk patients without evidence of being able to reduce incidence of adverse reactions.

While the pharmacology associated with drugs in the crash cart/emergency trolley are detailed in Chapter 12, here we briefly examine key medications that may be employed in the event of a serious or anaphylactoid reaction to CT contrast agents. It should be noted that a crash cart/emergency trolley should be immediately available at all times in or immediately adjacent to the CT room where intravenous contrast is being used. One should also keep in mind that serious adverse effects may occur in the short period after the patient leaves the scanning room.

Salbutamol (albuterol), discussed in Chapter 8, functions as a β_2-receptor agonist to cause bronchodilation and relieve bronchospasm. The standard dose is 1 to 2 inhalations of 100 mcg each with a third inhalation if necessary 1 minute after the second. This same dose can be given prophylactically. Patients with bronchospasm should also be supported with 10 L/min of oxygen delivered via a mask. Atropine is a parasympatholytic agent that can be used to treat bradycardia in a vasovagal reaction. The standard dose is 0.6 to 1.0 mg intravenously, repeated every 3 to 5 min as needed to a maximum of 3 mg. Elevation of the patient's legs and delivery of oxygen (10 L/min) should be used to support the patient experiencing a self-limiting vasovagal reaction. Diphenhydramine (Benadryl) is a histamine-1 (H_1) inhibitor, but antihistamines block further histamine-mediated reactions but do not stop histamine-mediated reactions already underway. It should be used only for mild urticaria or prophylaxis with doses of 25 to 50 mg orally or intramuscularly or 25 mg intravenously being standard. This dose can cause drowsiness. Epinephrine (adrenaline) is a sympathetic agonist with alpha (α)- and beta (β)-receptor activity. α-Receptor agonism with epinephrine causes peripheral vasoconstriction, which can help with severe urticaria, facial edema, and laryngeal edema. β_1-Receptor agonism produces inotropic and chronotropic effects and so should be used with caution in known heart disease. β_2-Receptor agonism causes bronchodilation, so epinephrine can be used to treat bronchospasm. Doses of epinephrine are typically 0.1 to 0.3 mg (1 mg/mL or 1:1,000) subcutaneously, 0.3 mg intramuscularly via EpiPen if the patient is not hypotensive, or 0.1 mg (0.1 mg/mL or 1:10,000) intravenously over 3 to 5 minutes repeated as needed up to a maximum of 1 mg if the patient is hypotensive. Diazepam is a benzodiazepine that can be used to treat seizures, if necessary, using an intravenous dose of

5 to 10 mg to a maximum of 30 mg as required. Lorazepam is an alternative benzodiazepine for seizures, especially in pediatric patients, with a dose of 0.01 mg/kg intravenously. Nitroglycerin is a vasodilator that decreases oxygen demand, which can be used to treat acute angina. The dose can be any one of the following: one 300 to 600 mcg sublingual tablet under the tongue, one or two sprays of 400 mcg each directed onto or under the tongue, or 2 to 3 mg buccal tablet placed between the upper lip and gum. Sublingual tablet or spray doses can be repeated if necessary.

In the case of generalized anaphylaxis-like symptoms, epinephrine should be used. Doses are typically 0.1 to 0.3 mg (1 mg/mL or 1:1,000) subcutaneously, 0.3 mg intravenously via EpiPen if the patient is not hypotensive, or 0.1 mg (0.1 mg/mL or 1:10,000) intravenously over 3 to 5 minutes, repeated as needed up to a maximum of 1 mg if the patient is hypotensive. A β_2-agonist can be added for bronchospasm. Saline infusion should be used for hypotension.

Nausea and vomiting are self-limiting, and patients need to be observed for 30 minutes with intravenous access kept open. If nausea and vomiting continue, antiemetic medications could be considered. Antiemetics are a class of medication that block neurotransmitters (e.g., acetylcholine, histamine, dopamine, substance P, and 5-hydroxytryptamine) responsible for nausea and vomiting in the emetic center in the medulla, vestibular apparatus, chemoreceptor trigger zone in the fourth ventricle, and higher brain centers that relay sensory inputs. Specific examples of medications include metoclopramide for D_2-receptor antagonism, hyoscine hydrobromide for muscarinic receptor antagonism, promethazine for H_1 receptor antagonism, ondansetron for $5-HT_3$ receptor antagonism, and aprepitant for NK_1 receptor antagonism. The recumbent position helps minimize aspiration.

Extravasation

Extravasation of iodinated contrast agents involves delivery of the contrast extravascularly due to human error, cannula dislodgement, or leakage. While well-recognized, true incidence of extravasation is hard to reliably determine, but several large studies report an incidence less than 1%. Extravasation of iodinated contrast agents typically causes self-limiting symptoms such as pain, erythema, and swelling. In severe reactions, skin ulceration, necrosis, or compartment syndrome may occur. While more severe reactions tend to occur with larger volumes of extravasated HOCM or ionic contrast, they can occur with small volumes of LOCM and nonionic contrast. The peak reactions occur at 24 to 48 hours after intravenous contrast administration.

Once again, prevention is a better option than therapy. Key strategies to minimize the risk of extravasation include but are not limited to the following:

- Ensure that reliable intravenous access is tested prior to contrast administration.
- Decrease flow rates, if the protocol allows, in high-risk patients.
- Limit flow rates to 3 mL/sec for large veins and 1.5 mL/sec for the hand or wrist.
- Monitor the infusion site directly for the first 15 seconds of the infusion.
- Counsel the patient to report immediately any unusual sensations at the intravenous site during contrast administration.
- Immediately stop the infusion if there is concern regarding extravasation.

If extravasation of iodinated contrast agents does occur, management will depend on the patient's symptoms and volume of extravasation. The infusion should be stopped immediately and the intravenous site elevated with a cold compress applied. For small volumes and self-limiting symptoms, the patient should be monitored in the CT department for 2 to 4 hours. For large volumes (30–100 mL), blistering or ulceration, altered perfusion, a change in sensation, or worsening pain or swelling after the 2- to 4-hour monitoring window, the patient should be referred to the local emergency department for surgical consultation.

Interactions

Iodinated contrast agents are not highly active pharmacologically; however, interactions with medications the patient may be taking is possible. Prevention is a good practice and is facilitated by taking a thorough patient history, being aware of drugs needing precautions, and administering contrast through a separate line, *not* the same line as medications. Iodinated contrast agents have anticoagulant properties (less so for nonionic) and prolong coagulation time, so they can potentiate the effects of anticoagulant (e.g., heparin and warfarin), antiplatelet (e.g., aspirin and NSAIDs), and fibrinolytic medications (e.g., urokinase). Metformin can have additive effects associated with iodinated contrast toxicity. β-Blockers increase the risk and severity of anaphylactoid reactions. Calcium channel blockers can potentiate hypotensive effects of iodinated contrast agents. Diuretics can have a cumulative effect with iodinated contrast agents for diuresis and increase the risk of nephrotoxicity. Nephrotoxic medications such as NSAIDs and gentamicin can potentiate the renal effects of iodinated contrast. Adverse reactions to iodinated contrast agents are more likely if the patient is taking immunomodulator medications. Allergic reactions or symptoms of a similar nature are more likely in patients taking β-blockers, interleukins, and interferons. Patients taking β-blocker medications have a 3-fold increase in risk for anaphylactoid adverse reactions to iodinated contrast. Any medication that relies on renal elimination may have increased retention and activity, and medications with a narrow therapeutic index may be susceptible to toxicity. Synergistic effects between iodinated contrast media and calcium channel blockers and digoxin are possible, especially with ionic HOCM.

Contraindications and Precautions

A number of medications are relatively contraindicated with ionic contrast media because they will crystalize and form precipitates, including cimetidine, diazepam, diphenhydramine, ethanol, meperidine, papaverine, promethazine, and protamine sulfate. Some of these medications are prescribed for prophylaxis or management of adverse reactions, and so caution is suggested, especially if administered through the same intravenous line. Nonionic contrast agents do not share this incompatibility. Caution should also be exercised when using iodinated contrast agents in patients medicated with known nephrotoxic drugs, including angiotensin-converting enzyme inhibitors (ACEI), acyclovir, aminoglycosides, amphotericin, antineoplastics, cyclosporin, furosemide, lithium, metformin, methotrexate, NSAIDs, tacrolimus, and vancomycin. Creatinine levels may warrant assessment before progression with CT contrast in these patients. As outlined previously, there are numerous factors that identify a patient as having a higher risk of adverse reaction, and while caution should be exercised, none are absolute contraindications. Perhaps the highest-risk group are patients with a GFR less than 30 mL/min/1.73 m^2. In this group, iodinated CT contrast should not be administered unless the patient is on dialysis and anuric or the diagnostic benefits outweigh the risk. LOCM, nonionic, dimer-based contrast- with low iodine concentration are lower-risk options for patients at increased risk of adverse reactions when the benefit of the contrast procedure warrants iodinated contrast CT.

Summary

Iodinated CT contrast agents have unique interventions that demand an expanded skill set and understanding of basic and applied pharmacology. An insight into the complexities of iodinated contrast enhances practice and patient safety. Specifically, command of adverse reactions is a key skill required for capability in CT and ensures that medical radiation technologists meet the minimum capabilities for their scope of practice.

References

Ayre-Smith G. Tissue necrosis following extravasation of contrast material. *J Can Assoc Radiol*. 1982;33:104.

Bae KT. Intravenous contrast medium administration and scan timing at CT: considerations and approaches. *Radiology*. 2010;256:32–61.

Block JH, Beale JM. *Wilson and Gisvold's Textbook of Organic Medicinal and Pharmaceutical Chemistry*. 12th ed. Philadelphia, PA: Lippincott Williams & Wilkins; 2011.

Bourin M, Jolliet P, Ballereau F. An overview of the clinical pharmacokinetics of x-ray contrast media. Clin Pharmacokinet. 1997;32:180–193.

Bryant B, Knights K, Salerno E. *Pharmacology for Health Professionals*. 2nd ed. Sydney, Australia: Mosby Elsevier; 2007.

Cohan RH, Ellis JH, Garner WL. Extravasation of radiographic contrast material: recognition, prevention, and treatment. *Radiology*. 1996;200:593–604.

Costa N. Understanding contrast media. *J Infusion Nursing*. 2004;27:302–312.

Federle MP, Chang PJ, Confer S, Ozgun B. Frequency and effects of extravasation of ionic and nonionic CT contrast media during rapid bolus injection. *Radiology*. 1998;206:637–640.

Greenen RWF, Kingma HJ, van der Molen AJ. Contrast-induced nephropathy: pharmacology, pathophysiology and prevention. *Insights Imaging*. 2013;4:811–820.

Iyer RS, Schopp JG, Swanson JO, Thapa MM, Phillips GS. Safety essentials: acute reactions to iodinated contrast media. *Can Assoc Radiol*. 2013;64:193–199.

Jacobs JE, Birnbaum BA, Langlotz CP. Contrast media reactions and extravasation: relationship to intravenous injection rates. *Radiology*. 1998;209:411–416.

Meurer K, Kelsch B, Hogstrom B. The pharmacokinetic profile, tolerability and safety of the iodinated, nonionic, dimeric contrast medium Iosimenol 340 injection in healthy human subjects. *Acta Radiologica*. 2015;56:581–586.

Morcos SK, Thomsen HS, Exley CM. Contrast media: interactions with other drugs and clinical tests. *Eur Radiol*. 2005;15:1463–1468.

Morzycki A, Bhatia A, Murphy KJ. Adverse reactions to contrast material: a Canadian update. *Can Assoc Radiol*. 2017;68:187–193.

Namasivayam S, Kalra MK, Torres WE, Small WC. Adverse reactions to intravenous iodinated contrast media: a primer for radiologists. *Emerg Radiol*. 2006;12:210–215.

Namasivayam S, Kalra MK, Torres WE, Small WC. Adverse reactions to intravenous iodinated contrast media: an update. *Curr Probl Diagn Radiol*. 2006;35(4):164–169.

Pasternak JJ, Williamson EE. Clinical pharmacology, use, and adverse reactions of iodinated contrast agents: a primer for non-radiologists. *May Clin Proc*. 2012;87:390–402.

Rang H, Dale M, Ritter J, Flower R. *Rang and Dale's Pharmacology*. 6th ed. London, England: Churchill Livingston; 2008.

Seibert JA, Boone JM. X-ray imaging physics for nuclear medicine technologists. Part 2: x-ray interactions and image formation. *J Nucl Med Technol*. 2005;33:3–18.

Sweetman SC (Ed.). Martindale: *The Complete Drug Reference*. 26th ed. Chicago, IL: Pharmaceutical Press; 2009.

Wang CL, Cohan RH, Ellis JH, Adusumilli S, Dunnick NR. Frequency, management, and outcome of extravasation of nonionic iodinated contrast medium in 69,657 intravenous injections. *Radiology*. 2007;243:80–87.

CHAPTER 11

Gadolinium MRI Contrast

Chapter Objectives

Specific learning outcomes (page ix) of this text addressed in this chapter:

- Apply the principles of pharmacology to the safe and effective use of medicines.
- Recognize general, patient-specific, and scenario-specific risks, precautions, and contraindications for use of medicines.
- Apply the pharmacokinetic and pharmacodynamic principles of medications to identify and explain normal and adverse reactions to medications.
- Administer medications safely, effectively, and appropriately according to procedures and within regulatory and statutory parameters.
- Monitor patients for, identify, and manage adverse reactions.

After reading, digesting, reflecting on, and reviewing the content of this chapter, readers should be able to

1. Demonstrate command of key pharmacology terms.
2. Demonstrate enhanced understanding of the principles associated with the pharmacology of magnetic resonance imaging (MRI) contrast.
3. Demonstrate critical thinking to effect problem solving related to MRI contrast protocols and procedures.
4. Recognize, explain, and interpret clinical problems and evidence in relation to MRI contrast use and application.
5. Demonstrate understanding of the mode of action, pharmacokinetics, risks, precautions, contraindications, adverse effects, interactions, and appropriate dosages of MRI contrast.
6. Apply knowledge of the general principles and concepts in a translational manner to clinical practice.

Key Terms

chelation	dipole-dipole	lanthanide	paramagnetic	relaxation
chemotoxic	ferromagnetic	macrocyclic	phagocytosis	relaxivity
conjugated	gadolinium	nanoparticle	polarization	saturated
demetallation	heavy metal toxin	nephrotoxicity	proton	superparamagnetic
dipole moment	hyperpolarized	neurotoxicity	radiofrequency	

Some of the text, tables, and figures in this chapter were extracted from "Pharmacology Part 5: CT and MRI Contrast" by Geoff Currie (*J Nucl Med Technol.* 2019;47:189–202).

Introduction

In imaging, a contrast agent is any agent that is administered to the patient in order to improve the visualization of an organ, tissue, or pathology. Generally, contrast agents are positive (T1), but some negative contrast agents (T2) exist. In the context of this chapter, the positive contrast agents associated with gadolinium for magnetic resonance imaging (MRI) are discussed. It should be noted, however, that gadolinium contrast agents are used outside of MRI.

While contrast agents have become safer and better tolerated in recent decades, adverse reactions still occur to varying degrees. Consequently, it is essential that those administering contrast or monitoring patients after contrast administration are familiar with the pharmacology and adverse reactions associated with those contrast agents. Foundations of pharmacology and pharmacokinetics outlined in previous chapters are considered assumed knowledge. This insight and understanding facilitate early detection of adverse reactions and inform a response with the most appropriate management.

MRI Contrast

A number of different types of contrast media are employed in MRI; however, the vast majority used clinically and the focus of this chapter are the T1 *paramagnetic* contrast agents associated with gadolinium. Worldwide, 40% to 50% of MRI procedures are undertaken with contrast. Nonetheless, it is important to highlight key aspects of the five classes of MRI contrast agents:

- T1 agents are discussed in this chapter.
- T2/T2* agents are *superparamagnetic* nanoparticles composed of iron oxides that shorten the relaxation times of T2/T2*. While paramagnetic contrast agents increase proton signal, superparamagnetic and ferromagnetic contrast agents destroy the signal (negative contrast). For example, MRI contrast might be achieved by a T2/T2* contrast agent destroying the signal for liver but not from a liver metastases.
- Chemical exchange saturation transfer (CEST) agents are chemicals that create MRI contrast by transferring saturated protons to the bulk water pool.
- ^{19}F nuclei not only are naturally occurring fluorine but also are the most sensitive spin (resonance) in MRI after hydrogen. As a result, ^{19}F nuclei are readily detected by MRI. The barrier to using ^{19}F nuclei instead of ^{18}F nuclei in radiopharmaceuticals is that in nuclear medicine the tracer principle is adopted, while MRI requires large (potentially toxic) concentrations: 1 fluorine atom versus 20 or more per structure. Instead, ^{19}F nuclei are incorporated into perfluorocarbon nanoparticles (PFCs), avoiding toxicity by encapsulation of many perfluorocarbon molecules in phospholipid encapsulated nanoparticle.
- Hyperpolarized probes use polarization techniques (such as dynamic nuclear polarization) to increase (up to 5 orders of magnitude) sensitivity to the spin energy levels. Unfortunately, despite excellent sensitivity, these agents require fast injection and target accumulation to overcome signal decay.

Paramagnetic substances have one or more particles (protons, neutrons, or electrons) with a spin that is not canceled out by another similar particle with an opposite spin. Magnetic dipole moments of unpaired electrons are very much larger than those of protons or neutrons, so the local magnetic fields generated by unpaired electrons are very strong. Substances that have unpaired electrons, such as gadolinium, are very effective paramagnetic contrast enhancers. When paramagnetic ions are added to water, the relaxation of water molecules is enhanced in the vicinity of the paramagnetic substance. Both T1 and T2 relaxation times are then reduced. The actual contrast agent does not alter the intensity of the image; rather, the presence of the contrast agent alters the relaxation characteristics of adjacent protons, thus indirectly affecting the intensity. While gadolinium is technically a paramagnetic agent as a result of its unpaired electrons, this characteristic is not the basis of T1 contrast enhancement. It is the dipole-dipole interaction that influences T1 relaxation. Gadolinium contains 7 unpaired electrons, making these compounds strongly paramagnetic. Gadolinium is a lanthanide because the inner electron shells of its atomic structure are not filled. In its ionized form (Gd^{3+}), gadolinium donates electrons from other subshells, leaving the seven 4f electrons unpaired, and this property ensures paramagnetic behavior after chelation.

Properties of Gadolinium MRI Contrast

Gadolinium contrast agents have a number of key properties that influence their behavior, efficiency, and adverse reaction risk profile. There is an interplay among these properties that optimizes the degree of enhancement and the tolerability of gadolinium contrast agents (Table 11-1):

- Chemical structure
- Osmolality
- Viscosity
- Ionicity, not to be confused with demetallation (dechelation)
- Relaxivity
- Half clearance rate
- Dose

Gadolinium is tightly *chelated* into a complex chemical structure that can be linear or macrocyclic (Fig. 11-1). *Macrocyclic* chemical structures employ dodecane tetraacetic acid (DOTA) chelation. The chemical structure prevents heavy metal toxicity because the tight chelation prevents cellular uptake of the toxic-free gadolinium ion. Collectively, the chemical structure and chelation of gadolinium enhance renal elimination and maintain distribution in the extravascular space. Regardless of chemical structure, the pharmacodynamics and pharmacokinetics are the same. The standard gadolinium contrast dose is 0.1 mmol/kg. This dosage primarily influences the T1 relaxation time, but higher doses may increase effect of T2 relaxation.

Relaxivity measures the degree to which a given amount of contrast agent shortens T1 or T2, so higher relaxivity equates to better enhancement. Relaxivity refers to the contrast agent's change in relaxation rates with changes in concentration. Largely, the early generation gadolinium contrast agents shared the same T1 relaxivity, while later-generation contrast agents have up to 50% higher T1 relaxivity at 1.5T.

As with iodinated contrast agents, osmolality contributes to the incidence of non-anaphylactoid adverse reactions mediated by endothelial damage, movement of fluid among compartments, and cell deformation. Adverse effects attributable to osmolality include pain, flushing, nausea, and vomiting. Contrast osmolality higher than blood results in movement of water from interstitial spaces into the vascular compartment, which causes increased blood viscosity, endothelial damage, hypervolemia, vasodilation, edema with neurotoxicity, decreased myocardial contractility, and toxicity. Gadolinium contrast is administered in much lower doses than iodinated contrast in CT, and as such, the alteration to plasma osmolality is very low, reducing impact of adverse reactions by comparison. Nonetheless, when large gadolinium contrast doses are to be administered, low osmolality agents should be employed.

The viscosity of gadolinium contrast agents is the flow friction, resistance or thickness of the contrast media. Gadolinium contrast is generally of similar viscosity to blood at body temperature (37°C). Viscosity plays an important role in renal tolerance, with near serum viscosity reducing the risk of contrast-induced nephrotoxicity associated with iodinated contrast media. Viscosity of gadolinium contrast agents is not considered a significant concern for adverse reactions.

TABLE 11-1 Comparison of Key Properties of the Main Gadolinium Contrast Agents*

Contrast Agent	Structure	Ionicity	Clearance $T_{0.5}$ (h)	Osmolality (mOsm/kg Water)	Viscosity at 37°C (cps)	T1 Relaxivity (L/mmol-s)
Gadopentetate dimeglumine (Magnevist, Gd-DTPA)	Linear	Ionic	1.6	1,960	2.9	4.1
Gadoteridol (ProHance, Gd-HP-DO3A)	Macrocyclic	Nonionic	1.57	630	1.3	4.1
Gadodiamide (Omniscan, Gd-DTPA-BMA)	Linear	Nonionic	1.3	789	1.4	4.3
Gadoversetamide (OptiMARK, Gd-DTPA-BMEA)	Linear	Nonionic	1.73	1,110	2.0	5.2
Gadobenate dimeglumine (MultiHance, Gd-BOPTA)	Linear	Ionic	1.2–2	1,970	5.3	6.3
Gadoterate (Dotarem, Gd-DOTA)	Macrocyclic	Ionic	1.6	1,350	2.4	3.6
Gadobutrol (Gadavist, Gd-BT-DO3A)	Macrocyclic	Nonionic	1.81	1,603	5.0	5.2
Gadoxetate (Eovist or Primovist, Gd-EOB-DTPA)	Linear	Ionic	0.93	688	1.2	6.9
Gadofosveset (Ablavar)	Linear	Ionic		1,110	3.0	19
Blood				290	1.5–2	

*With the exception of Primovist, the dosage is 0.1 mmol/kg. Primovist dosage is 0.025 mmol/kg.

Ionic gadolinium CT contrast agents dissociate into ion pairs, while nonionic agents do not. Ionic contrast may increase the risk of some adverse reactions, such as cardiac arrhythmia. A combination of ionic and high-osmolar gadolinium contrast increases the adverse cardiovascular effects, and the hemodynamic changes present a risk to patients with coronary artery disease. Like the effects of osmolality, the low dose of gadolinium contrast compared to iodinated CT contrast, even with ionic MRI contrast, the ionic charge of the gadolinium complex is not considered significant in terms of safety and risk of adverse reactions.

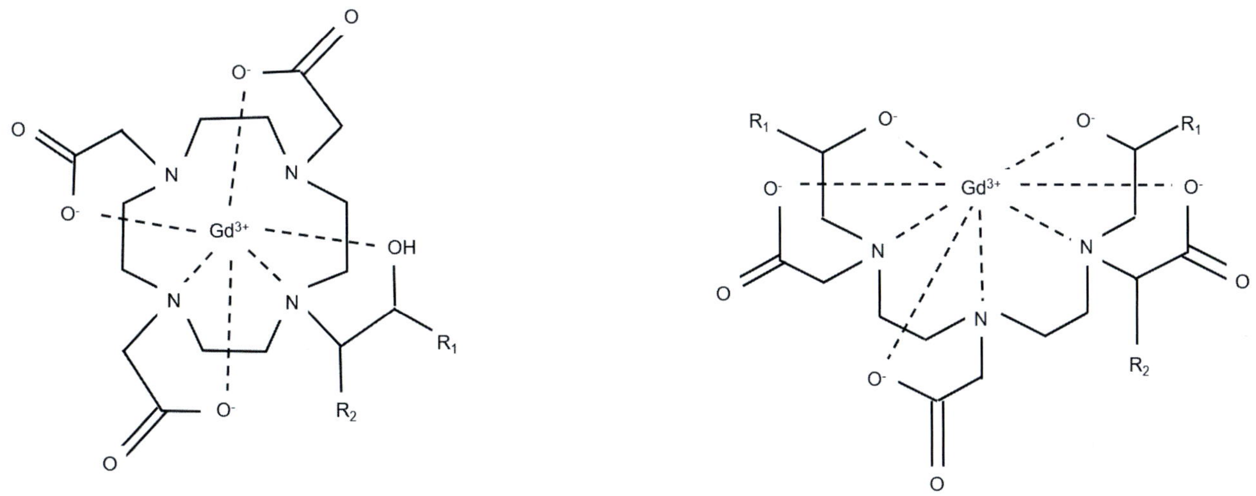

FIGURE 11-1 The chemical structure of gadolinium contrast agents adopts either a macrocyclic base (left) or a linear base (right) with the major differences between each agent being changes to the R groups.

Mechanism of Action

As with iodinated CT contrast, MRI contrast agents provide image contrast without altering biological function. Unlike iodinated contrast agents in CT, MRI contrast agents are detected not directly but indirectly by influencing the nuclear magnetic relaxation time of water. While gadolinium shortens the relaxation time constants for T1, T2, and T2* in adjacent protons (water) in tissues, it is the shortening of T1 that is the target of MRI imaging. As a result, rapid acquisition of T1-weighted MRI images will have an increased signal from contrast-enhanced tissues. MRI physics is too complex to describe in the context of this chapter, but some assumed knowledge is necessary to understand the mechanism of action. Nonetheless, Figure 11-2 provides a schematic representation of T1 and T2 contrast enhancement. Specifically, gadolinium causes T1 shortening through dipole-dipole interactions with protons.

Pharmacokinetics

Gadolinium is a heavy metal toxin when free in vivo as an ion, yet the risk of adverse reaction is low and the majority of adverse reactions are mild. This is primarily the result of the chemical stability associated with gadolinium chelation (much the same way ^{68}Ga, ^{99m}Tc, and other radiometals are chelated in radiopharmaceuticals). These chelates also overcome the potential consequences of the long biological half-life of free gadolinium. Consequently, gadolinium contrast agents are almost exclusively eliminated unchanged (no metabolism) via the kidneys with a half clearance time in normal renal function of 1.5 to 2 hours. Renal clearance occurs without secretion or reabsorption. Gadolinium contrast demonstrates 85% elimination by 4 hours after intravenous administration, 98% elimination by 24 hours, and 100% by 48 hours after administration, but renal dysfunction prolongs retention.

Extracellular gadolinium chelates have pharmacokinetic properties similar to iodinated CT contrast media. After intravenous administration, gadolinium contrast agents are rapidly cleared from intravascular space to extravascular space with a distribution equivalent to extracellular water. They show no plasma protein binding, and they do not cross intact blood-brain barrier. Like iodinated contrast, gadolinium clearance is biphasic, with initial distribution with a 4-minute half-life followed by the aforementioned 1.5- to 2-hour elimination half-life. Gadolinium contrast is best illustrated with a two-compartment model, as illustrated for iodinated contrast (Fig. 11-3). Gadolinium contrast can enter and wash out of normal tissues and diseased tissues at different rates, which will change T1 and T2 relaxation times between those tissues.

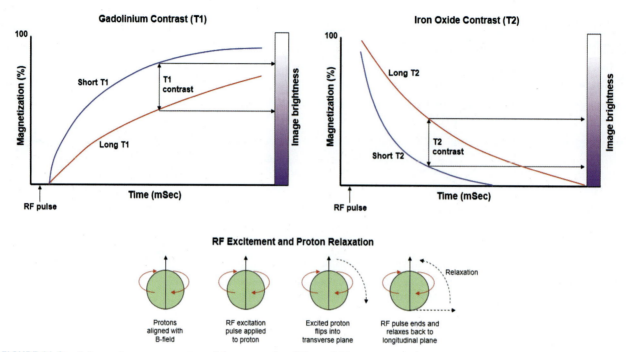

FIGURE 11-2 Schematic representation of the principle of T1 and T2 contrast enhancement in MRI. As represented at the bottom of the figure, hydrogen (protons) initially aligns with the magnetic field. A radiofrequency (RF) excitation pulse is applied to the proton, which flips into the transverse plane. The RF pulse ends, allowing the proton to relax back to the longitudinal plane. The T1 plot (top left) shows the effect of shortening the relaxation time with gadolinium contrast and resultant positive enhancement of the contrast. Likewise, the T2 plot (top right) shows the effect of shortening relaxation time with iron oxide contrast and resultant negative enhancement of the contrast.

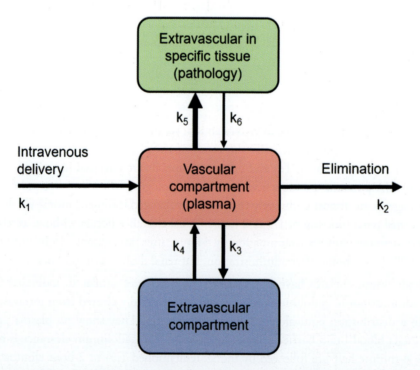

FIGURE 11-3 Modified two-compartment model for iodinated CT contrast or gadolinium MRI contrast administered intravenously. The second extravascular compartment represents pathological tissue that may enhance with contrast administration and therefore be differentiated by surrounding normal tissue by a greater rate constant (k_5 over k_3 or k_4 over k_6).

Contraindications and Precautions

Gadolinium contrast agents cross the placenta and undergo fetal excretion via the kidneys. The excreted contrast remains in the amniotic fluid for a protracted period of time, where it could undergo demetallation (dechelation) into free gadolinium and expose the fetus's lungs and gut. Consequently, gadolinium contrast is contraindicated during pregnancy, especially the first trimester. If gadolinium contrast is to be used during pregnancy, macrocyclic varieties should be employed. While gadolinium contrast agents are also excreted in breast milk, the dose to the infant is a fraction of that of the mother and is excreted after oral absorption in feces. There is no need for cessation of breast-feeding, although a cautious approach would include expressing and discarding for 6 hours after intravenous gadolinium contrast.

While gadolinium contrast agents are considered safe and biologically inert, they are more nephrotoxic than iodinated contrast agents in the equivalent dosage. High doses in impaired renal function is contraindicated. Acute renal failure occurs in 3.5% of cases of abnormal creatinine levels. Gadolinium contrast is contraindicated in patients with a glomerular filtration rate (GFR) below 30 mL/min/1.73m^2 or where renal function is acutely deteriorating. Previous anaphylactoid and hypersensitivity reactions to gadolinium contrast should be treated with caution. Preexisting nephrogenic systemic fibrosis (NSF) is also a contraindication. Caution should be exercised in gadolinium contrast use in patients with moderate renal dysfunction, epilepsy, hypotension, a history of hypersensitivity, asthma, or allergic respiratory disorders. Caution should be exercised in patients with severe cardiovascular disease or drug-induced arrhythmia.

Adverse Reactions

Adverse effects to gadolinium contrast agents are very uncommon, with an incidence generally reported in the range 1.5% to 2.4%. Most adverse reactions are considered mild and more commonly include mucosal reactions, urticaria, vomiting, change in taste, local warmth, local pain, headache, paresthesia, and dizziness (Fig. 11-4). Vasodilation and injection site discomfort are also possible. The risk of an adverse reaction increases in patients with asthma, allergies, and a history of contrast reaction to gadolinium or iodine.

In a study of 17,767 patients undergoing cardiac MRI with gadolinium contrast, only 0.17% of patients experienced adverse reactions, and 100% of those were mild in nature. Furthermore, the adverse reaction rate between different agents varied between 0.06% and 0.47%. In another study involving 194,400 ionic, linear gadolinium contrast injections, there was a 0.1% incidence of adverse reactions of which 83.8% were classified as mild, 13.7% as moderate, and 2.4% as severe (5 cases).

Acute hypersensitivity reactions occur within 1 hour of contrast administration and in 0.1% of patients, and they include mild pruritus (itching) and urticaria (hives). It should be noted that a prior gadolinium contrast agent hypersensitivity reaction is associated with 30% risk of reaction to subsequent gadolinium administrations and with greater severity. Patients can experience moderate hypersensitivity reactions, including bronchospasm, laryngeal edema, facial edema, tachycardia, angioedema, hypotension, arrhythmia, and widespread urticaria. Severe anaphylactoid reaction has an incidence of 0.005%, and fatal reaction, 0.0003%. An increased risk of a hypersensitivity reaction to gadolinium contrast is associated with females, those with allergies or asthma, and those having prior gadolinium contrast administrations.

The adverse reaction profile of gadolinium contrast agents is uniform across the range of agents. This may seem a little surprising given the variability in ionicity, viscosity, and osmolality known to be major contributors to adverse reactions in iodinated contrast media. This is likely to reflect actual differences that cannot be distinguished statistically. For example, there is a 10-fold difference in the incidence of urticaria across a range of gadolinium contrast media from 0.2% to 2%, but data does not permit a statistically significant difference to be reported. Likewise, the incidence of nausea ranges from 1.2% to 3.2% across the range of contrast agents. Faster injection rates (e.g., MRI angiography) have been reported to demonstrate higher incidence of nausea. Acute reactions occur even with antihistamine or corticosteroid premedication.

144 Pharmacology Primer for Medications

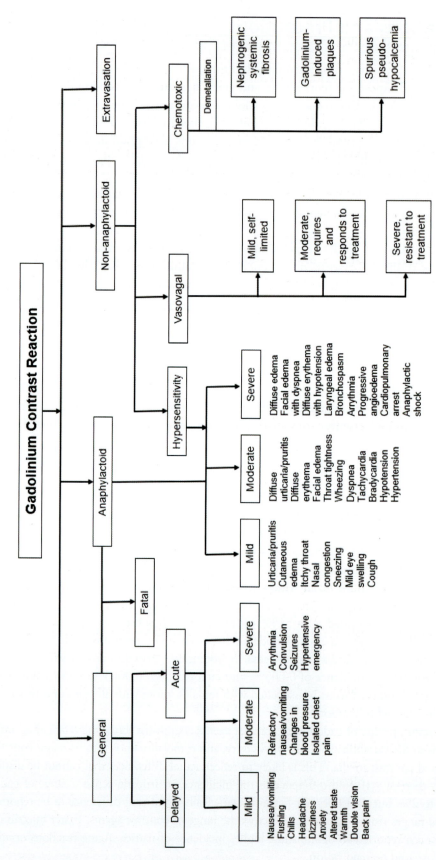

FIGURE 11-4 Flow chart of gadolinium contrast reaction classification.

Gadolinium MRI contrast is not generally considered nephrotoxic, and this relates to the low viscosity and comparative low dose. Contrast-induced nephrotoxicity for iodinated contrast agents (Fig. 10-5) is driven by viscosity and osmolality. Gadolinium contrast has near serum viscosity and sufficiently low doses that blood and tissues remain isotonic after contrast. Gadolinium contrast does, however, have higher nephrotoxicity than iodinated CT contrast for equivalent dosage.

Free gadolinium (Gd^{3+}) is highly toxic, and this relates, in part, to cellular inhibition of calcium (Ca^{2+}) at calcium channels. As outlined in Chapters 3 and 8, alteration to influx of calcium interferes with muscle contraction (e.g., cardiac force of contraction), vascular smooth muscle vasoconstriction, and bronchial smooth muscle bronchoconstriction. Free gadolinium can also depress the reticuloendothelial system, including inhibition of phagocytosis. The LD_{50} for nonchelated gadolinium is 0.35 mmol/kg while DOTA chelation increases LD_{50} to 10.6 mmol/kg.

Nephrogenic Systemic Fibrosis

Gadolinium has an excellent safety record, but patients are at risk of developing NSF. Unfortunately, NSF is irreversible with no treatment and is associated with progressive movement, swallowing, and breathing difficulties. NSF patients may develop subcutaneous edema, causing hard, erythematous plaques of skin with or without hyperpigmentation, papules, blistering, and ulceration. Patients present with symptoms of pain, severe pruritus, paresthesia, flexion contractures, and unstable hypertension. The incidence of NSF is very low and has decreased substantially since awareness to the risk was uncovered. An evaluation of more than 185 million gadolinium contrast injections revealed less than 1,000 cases of NSF (0.0005%). This rate varied among contrast agents from a 1 in 2 million risk to a 1 in 50,000 risk. Linear nonionic chelates are considered the highest risk, while macrocyclic chelates are considered low risk, and linear ionic chelates are considered the middle ground of risk. Macrocyclic gadolinium contrast exhibits less demetallation, and ionic gadolinium contrast also tends to be more tightly bound.

A history of renal dysfunction or significant infirmity increases the risk of developing NSF. Gadolinium contrast is contraindicated in patients at high risk of NSF. High-risk patients meet one or more of the following criteria:

- Kidney or liver transplant with GFR less than 60 mL/min/1.73 m^2
- GFR less than 30 mL/min/1.73 m^2
- Acute renal failure
- One or more of the following comorbid conditions: major infection, vascular ischemia of extremities, vascular thrombosis, major surgery, major vascular procedure, or multiorgan system failure

Given the long biological half-life of free gadolinium and the very long retention of lanthanides in bone, it is important to consider the life-long burden of gadolinium, especially in those who have multiple contrast studies over their life span.

Most, if not all, NSF cases after gadolinium contrast have significant renal dysfunction prior to administration. The worse the renal function at the time of administration, the higher the risk of NSF. The greater the total contrast dose, the greater the risk and severity of NSF. The vast majority of patients who received gadolinium contrast, despite having significant renal dysfunction, do not get NSF.

NSF usually develops clinically within days to months following gadolinium exposure, although rare cases have been reported years later. Renal dysfunction causes a prolonged elimination half-life, and the retention of gadolinium increases the predisposition of the Gd^{3+} to be displaced in the chelate by other metal cations, such as iron (Fe^{3+}), copper (Cu^{2+}), zinc (Zn^{2+}), or Ca^{2+}, in a process called *transmetallation*. At the same time, a number of anions, including phosphate, carbonate, hydroxide, and citrate, can compete for the Gd^{3+} ligand. Gd^{3+} can then be deposited in skin and soft tissue to precipitate NSF. Procedural changes, improved contrast agents, and prescreening high-risk patients have virtually eliminated this iatrogenic condition. In the absence of severe renal dysfunction, free gadolinium can manifest as gadolinium-induced plaques in the extremities. Transmetallation of the cation and exchange of the anion may cause spurious pseudo-hypocalcemia.

Management of Adverse Reactions

Given the absence of treatment for NSF, the remainder of the adverse reactions can and should be managed in the same way outlined in Chapter 10 for iodinated contrast based on the type of adverse reaction and symptoms (Fig. 11-4). While the pharmacology associated with drugs in the crash cart/emergency trolley are detailed in Chapter 12, here we briefly examine key medications that may be employed in the event of a serious or anaphylactoid reaction to MRI (and CT) contrast agents. It should be noted that a crash cart/emergency trolley should be immediately available at all times in or immediately adjacent to the MRI/CT room where intravenous contrast is being used. One should also keep in mind that serious adverse effects may occur in the short period after the patient leaves the scanning room. For details, refer to Chapter 10:

- Salbutamol (albuterol) functions as a beta-2 (β_2) receptor agonist to cause bronchodilation and relieve bronchospasm. The standard dose is 1 to 2 inhalations of 100 mcg each, with a third inhalation if necessary 1 minute after the second.

- Atropine is a parasympatholytic agent that can be used to treat bradycardia in a vasovagal reaction. The standard dose is 0.6 to 1.0 mg intravenously, repeated every 3 to 5 minutes as needed, to a maximum of 3 mg.

- Diphenhydramine (Benadryl) is a histamine-1 (H_1) inhibitor to be used for mild urticaria or prophylaxis, with doses of 25 to 50 mg orally or intramuscularly or 25 mg intravenously being standard.

- Epinephrine (adrenaline) is a sympathetic agonist with alpha (α)- and beta (β)-receptor activity. Doses of epinephrine are typically 0.1 to 0.3 mg (1 mg/mL or 1:1,000) subcutaneously, 0.3 mg intramuscularly via EpiPen if the patient is not hypotensive, or 0.1 mg (0.1 mg/mL or 1:10,000) intravenously over 3 to 5 minutes, repeated as needed up to a maximum of 1 mg if the patient is hypotensive.

- Diazepam is a benzodiazepine that can be used to treat seizures, if necessary, using an intravenous dose of 5 to 10 mg to a maximum of 30 mg as required.

- Lorazepam is an alternative benzodiazepine for seizures, especially in pediatric patients, with a dose of 0.01 mg/kg intravenously.

- Nitroglycerin is a vasodilator given as any one of the following: one 300 to 600 mcg sublingual tablet under the tongue, one or two sprays of 400 mcg each directed onto or under the tongue, or 2 to 3 mg buccal tablet placed between the upper lip and gum.

- In the case of generalized anaphylaxis-like symptoms, epinephrine should be used.

- Nausea and vomiting are self-limiting, and patients need to be observed for 30 minutes with intravenous access kept open.

Extravasation

Fast mechanical injectors with large volumes for MRI contrast agents increase the risk of full- or partial-dose extravasation. Given the hypertonic nature of gadolinium contrast media, the effects and treatment are the same as those outlined in the previous chapter for iodinated CT contrast. The prevention strategies and risk factors are also similar.

Extravasation of gadolinium contrast agents involves delivery of the contrast extravascularly due to human error, cannula dislodgement, or leakage. Extravasation of contrast agents typically causes self-limiting symptoms such as pain, erythema, and swelling. In severe reactions, skin ulceration and necrosis or compartment syndrome may occur. The peak reactions occur at 24 to 48 hours after intravenous contrast administration.

As detailed in Chapter 10 for CT contrast, key strategies to minimize the risk of extravasation include but are not limited to the following:

- Ensure reliable intravenous access.
- Decrease/limit flow rates.
- Monitor the infusion site.
- Communicate with the patient.
- Immediately stop the infusion if there is concern regarding extravasation.

If extravasation of contrast agents does occur, management will depend on the patient's symptoms and volume of extravasation, as outlined in Chapter 10.

Interactions

Specific interactions between gadolinium contrast agents and medications have not been widely evaluated or reported. The common properties of gadolinium contrast and iodinated contrast (iconicity, osmolality) present a similar interaction profile, although the lower doses of gadolinium truncate interaction risk. Like iodinated contrast agents, gadolinium contrast agents are not highly active pharmacologically. Prevention relies on a thorough patient history, an awareness of drugs needing precautions, and administering contrast through a separate line, not the same line as medications. Ionic gadolinium contrast agents have anticoagulant properties, and both ionic and nonionic can prolong coagulation time, which can potentiate the effects of anticoagulants (e.g., heparin and warfarin), antiplatelet (e.g., aspirin and NSAIDs), and fibrinolytic medications (e.g., urokinase).

Gadolinium contrast agents are not considered to present a high risk of nephrotoxicity, so they do not substantially increase the bioavailability of renally eliminated medications. However, nephrotoxic medications such as NSAIDs and gentamicin can compound renal dysfunction to increase the risk of NSF. Adverse reactions to gadolinium contrast agents are more likely if the patient is taking immunomodulator medications. Allergic reactions or symptoms of a similar nature are more likely in patients taking β-blockers, interleukins, and interferons. Synergistic effects between gadolinium contrast media and calcium channel blockers and digoxin are possible. Higher-osmolality gadolinium contrast agents used for cerebral angiography lower the seizure threshold of antipsychotics, thioxanthenes, antidepressants, and analeptics.

From a nuclear medicine perspective, gadolinium contrast agents in the 72 hours prior to ^{67}Ga-citrate administration is known to alter biodistribution, evident in more defined skeletal accumulation of the ^{67}Ga. Gallium is an iron analog and can readily undergo transmetallation with gadolinium and exchange between citrate and the chelate can also occur.

Summary

MRI contrast offers unique interventions that demand an expanded skill set and understanding of basic and applied pharmacology. An insight into the complexities of gadolinium contrast enhances practice and patient safety. Specifically, command of adverse reactions is a key skill required for capability in MRI and ensures that medical radiation technologists meet the minimum capabilities for their scope of practice.

References

Abraham JL, Thakral C. Tissue distribution and kinetics of gadolinium and nephrogenic systemic fibrosis. *Euro J Radiol.* 2008;66:200–207.

Aran S, Shaqdan KW, Abujudeh HH. Adverse allergic reactions to linear ionic gadolinium-based contrast agents: experience with 194,400 injections. *Clin Radiol.* 2015;70:466–475.

Ayre-Smith G. Tissue necrosis following extravasation of contrast material. *J Can Assoc Radiol.* 1982;33:104.

Behzadi AH, Zhao Y, Farooq Z, Prince MR. Immediate allergic reactions to gadolinium-based contrast agents: a systemic review and meta-analysis. *Radiology.* 2018;286:471–482.

Bellen MF, van der Molen. Extracellular gadolinium-based contrast media: an overview. *Euro J Radiol.* 2008;66:160–167.

Bourin M, Jolliet P, Ballereau F. An overview of the clinical pharmacokinetics of x-ray contrast media. *Clin Pharmacokinet.* 1997;32:180–193.

Bruder O, Schneider S, Nothnagel D, et al. Acute adverse reactions to gadolinium-based contrast agents in CMR. *JACC Cardiovasc. Imaging.* 2011;4:1171–1176.

Bryant B, Knights K, Salerno E. *Pharmacology for Health Professionals.* 2nd ed. Sydney, Australia: Mosby Elsevier; 2007.

Cohan RH, Ellis JH, Garner WL. Extravasation of radiographic contrast material: recognition, prevention, and treatment. *Radiology.* 1996;200:593–604.

Costa N. Understanding contrast media. *J Infusion Nursing.* 2004;27:302–312.

Greenen RWF, Kingma HJ, van der Molen AJ. Contrast-induced nephropathy: pharmacology, pathophysiology and prevention. *Insights Imaging.* 2013;4:811–820.

Jacobs JE, Birnbaum BA, Langlotz CP. Contrast media reactions and extravasation: relationship to intravenous injection rates. *Radiology.* 1998; 209:411–416.

Jung JW, Kang HR, Kim MH, et al. Immediate hypersensitivity reaction to gadolinium-based MR contrast media. *Radiology.* 2012;264:414–422.

Kanal E. Gadolinium based contrast agents (GBCA): safety overview after 3 decades of clinical experience. *Magn Reson Imaging.* 2016;34:1341–1345.

Khawaja AZ, Cassidy DB, Shakarchi JA, McGrogan DG, Inston NG, Jones RG. Revisiting the risks of MRI with gadolinium based contrast agents—review of literature and guidelines. *Insights Imaging.* 2015;6:553–558.

Lin SP, Brown JJ. MR contrast agents: physical and pharmacologic basics. *J MRI.* 2007;25:884–899.

Morcos SK, Thomsen HS, Exley CM. Contrast media: interactions with other drugs and clinical tests. *Eur Radiol.* 2005;15:1463–1468.

Morzycki A, Bhatia A, Murphy KJ. Adverse reactions to contrast material: a Canadian update. *Can Assoc Radiol.* 2017;68:187–193.

Rang H, Dale M, Ritter J, Flower R. *Rang and Dale's Pharmacology.* 6th ed. London, England: Churchill Livingston; 2008.

Sweetman SC (Ed.). *Martindale: The Complete Drug Reference.* 26th ed. Chicago, IL: Pharmaceutical Press; 2009.

Terreno E, Aime S. MRI contrast agents in pharmacological research. *Front Pharmacol.* 2015;6:290.

CHAPTER 12

The Crash Cart/Emergency Trolley

Chapter Objectives

Specific learning outcomes (page ix) of this text addressed in this chapter:

- Apply the principles of pharmacology to the safe and effective use of medicines.
- Recognize general, patient-specific, and scenario-specific risks, precautions, and contraindications for use of medicines.
- Apply the pharmacokinetic and pharmacodynamic principles of medications to identify and explain normal and adverse reactions to medications.
- Administer medications safely, effectively, and appropriately according to procedures and within regulatory and statutory parameters.
- Monitor patients for, identify, and manage adverse reactions.

After reading, digesting, reflecting on, and reviewing the content of this chapter, readers should be able to

1. Demonstrate command of key pharmacology terms.
2. Demonstrate enhanced understanding of the principles associated with the pharmacology of drugs in the crash cart/emergency trolley.
3. Demonstrate critical thinking to effect problem solving related to drugs in the crash cart/emergency trolley.
4. Demonstrate understanding of the mode of action, pharmacokinetics, risks, precautions, contraindications, adverse effects, interactions, and appropriate dosage of key drugs in the crash cart/emergency trolley.
5. Apply knowledge of the general principles and concepts in a translational manner to clinical practice.

Key Terms

adrenergic	anaphylactoid	anxiolytic	diuretic	tolerance
adverse reaction	antiarrhythmia	bronchodilator	drug interaction	vasovagal
analgesic	anticholinergic	beta-agonist	inotropic	vasodilator
anaphylaxis	antihistamine	beta-blocker	stimulant	vasoconstrictor
anaphylactic	antihypertensive	dependence		

Introduction

The crash cart, or emergency trolley, is an essential resource in a medical imaging department. The location of the crash cart may depend on department activities. If contrast computed tomography (CT) is undertaken, the crash cart is generally located in or immediately outside the CT room. Departments performing cardiac stress testing require that a crash cart be immediately accessible. Large departments of radiology and nuclear medicine modalities may have more than one crash cart to accommodate these diverse needs. Furthermore, magnetic resonance imaging (MRI)–compatible crash carts are available for dedicated use inside the magnetic field. The specific size and contents of a crash cart vary among hospitals, hospital departments, and outpatient clinics and are based on the cross section of patients serviced. An adult crash cart is set up differently than a pediatric crash cart. A medical imaging department crash cart differs from that of the emergency or the intensive care department. The crash cart is comprised of a variety of equipment, and all medical radiation scientists are encouraged to familiarize themselves with both the location and use of the contents of the crash cart. In this chapter, the medications stored in the crash cart, generally in drawers 1 and 2, are detailed. While beyond the scope of this chapter, it is critical that medical radiation scientists familiarize themselves with medications, locations, and dosages for the crash cart used in their facility to avoid confusion, delays, or error during an emergency (Fig. 12-1).

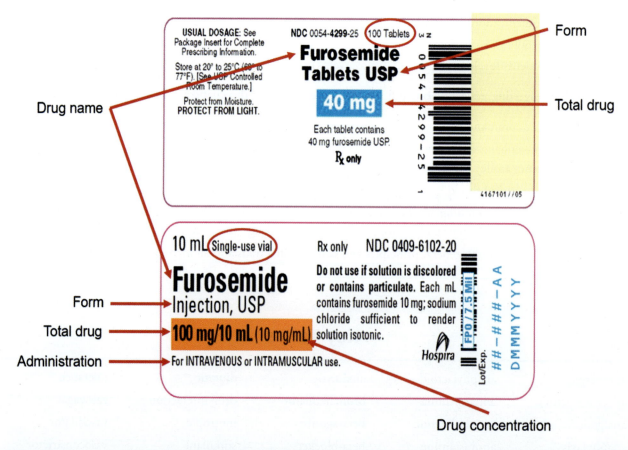

FIGURE 12-1 It is crucial to be able to identify the medication in an emergency quickly and accurately. Specific labeling varies across manufacturers, countries, and institutions, so it is critical to be familiar with the specific crash cart and contents in use. For each medication, it is critical to be able to quickly and accurately identify the drug, form, dose, concentration, and expiry date on the label. This can be difficult on a small vial, but the boxing label should be used only as a guide. The contents must be rigorously confirmed as the correct medication and form.

Medications

Crash cart medications need to be readily accessible during an emergency. Consequently, they need to be organized, in a form that is easy to measure, and able to be dispensed quickly. The specific contents of the crash cart depend on the type of emergencies likely to be confronted. When we consider medications and their pharmacology, consideration needs to be given to the specific circumstances of the emergency and what medications will address specific patient conditions. For the purposes of the medical imaging department, we can generally consider the likely emergencies to be classified into one or more of the following:

- *Anaphylaxis* (e.g., contrast media), *anaphylactoid* (e.g., monoclonal antibodies), allergic responses (e.g., radiopharmaceuticals or contact allergy), and, while not an allergy, *vasovagal* responses to injections.
- Cardiovascular emergencies, including arrest, shock, angina, arrhythmia, pulmonary edema, and hypertensive states. These may occur organically in any patient in response to their therapy or as a direct result of the procedure performed in the imaging department (e.g., stress test).
- Respiratory emergencies may be associated with preexisting conditions (e.g., asthma, chronic obstructive airways disease), allergic response (e.g., contrast), adverse reactions to imaging medications (e.g., dipyridamole), or pathology (e.g., pulmonary embolism).
- Neurological emergencies are less likely but include seizures and potentially severe anxiety. These may be preexisting or exacerbated by the imaging procedure (e.g., claustrophobia or trypanophobia).
- Endocrine emergencies may include thyroid storm and hypoglycemia (e.g., fasting patients).
- It is possible that patients present with fluid or electrolyte emergencies, especially in patients with massive blood loss (e.g., gastrointestinal tract bleed leading to hypovolemic shock) or those presenting dehydrated due to fluid fasting or heat conditions.
- Trauma associated with falls or incidents within the imaging department or preexisting injuries exacerbated by the procedure or positioning during imaging.
- Poisoning and overdose are unlikely to require an emergency response in the imaging department.

Consideration of likely emergencies provides an insight into the classes of medications required to manage emergencies in the radiology or nuclear medicine department:

- Anticholinergic
- Antiarrhythmic
- Antihistamine
- Antihypertensive
- Vasodilator
- Vasoconstrictor
- Beta-blocker
- Beta-agonist
- Calcium channel blocker
- Inotropic agents
- Adrenergic stimulant
- Diuretic
- Bronchodilator
- Analgesic
- Anxiolytic

It should be kept in mind that for acute emergency management of a condition or symptom, both the medication and the dosage may vary substantially from medications and dosages used in an ongoing fashion. For example, angiotensin-converting enzyme (ACE) inhibitors lack the immediate effect required for emergency management of hypertensive states, and intravenous lidocaine is not a suitable antiarrhythmic for ongoing patient management.

Medication Use in an Emergency

As discussed, the specific contents of a crash cart vary depending on the patients and circumstances likely to be served. In the nuclear medicine and radiology departments, the range of emergency situations is quite different from those in an emergency department, trauma unit, intensive care unit, and so on. In nuclear medicine, cardiac emergencies associated with stress testing are the most likely to be encountered, and anaphylaxis is most commonly seen in the radiology department. That does not preclude other emergencies or the need to be prepared for them. The essential medications in an imaging department crash cart are summarized in Table 12-1.

TABLE 12-1 Principal Medications for an Imaging Department Crash Cart, Their Indications, Dose, and Precautions Required*

Medication	Indication	Dose (Pediatric Dose)	Frequency (Pediatric Dose)	Precautions/Contraindications (Other than Allergy)
Adenosine (6 mg/2 mL)	SVT	3 mg rapid IV (0.1 mg/kg rapid IV to maximum of 6 mg)	2nd dose of 6 mg if required after 1–2 min and 3rd dose of 12 mg (0.2 mg/kg up to 12 mg if required)	Caution: hypotension, unstable angina Avoid: AV block, severe bronchospasm
Amiodarone (150 mg/3 mL)	VF, VT (with or without a pulse), and supraventricular tachycardia	150–300 mg IV over 1–3 min (4 mg/kg)	May use 2nd dose of 150 mg for recurrent VF or VT (5 mg/kg doses to a total of 15 mg/kg)	Caution: heart failure, liver dysfunction, thyroid dysfunction Avoid: bradycardia, 2nd or 3rd degree heart block
Atenolol (50 mg tablet)	SVT and myocardial infarction	25–100 mg orally		Caution: asthma, airways disease, metabolic acidosis, cardiogenic shock, hypotension, severe peripheral vascular disease, sinus bradycardia, AV block Avoid: severe bronchospasm, severe bradycardia, overt LV failure
Atropine (0.6 mg/1 mL or 1.2 mg/1 mL)	Bradycardia and asystole	1 mg IV (20 μg/kg IV)	Repeat every 3–5 min until target heart rate is achieved or to a maximum dose of 3 mg (1 mg maximum)	Nil in cardiac arrest or hypotensive bradycardia but can worsen ischemia

TABLE 12-1 Principal Medications for an Imaging Department Crash Cart, Their Indications, Dose, and Precautions Required*

Medication	Indication	Dose (Pediatric Dose)	Frequency (Pediatric Dose)	Precautions/Contraindications (Other than Allergy)
Promethazine (Phenergan) (50 mg/2 mL)	Allergic reaction	25–50 mg IM at 25 mg/min (0.125 mg/kg IM)	Single dose	Caution: epilepsy, respiratory depression, closed-angle glaucoma Avoid: elderly or reduce dose
Diazepam (10 mg/2 mL)	Severe anxiety Seizures	5–10 mg IV over 1–2 min (0.2–0.3 mg/kg to maximum of 10 mg) 10 mg by slow IV or 10–20 mg rectally	Repeat every 5–10 min to maximum of 30 mg as necessary (repeat once in pediatrics) Repeat once if necessary	Caution: dependence, glaucoma, liver or kidney dysfunction, depression, pregnancy, lactation Avoid: cardiorespiratory failure, CNS depression
Verapamil (5 mg/2 mL)	SVT	5 mg over 2–3 min (0.1–0.3 mg/kg to maximum of 5 mg)	Repeat after 5–10 min	Caution: heart failure, severe LV dysfunction Avoid: severe bradycardia, sick sinus syndrome, 2nd and 3rd degree block, hypotension
Dobutamine (250 mg/20 mL)	Hypotension	2–20 µg/kg/min IV	Titrate to effect	Caution: β-blocker use, myocardial infarction, cardiogenic shock Avoid: uncontrolled hypertension, unstable angina, atrial fibrillation, ventricular arrhythmia, pheochromocytoma
Dopamine (200 mg/5 mL)	Hypotension and shock	5–20 µg/kg/min IV to maximum of 60 µg/kg/min	Low doses are predominantly beta, higher Doses become predominantly alpha	Caution: pulmonary hypertension, vascular disease Avoid: pheochromocytoma, tachycardia
Epinephrine (adrenaline) (1 mg/1 mL or 1:1,000) (1 mg/10 mL or 1:10,000)	Any pulseless arrhythmias Anaphylaxis	0.5–1 mg slow IV (0.01 mg/kg IV) 50 µg slow IV (1 µg/kg IV)	Repeat every 3–5 min if required Repeat using IV infusion if required	Caution: tachyarrhythmia, pulmonary hypertension Avoid: nil in cardiac arrest and anaphylaxis

(continued)

154 Pharmacology Primer for Medications

TABLE 12-1 Principal Medications for an Imaging Department Crash Cart, Their Indications, Dose, and Precautions Required*

Medication	Indication	Dose (Pediatric Dose)	Frequency (Pediatric Dose)	Precautions/Contraindications (Other than Allergy)
EpiPen (300 µg/0.3 mL) EpiPen Junior (150 µg/0.3 mL)	Anaphylaxis	0.3 mg IM >20 kg (0.15 mg IM 10–20 kg)	Repeat every 3–5 minutes if no response	Caution: not to be administered into buttock, digits, hands, feet, or by IV Avoid: there are no absolute contraindications to the use of EpiPen in a life-threatening allergic situation
Frusemide (20 mg/2 mL)	LV failure, acute pulmonary edema, and hypertension	20–40 mg IV or IM (0.5–1 mg/kg)		Caution: kidney or liver disease, diabetes, gout, SLE, pregnancy, and after urologic procedures Avoid: sulfonamide allergy, anuria, sodium or fluid depletion
Lidocaine (lignocaine) (100 mg/5 mL)	VF, pulseless VT, and SVT	1 mg/kg IV over 1–2 min	Repeat after 5 min if required	Caution: bradycardia, heart failure, severe renal impairment, severe hepatic dysfunction Avoid: 2nd or 3rd degree block
Metoprolol (5 mg/5 mL)	SVT and myocardial infarction	5 mg IV over 3 min	Repeat every 5 min as required to a maximum dose of 20 mg	Caution: asthma, airways disease, metabolic acidosis, cardiogenic shock, hypotension, severe peripheral vascular disease, sinus bradycardia, AV block Avoid: severe bronchospasm, severe bradycardia, overt LV failure
Metoclopramide (10 mg/2 mL)	Nausea and vomiting	10 mg IV or IM for ≥60 kg; 5 mg for <60 kg	Maximum of 0.5 mg/kg/d	Acute complete bowel obstruction
Morphine sulphate (15 mg or 30 mg/1 mL)	Severe pain	SC or IM based on age: <40 y, 7.5 mg; 40–59 y, 5 mg; 60–85 y, 2.5 mg; >85 y, 2 mg (0.05 mg/kg SC or IM >1 y up to 50 kg)		Caution: renal or liver impairment, pregnancy, seizures, head injuries, asthma, hypotension, hypothyroidism, pheochromocytoma, addiction, dyspnea Avoid: respiratory or CNS depression
Naloxone (2 mg/5 mL)	Opioid overdose	0.4–0.8 mg IV, IM, or SC	Repeat as required	Nil (other than known hypersensitivity) during emergency (opioid overdose)

TABLE 12-1 Principal Medications for an Imaging Department Crash Cart, Their Indications, Dose, and Precautions Required*

Medication	Indication	Dose (Pediatric Dose)	Frequency (Pediatric Dose)	Precautions/ Contraindications (Other than Allergy)
Nitroglycerin spray (glyceryl trinitrate or GTN) (400 µg/dose)	Acute angina and acute LV failure	1–2 sprays of 400 µg each onto or under the tongue 300–600 µg SL tablet or 2–3 mg buccal tablet are alternatives	Repeat after 5 min if required to a maximum of 3 sprays	Caution: phosphodiesterase-5 inhibitors (e.g., Viagra) potentiate the effects of nitric oxide in the corpora cavernosa Avoid: hypotension, hypovolemia, increased intracranial pressure
Norepinephrine (2 mg/2 mL or 1:1,000)	Hypotension and shock	Start at 8–12 µg/min, then titrate to 2–4 µg/min for maintenance; maximum dose of 30 µg/min if hypotension unresponsive to lower doses (0.02–0.1 µg/kg/min)	Titrate to effect	Caution: hypovolemia, hyperthyroidism Avoid: hypertension
Procainamide (100 mg/mL or 500 mg/mL)	VT	17 mg/kg IV slow bolus (20–30 min) at maximum rate of 50 mg/min (15 mg/kg IV load; 3–6 mg/kg over 5 min, to a maximum of 100 mg/kg)	Continue infusion (4 mg/min) until QRS widening >50%, dysrhythmia terminated, onset of hypotension, or 17 mg/kg infused	Caution: heart failure, hypotension Avoid: heart block, SLE
Salbutamol (100 µg/dose inhaler or 5 mg/2.5 mL nebulizer)	Acute asthma and bronchospasm Anaphylaxis	4 inhalations of 100 µg each via spacer (Same) 2.5–5 mg by nebulizer (same >2 y) 5 mg by nebulizer	Repeat every 4 minutes as required Repeat if required Repeat if required	Nil in emergency

Abbreviations: AV, atrioventricular; CNS, central nervous system; IM, intramuscular; IV, intravenous; LV, left ventricular; SC, subcutaneous; SL, sublingual; SLE, systemic lupus erythematosus; SVT, supraventricular tachycardia; VF, ventricular fibrillation; VT, ventricular tachycardia.

*It should be kept in mind that precautions and contraindications are relative to the nature of the emergency and, in many cases, are nullified by the life-threatening nature of the circumstances.

Emergency Medication Pharmacology

An insight into the pharmacology of each class of medication provides useful understanding that could translate to capability and problem solving. The general pharmacokinetic information, mode of action, potential adverse reactions, potential interactions, and drug class are summarized in Table 12-3.

Acetylcholine (ACh) activation of M_2 muscarinic receptors produces cardiac activity. Endogenous ACh produces decreased heart rate, decreased cardiac output, vasodilation, hypotension, and arrhythmias. Muscarinic antagonists (parasympatholytic) include belladonna alkaloids (e.g., atropine) and synthetic atropine substitutes. The effects include an increased heart rate, vasoconstriction, hypertension, smooth muscle relaxation, bronchodilation, decreased exocrine secretion (sweat, tears, saliva, etc.), pupil dilation (mydriasis), increased intraocular pressure, cycloplegia, depression, restlessness, agitation, hyperactivity, and increased body temperature. Atropine is the most widely known muscarinic antagonist and is used intravenously to treat sinus bradycardia, as a preanesthetic, as a low-risk and long-lasting sedative, to treat tremor and rigidity in Parkinson disease, to treat motion sickness, as an antispasmodic, and as a mydriatic to counter miosis. Cholinesterase inactivates ACh by breaking it down into choline and acetate (Fig. 12-2). The effects of anticholinesterase are to inhibit that breakdown and increase ACh.

Endogenous catecholamines include norepinephrine (noradrenaline), epinephrine (adrenaline), and dopamine, which is the precursor for norepinephrine (NE) synthesis (Fig. 12-3). As previously outlined, NE acts as a neurotransmitter via activation of alpha (α)- and beta (β)-adrenoreceptors. NE (to treat severe hypotension) and epinephrine (to treat bronchospasm and anaphylaxis) are direct-acting nonselective α-agonists. Agonism of β_1-receptors increases heart rate, cardiac contraction force, cardiac output, and myocardial oxygen use but can cause arrhythmia (Fig. 12-4). Agonism of β_2-receptors relaxes smooth muscle (bronchodilation, vasodilation), increases glycolysis in liver and muscle, and decreases histamine release. Agonism of β_3-receptors releases fatty acids (lipolysis). Dobutamine is a selective β_1-receptor agonist that is used to treat hypotension. Salbutamol and salmeterol are selective β_2-receptor agonists largely used as bronchodilators (Fig. 12-5). Epinephrine is a nonselective β-receptor agonist. Antagonists of the β-adrenergic receptors are referred to as *β-blockers* and function by competitive blockade of the actions of catecholamines. Atenolol and metoprolol are a β-blocker selective for β_1, resulting in decreased heart rate, decreased contraction force, decreased oxygen demand, peripheral vasoconstriction, and bronchospasm. Consequently, β-blockers are used to treat hypertension, arrhythmia, and angina.

Purine pharmacology is discussed in Chapter 8. Adenosine is a natural regulator of blood flow and coronary demand, acting directly on adenosine cell surface receptors (Fig. 12-6). There are four main adenosine receptor subtypes. A_1 blocks AV conduction, reduces force of cardiac contraction (negative inotropic and chronotropic action), produces cardiac depression, and causes bronchoconstriction. A_{2A} causes potent vasodilation, decreased blood pressure, and bronchodilation. A_{2B} stimulates release of mast cell mediators, and A_3 contributes to bronchoconstriction. The principle agonists include the neurotransmitter adenosine, adenosine phosphates—adenosine monophosphate (AMP), adenosine diphosphate (ADP), and adenosine triphosphate (ATP)—and dipyridamole, which is an indirect agonist that blocks adenosine metabolism and thus increases bioavailability of adenosine.

Nitroglycerin (glyceryl trinitrate) is another potent vasodilator that enhances oxygen delivery and reduces oxygen demand. Nitrites and nitrogen compounds enter the endothelial cell and are converted from arginine to nitric oxide (and citrulline), which in turn stimulates guanylate cyclase metabolism in smooth muscle cells (Fig. 12-7). Vasodilation is associated with reduction in calcium concentration and dephosphorylation of myosin. Nitroglycerin results in pooling of blood in veins, and by reducing the amount of blood returned to the heart, it decreases preload (left ventricular end-diastolic volume) and decreases myocardial oxygen demand. Nitroglycerin also causes dilation of coronary (and collateral) vessels to more efficiently distribute blood and oxygen to ischemic tissues. Two important relationships need to be outlined for nitroglycerin. First, nitric oxide reacts with metals, thiols, and oxygen and can thereby modify proteins, lipids, and DNA. Second, phosphodiesterase-5 inhibitors used for erectile dysfunction, such as sildenafil (Viagra), function by potentiating the effects of nitric oxide in the corpora cavernosa.

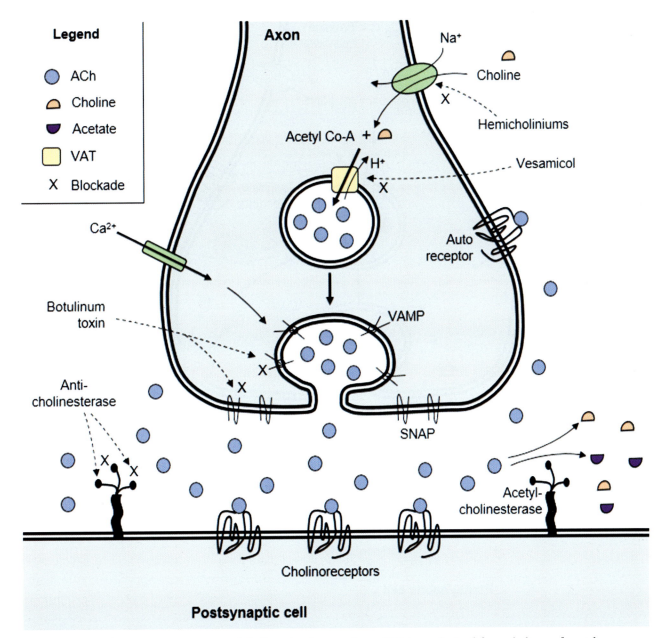

FIGURE 12-2 Schematic representation of cholinergic pharmacology. ACh is synthesized from choline and acetyl coenzyme A, transported into the vesicle through the vesicle-associated transporter (VAT), and released from the vesicle. Anticholinesterase medications such as atropine can block synaptic breakdown of ACh to choline and acetate.

Histamine release from the mast cell is mediated by an interaction between the antigen and the immunoglobulin E (IgE) antibody (Fig. 12-8) or in response to substance P, as outlined in Chapter 1. Histamine has been implicated in 3 common conditions: peptic ulcer associated with H_2, H_1-mediated type 1 sensitivity (urticarial, hay fever), and asthma (bronchoconstriction). Antihistamine refers to H_1 medications that, rather than being antagonists of the receptor, are inverse agonists of the H_1 receptor. That is, antihistamines not only block the receptor but also produce an effect that opposes the normal histamine agonistic effect. First-generation antihistamines, such as diphenhydramine (Benadryl) and promethazine (Phenergan), are often referred to as *sedating antihistamines*. Second-generation antihistamines, such as loratadine, cetirizine, and fexofenadine, are less-sedating antihistamines. Both first- and second-generation antihistamines are used for allergic reactions.

158 Pharmacology Primer for Medications

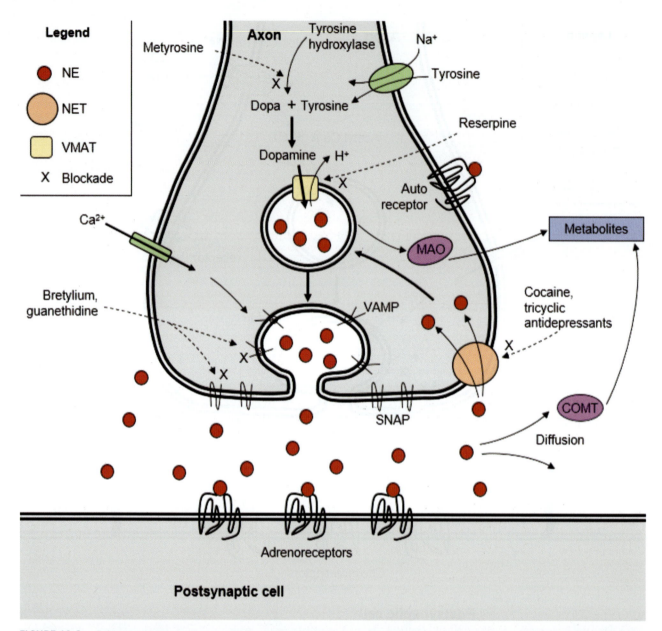

FIGURE 12-3 Schematic representation of adrenergic pharmacology. Tyrosine is transported into the presynaptic nerve it is synthesized with dopa into dopamine. NE is synthesized from dopamine transported inside the vesicle via the vesicular monoamine transporter (VMAT). Release of NE from the vesicle is dependent on calcium and modulation by synaptosome-associated proteins (SNAP) and vesicle-associated membrane proteins (VAMP). NE can be recycled to the axon via NE transporters (NET), metabolized by catechol-O-methyltransferase (COMT) from the cleft, and metabolized by monoamine oxidase (MAO) from the vesicle.

Diuretics generally increase urine volume by inhibiting reabsorption of sodium and chloride in the nephron. There are four classes of diuretics (Fig. 12-9):

1. Loop diuretics (e.g., furosemide)
2. Thiazide diuretics (e.g., hydrochlorothiazide)
3. Potassium-sparing diuretics (e.g., amiloride)
4. Carbonic anhydrase inhibitors (e.g., acetazolamide)

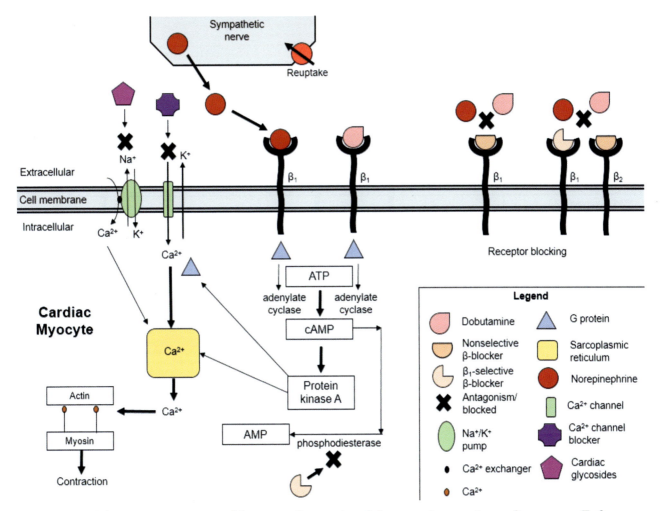

FIGURE 12-4 Schematic representation of the action of inotropic and chronotropic agents in a cardiac myocyte. Endogenous norepinephrine is released from the sympathetic nerve. In the extracellular space, endogenous norepinephrine and exogenous dobutamine can couple with β1-receptors. Receptor β1 can be antagonized by a β-blocker either nonselective (e.g., propranolol) or selective for β1 (e.g., atenolol). Calcium channel blockers (e.g., verapamil) act to antagonize the voltage-dependent calcium channel to block the inotropic and chronotropic contraction response.

Antiarrhythmic medications tend to be classified into four groups (Figs. 12-10 and 12-11). Class I antiarrhythmics act on sodium channels (sodium channel blockers) during rapid depolarization by interfering with sodium influx (Fig. 12-12). This decreases the rate of depolarization, decreases atrioventricular (AV) conduction and decreases contractility. Class Ib antiarrhythmics, such as lidocaine, also decrease the action potential duration and increase the effective refractory period. Class II antiarrhythmics are β-blockers (β-adrenoreceptor antagonists) that act at the pacemaker (automaticity) potential at the end of the cardiac action potential cycle to decrease AV conduction and decrease contractility, as previously described (e.g., atenolol, metoprolol). Class III antiarrhythmics such as amiodarone are potassium channel blockers and act during repolarization to increase the action potential duration, increase the effective refractory period, and decrease AV conduction (Fig. 12-12). Class IV antiarrhythmics such as diltiazem are calcium channel blockers that act on the plateau prior to repolarization to decrease the action potential duration, decrease AV conduction, and decrease contractility (Fig. 12-12). It is worth noting that a number of other medications have antiarrhythmic effects but are not classified in this system; they include but are not limited to adenosine, atropine, and epinephrine. In an emergency situation, antiarrhythmic medications are designed to prevent life-threatening arrhythmia, prevent sudden cardiac death, and control the ventricular contraction rate, but paradoxically, all antiarrhythmic medications can worsen arrhythmia and cause sudden cardiac death.

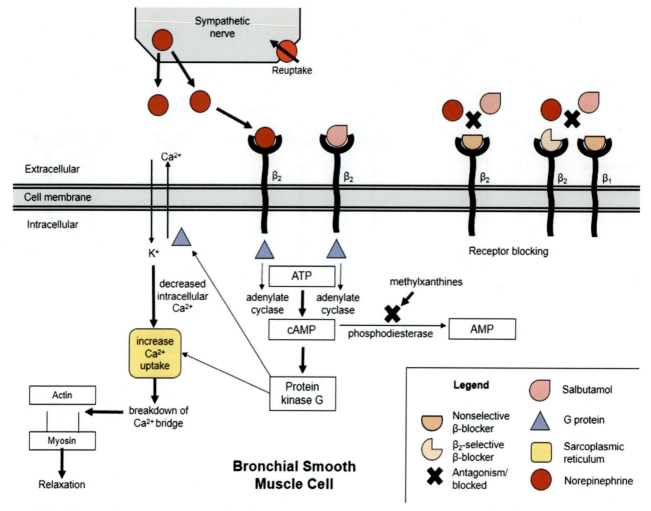

FIGURE 12-5 Schematic representation of the action of β-agonism in a bronchial smooth muscle (e.g., salbutamol). Inhibition of phosphodiesterase conversion of cyclic adenosine monophosphate (cAMP) to AMP by methylxanthines (e.g., caffeine, theobromine, theophylline) further decreases intracellular calcium. This response can be antagonized by a β-blocker either nonselective (e.g., labetalol) or selective for β2 (e.g., butoxamine).

Analgesic medications are important in an emergency to manage pain. Pain may be associated with traumatic injuries that patients present for evaluation rather than with injuries occurring in the department. Nonetheless, patients under our care present with a variety of comorbidities and risks that could result in an acute episode of pain. Consider the level of pain associated with older, diseased, and injured patients who have a fall in our department, creating an urgent situation. In some cases, our procedure or positioning may exacerbate already high pain levels. While general pain management is covered in more detail in Chapter 13, some discussion is required of analgesics used under emergency conditions via the crash cart. The crash cart may contain morphine for the purpose of managing severe pain. Morphine has significant potential for abuse and therefore may be stored remotely and more securely from the crash cart itself.

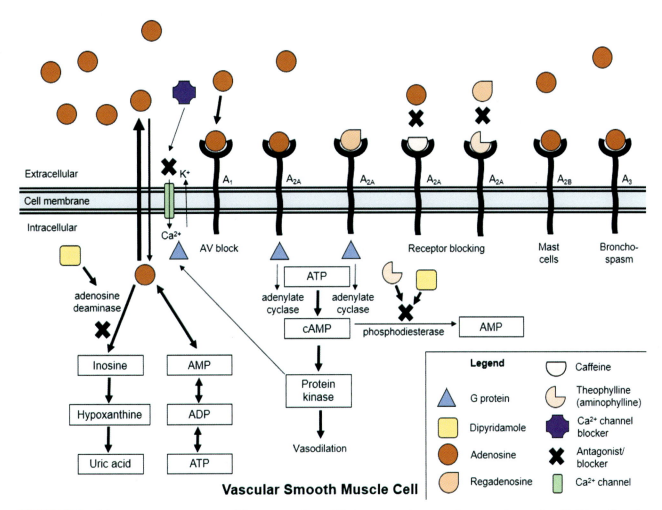

FIGURE 12-6 Schematic representation of the action of vasodilating agents in a vascular smooth muscle cell. Dipyridamole antagonizes adenosine deaminase, which reduces adenosine metabolism and thus increases availability of adenosine in the extracellular space. Dipyridamole is also a phosphodiesterase inhibitor, so it blocks conversion of cAMP to AMP, further increasing vasodilation. Calcium channel blockers act to antagonize the voltage-dependent calcium channel to block vasodilation.

Morphine is the classic or prototype opioid analgesic and, as such, is the focus of this discussion. Nonetheless, a number of morphine derivatives or other opioid medications are used routinely. Pharmacological principles are largely transferrable. Morphine acts on the opioid receptor and is considered a strong agonist (as is methadone and meperidine). Moderate efficacy opioid agonists include codeine and oxycodone, while propoxyphene is a weak agonist. Naloxone and naltrexone are antagonists, whereas buprenorphine has mixed agonist and antagonist activity. Morphine is an opioid agonist that is mostly selective for μ-opioid receptor (OP_3) but can interact with other opioid receptors (κ and δ) at high doses. **Since naloxone has a short duration of action (1–2 h), multiple doses are used in opioid analgesic overdose. Naltrexone has a longer half-life and can be used to block opioid effects for up to 48 hours, but it is more commonly associated with decreasing craving for alcohol.**

As an analgesic, the mechanism of action of opioids is outlined in Chapter 13. Morphine has both central and peripheral effects. Centrally, opioids provide analgesia but can suppress the cough reflex (hence the use of codeine in dry cough mixtures) and cause respiratory depression, sedation, euphoria and dysphoria, miosis, nausea, hypotension, and bradycardia. Peripherally, opioids can cause constipation, sphincter spasm, suppression of spinal reflexes, and release of histamine. Tolerance and dependence can develop quickly. A summary of the various opioid medications is provided in Table 12-2.

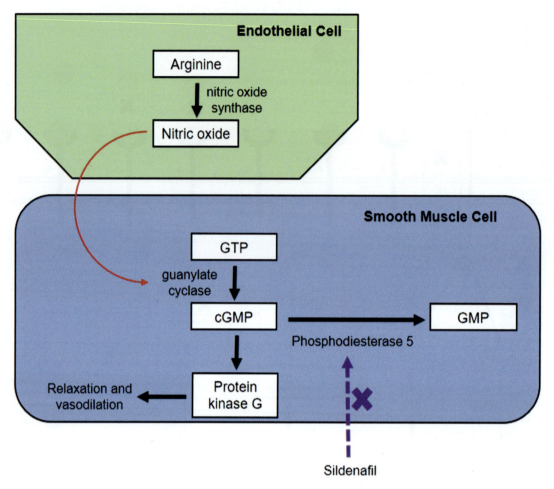

FIGURE 12-7 Schematic representation of the production of nitric oxide in endothelial cells with subsequent activation of guanylate cyclase in smooth muscle cells. This facilitates the conversion of guanine triphosphate (GTP) to cyclic guanosine monophosphate (cGMP), activating protein kinase G, which leads to smooth muscle relaxation and vasodilation.

Anxiolytic or antianxiety medication may be useful in the crash cart for managing situations in which a conscious patient in an emergency may be sufficiently anxious about his or her condition that it prohibits adequate, safe management of that condition. It may also be appropriate for use in seizure disorders or during acute episodes of muscle spasm. Benzodiazepines are widely used as hypnotics or anxiolytics because of their superior safety profile, which includes dose-related effects, less fatality from toxicity and overdose, lower abuse potential, less adverse effects, and less serious drug interactions. Diazepam, which is the prototype diazepam, is a CNS depressant that has specific functions to reduce anxiety. Diazepam acts on the gamma-aminobutyric acid (GABA) receptor. GABA is an endogenous inhibitory neurotransmitter that causes increased chloride permeability, hyperpolarization, and decreased excitability of the neuron. Diazepam is not a GABA agonist, but rather, it modulates the binding of GABA to the GABAA receptor, further inhibiting the neuron.

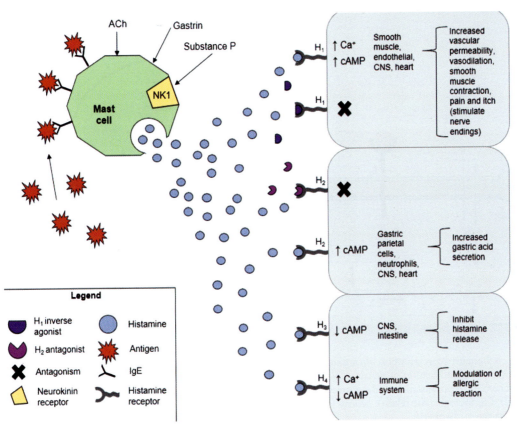

FIGURE 12-8 Schematic representation of the release of histamine from a mast cell mediated by antigen, IgE, and substance P activity.

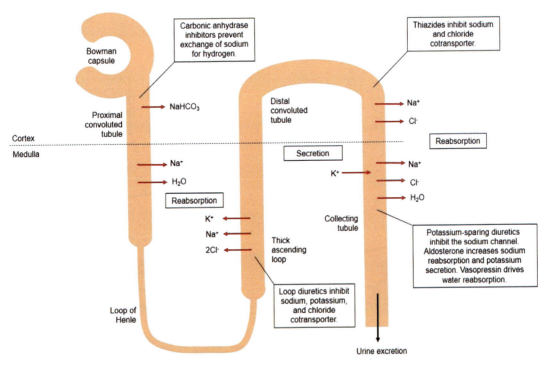

FIGURE 12-9 Schematic representation of the sites of action of different classes of diuretics. Furosemide is a loop diuretic acting on the thick ascending loop of the loop of Henle in the nephron.

164   Pharmacology Primer for Medications

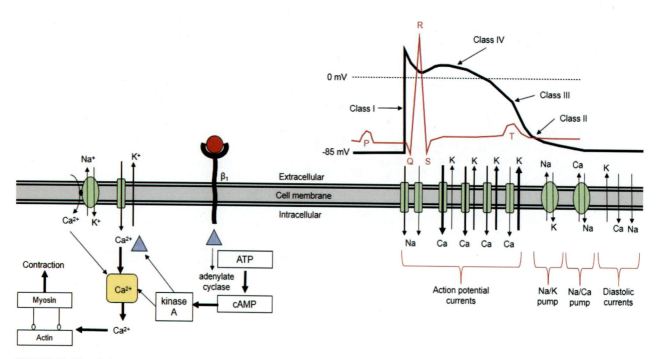

FIGURE 12-10   Schematic representation of cardiac electrical activity with the electrocardiogram (ECG; red) overlaid on action potentials (black) with identification of phases of action for the different classes of antiarrhythmic medications. On the left, a more detailed schematic representation of the 4 mechanisms is summarized (sodium channel, β-receptor, potassium channel, and calcium channel). On the right, the relative actions (influx and efflux) of sodium, calcium, and potassium, plus their mechanisms, are mapped across the cardiac cycle.

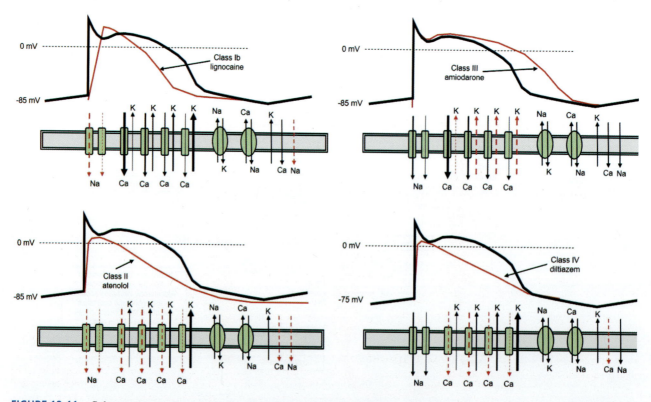

FIGURE 12-11   Schematic representation of cardiac electrical activity with the resulting change in action potential (red) overlaid on normal action potentials (black) for the different classes of antiarrhythmic medications.

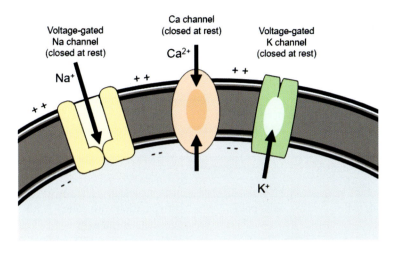
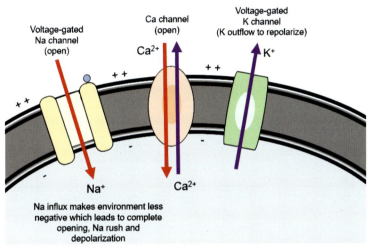
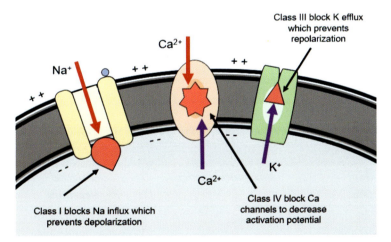

FIGURE 12-12 Schematic representation of the effects of anti-arrhythmia drugs. The top image represents the sodium, calcium, and potassium channels closed at rest. In response to stimulus, as depicted in the middle image, the sodium channel opens, allowing rapid influx of sodium and change of charge of the internal environment. This prompts the potassium channel to efflux potassium for repolarization. The calcium channel allows influx (red) and efflux (purple) associated with depolarization and repolarization respectively. The bottom image represents the effects of various antiarrhythmics, with class I blocking the open sodium channel, class III preventing opening of the potassium channel, and class IV blocking the calcium channel.

TABLE 12-2 Comparison of Various Opioid Medications

Medication	Administration	Use	Comment	Plasma Half Clearance	Potency Relative to Morphine
Morphine	Oral, IM, IV, SC, epidural	Moderate to severe acute and chronic pain	Sustained-release formulations available	2–3.5 h	1×
Buprenorphine	IM, SL, transdermal patch	Moderate to severe pain		3–5 h	80×
Codeine	Oral, IM	Mild pain	Preparation with cough medicines and with paracetamol of ibuprofen are subanalgesic	3 h	0.1×
Fentanyl	IV, SC, transdermal patch, lozenge	Palliation, moderate to severe acute and chronic pain, including in renal impairment	Lozenge for breakthrough pain	3–4 h	100×
Hydromorphone	Oral, IM, IV, SC	Severe pain	Less sedation	2–3 h	4–5×
Methadone	Oral, IM, IV	Severe chronic pain	Long half-life, so daily for narcotic rehabilitation	24 h	5–10×
Oxycodone	Oral, IV, SC, rectal	Moderate to severe acute and chronic pain, including in renal impairment	Oral is controlled release for longer action	2–3 h	1.5×
Pethidine	IM, IV, SC	Renal and colic pain or in labor	Can cause paradoxical excitement	3–4 h	0.125×
Tramadol	Oral, IM	Neuropathic pain	Lower abuse risk	4–6 h	

Abbreviations: IM, intramuscular; IV, intravenous; SC, subcutaneous; SL, sublingual.

TABLE 12-3 General Pharmacokinetic Information, Mode of Action, Potential Adverse Reactions, Potential Interactions, and Drug Class

Medication (Drug Class)	Mode of Action	Pharmacokinetics	Adverse Reactions	Interactions
Adenosine (purine vasodilator)	Depresses the sinus node activity and slows conduction	◆ Rapid onset ◆ Peak <1 min ◆ Half-life <10 sec ◆ Duration <1 min constant infusion ◆ No plasma protein binding	Resolve rapidly with cessation but include chest, neck, jaw, or arm pain; headache; flushing; dyspnea; ECG changes. Bronchospasm is possible, especially in patients with asthma.	Caffeine or xanthine drugs or foods

TABLE 12-3 General Pharmacokinetic Information, Mode of Action, Potential Adverse Reactions, Potential Interactions, and Drug Class

Medication (Drug Class)	Mode of Action	Pharmacokinetics	Adverse Reactions	Interactions
Amiodarone (antiarrhythmic)	Decreases sinus node and junctional automaticity to slow AV node conduction	◆ Onset IV: 1–30 min ◆ Duration of effect: 1–3 h ◆ Half-life: 14–59 d ◆ 96% plasma protein bound	Dizziness, headache, nausea, vomiting, constipation, ataxia, bitter taste	Digoxin, phenytoin, warfarin, other antiarrhythmic medications
Atenolol (selective β_1-receptor blocker)	Competitive antagonism of β-receptors in the heart	◆ 50% absorbed orally ◆ Peak plasma concentrations 2–4 h ◆ Half-life 6–7 h ◆ 6%–16% plasma protein bound	Headache, nausea, hypotension, dizziness, confusion, heart failure, heart block, bradycardia, dyspnea, bronchospasm	Reserpine, other β-blockers, calcium channel blockers, disopyramide, amiodarone
Atropine (anticholinergic)	Competitively blocks acetylcholine at muscarinic receptors	◆ Onset 3 min ◆ Half-life 3 h (substantially shorter in children and longer in elderly) ◆ 14%–22% plasma protein bound	α- and β-agonist actions and its interactions are complex and may be hazardous. Particular caution is needed if adrenaline is given to patients taking β-blockers, since severe hypertension may result; patients taking β-blockers may also have an impaired response to adrenaline if it is needed for anaphylaxis.	Benztropine, digoxin, bronchodilators, pralidoxime
Promethazine (Phenergan) (antihistamine)	Antagonize histamine at H_2 receptors to decrease histamine release	◆ Onset 5 min IV; 20 min IM ◆ Half-life 9–10 h ◆ Duration of action 4–6 h ◆ 76%–93% plasma protein bound	Pain and inflammation at injection site, dizziness, sedation, hypotension, confusion; can cause paradoxical stimulation	CNS depressants, epinephrine, anticholinergics, MAOIs
Diazepam (anxiolytic)	Benzodiazepine that activates GABA for CNS inhibition	◆ Onset 15–45 min ◆ Peak 30–90 min ◆ Half-life 46 h ◆ Duration can be prolonged ◆ 100% bioavailability orally ◆ 98%–99% plasma protein bound ◆ Biphasic elimination with rapid component followed by slower 1–2 d half-life	Drowsiness, sedation, muscle weakness, ataxia, vertigo, headache, confusion, paradoxical excitement, all with increased risk in elderly	CNS depressants, including antihistamines, and drugs metabolized by the liver

(continued)

TABLE 12-3 General Pharmacokinetic Information, Mode of Action, Potential Adverse Reactions, Potential Interactions, and Drug Class

Medication (Drug Class)	Mode of Action	Pharmacokinetics	Adverse Reactions	Interactions
Verapamil (calcium channel blocker)	Blocks calcium influx to reduce cardiac conduction and contractility	◆ 3–6 min onset after IV bolus ◆ Half-life biphasic at 4 min and 2–5 h ◆ 90% plasma protein bound	Peripheral edema, rash, headache, dizziness, nausea, bradycardia, constipation	Other antiarrhythmics, β-blockers, dabigatran, lithium, cimetidine, rifampin, phenobarbital, cyclosporin, carbamazepine
Dobutamine (β_1-agonist)	Inotropic vasodilator	◆ 1–2 min onset ◆ Duration 10 min ◆ Half-life 2–3 min ◆ 40% plasma protein bound	Angina, palpitations, headache, nausea, hypertension, tachycardia. Adverse reactions reversed with cessation of infusion or β-blockers	Blood pressure medications, β-blockers, tricyclic antidepressants, MAOIs, CNS stimulants, potassium-depleting drugs
Dopamine (adrenergic stimulant)	Vasoconstriction, positive inotropic, and chromotropic action at high dose; vasodilation at low doses	◆ 5 min onset IV ◆ Duration <10 min ◆ Half-life 2 min ◆ 13% plasma protein bound	Ectopic beats, tachycardia, nausea, angina, dyspnea, hypotension, hypertension	Ergot alkaloids, halogenated hydrocarbon gas, MAOIs, tricyclic antidepressants, diuretics, phenytoin, β-blockers
Epinephrine (adrenergic stimulant)	Positive inotropic and chromotropic action, vasodilation at low doses but vasoconstriction at high doses, mast cell stabilizer, relaxes bronchial smooth muscle	◆ Rapid onset IV ◆ Duration 2–5 min ◆ Steady state in 10–15 min for infusion ◆ Half-life <5 min ◆ 15%–20% plasma protein bound	Anxiety, dyspnea, hyperglycemia, restlessness, palpitations, tachycardia (sometimes with anginal pain), tremors, sweating, hypersalivation, weakness, dizziness, headache, coldness of extremities	α- and β-agonist, digitalis, diuretics, antiarrhythmics, tricyclic antidepressants, MAOIs, sodium levothyroxine, chlorpheniramine, tripelennamine, diphenhydramine. Patients taking β-blockers may also have an impaired response to epinephrine if it is needed for anaphylaxis.

TABLE 12-3 General Pharmacokinetic Information, Mode of Action, Potential Adverse Reactions, Potential Interactions, and Drug Class

Medication (Drug Class)	Mode of Action	Pharmacokinetics	Adverse Reactions	Interactions
EpiPen (adrenergic stimulant)	Positive inotropic and chromotropic action, vasodilation at low doses but vasoconstriction at high doses, mast cell stabilizer, relaxes bronchial smooth muscle	◆ Rapid onset IM ◆ Short duration ◆ Half-life <5 min ◆ 15%–20% plasma protein bound	Transient effects include anxiety, overstimulation, restlessness, tremor, weakness, dizziness, sweating, tachycardia, palpitations, pallor, nausea, headache, respiratory difficulties. Ventricular arrhythmias can occur.	α- and β-agonist, digitalis, diuretics, antiarrhythmics, tricyclic antidepressants, MAOIs, sodium levothyroxine, chlorpheniramine, tripelennamine, diphenhydramine. Patients taking β-blockers may also have an impaired response to epinephrine if it is needed for anaphylaxis.
Frusemide (loop diuretic)	Inhibition of sodium and chloride reabsorption in the ascending loop of Henle.	◆ 5 min onset ◆ Peak 15–30 min ◆ Half-life 1.5–2 h ◆ Duration 2–3 h ◆ 99% plasma protein bound	Tinnitus, allergic reaction, nausea, vomiting, dizziness, blurred vision, headache, hypotension, dehydration	Aspirin, diuretics, digoxin, lithium, antihypertensives, NSAIDs
Lidocaine (antiarrhythmic)	Reduces automaticity without changing contractility (class Ib)	◆ Onset of action 1 min V or 3–15 min IM ◆ Duration 10–20 min IV ◆ Half-life is biphasic at 1.5 and 2 h ◆ Plasma protein binding is inversely proportional to concentration but 60%–80% range	Serious adverse effects including the potential to worsen arrhythmia and cardiac failure. Do not use outside of hospital.	Flecainide, disopyramide
Metoprolol (selective β$_1$-receptor blocker)	Competitive antagonism of beta receptors in the heart	◆ Onset 10–20 min ◆ Half-life 3–4 h ◆ 10%–12% plasma protein bound	Headache, nausea, hypotension, dizziness, confusion, heart failure, heart block, bradycardia, dyspnea, bronchospasm	Reserpine, other β-blockers, calcium channel blockers, disopyramide, amiodarone
Morphine sulphate (analgesic)	Opioid receptor agonist	◆ 5 min onset ◆ Peak 20 min ◆ Half-life 2 h ◆ Duration 20–50 min ◆ 35% plasma protein bound	Respiratory depression, hypotension, vomiting, dysphoria, urinary retention, dizziness, sedation, nausea, constipation	Narcotic analgesics, CNS depressants, benzodiazepines, MAOIs

(continued)

TABLE 12-3 General Pharmacokinetic Information, Mode of Action, Potential Adverse Reactions, Potential Interactions, and Drug Class

Medication (Drug Class)	Mode of Action	Pharmacokinetics	Adverse Reactions	Interactions
Naloxone (opioid antagonist)	Opioid antagonist displaces agonists at the receptor due to higher affinity for µ-opioid receptors	◆ 2 min onset IV, 5 min IM ◆ Half-life 1–1.5 h ◆ Duration 30–60 min ◆ Weak plasma protein binding	Hypotension, hypertension, ventricular tachycardia, ventricular fibrillation, dyspnea, pulmonary edema	Buprenorphine, methohexital
Nitroglycerin (vasodilator)	Increases exogenous nitric oxide for venodilation	◆ 1–3 min onset ◆ Half-life 2–3 min ◆ Duration 30–60 min	Flushing, dizziness, tachycardia, headache	Phosphodiesterase inhibitors, alcohol, antihypertensives, vasodilators
Norepinephrine (adrenergic vasoconstrictor)	Vasoconstrictor without major cardiac effects	◆ Rapid onset IV ◆ Short duration ◆ Half-life <5 min ◆ Minimally plasma protein bound	Anxiety, palpitations, headache	Cyclopropane, halothane, MAOIs, amitriptyline or imipramine antidepressants
Procainamide (antiarrhythmic)	Class Ia antiarrhythmic inhibits post-repolarization recovery to decrease conduction velocity and excitability	◆ Peak 15–60 min IM ◆ Half-life 2.5–5 h ◆ 15%–20% plasma protein bound	Rapid IV dosage may result in severe hypotension, ventricular fibrillation, and asystole. High plasma concentrations are also associated with impaired cardiac conduction.	Enhance effects of antihypertensives, other antiarrhythmics and arrhythmogenic drugs, antimuscarinics, and neuromuscular blockers; diminish effects of parasympathomimetics
Salbutamol (bronchodilator β_2-receptor agonist)	Activates B_2-receptors in the lungs to produce smooth muscle relaxation	◆ 5 min onset ◆ Peak 60 min ◆ Half-life 4–6 h ◆ Duration 3–6 h	Tremor, palpitations, tachycardia, anxiety, headaches, peripheral vasodilation, muscle cramps, hyperglycemia, hypersensitivity	Other β_2-agonists, corticosteroids, diuretics, xanthines, β-blockers, antidepressants

Abbreviations: IM, intramuscular; IV, intravenous; MAOI, monoamine oxidase inhibitor; SC, subcutaneous; SL, sublingual.

References

Asperheim K, Favaro J. *Introduction to Pharmacology*. 12th ed. St Louis, MO: Elsevier; 2012.

Block JH, Beale JM. *Wilson and Gisvold's Textbook of Organic Medicinal and Pharmaceutical Chemistry*. 12th ed. Philadelphia, PA: Lippincott Williams & Wilkins; 2011.

Bryant B, Knights K, Salerno E. *Pharmacology for Health Professionals*. 2nd ed. Sydney, Australia: Mosby Elsevier; 2007.

Golan DE, Tashjian AH, Armstrong EJ, Armstrong AW. *Principles of Pharmacology: The Pathophysiologic Basis of Drug Therapy*. 3rd ed. Philadelphia, PA: Lippincott Williams & Wilkins; 2012.

Greenstein B. *Rapid Revision in Clinical Pharmacology*. New York, NY: Radcliffe Publishing; 2008.

Hacker M, Messer W, Bachmann K. *Pharmacology: Principles and Practice*. London, England: Elsevier; 2009.

Jambhekar SS, Breen PJ. *Basic Pharmacokinetics*. London, England: Pharmaceutical Press; 2009.

Katzung BG, Masters SB, Trevor AJ. *Basic and Clinical Pharmacology*, 12th ed. New York, NY: McGraw Hill; 2012.

Rang H, Dale M, Ritter J, Flower R. *Rang and Dale's Pharmacology*. 6th ed. London, England: Churchill Livingston; 2008.

Waller D, Renwick A, Hillier K. *Medical Pharmacology and Therapeutics*. 2nd ed. London, England: Elsevier; 2006.

CHAPTER 13

Pain Management

Chapter Objectives

Specific learning outcomes (page ix) of this text addressed in this chapter:

- Apply the principles of pharmacology to the safe and effective use of medicines.
- Recognize general, patient-specific, and scenario-specific risks, precautions, and contraindications for use of medicines.
- Apply the pharmacokinetic and pharmacodynamic principles of medications to identify and explain normal and adverse reactions to medications.
- Administer medications safely, effectively, and appropriately according to procedures and within regulatory and statutory parameters.
- Monitor patients for, identify, and manage adverse reactions.

After reading, digesting, reflecting on, and reviewing the content of this chapter, readers should be able to

1. Demonstrate command of key pharmacology terms.
2. Demonstrate enhanced understanding of the principles associated with the pharmacology of pain medications.
3. Demonstrate critical thinking to effect problem solving related to pain medications.
4. Demonstrate understanding of the mode of action, pharmacokinetics, risks, precautions, contraindications, adverse effects, interactions, and appropriate dosage of pain medications.
5. Apply knowledge of the general principles and concepts in a translational manner to clinical practice.

Key Terms

action potential	anti-inflammatory	dependence	neurotransmitter	repolarization
acute pain	antipyretic	depolarization	nociceptive pain	tolerance
agonist	chronic pain	drug interaction	nonopioid	topical
analgesic	COX-1	hypersensitivity	opioid	trypanophobia
anesthetics	COX-2	neuropathic pain	prostaglandin	voltage-gated
antihistamine				

Introduction

Pain management is a complex topic and beyond the scope of a single chapter. The purpose of this chapter is to explore the mechanisms of pain and pain management from the context of patients encountered in the medical imaging department. This broad list includes

- Patients with onset of pain during their visit to the department requiring intervention.
- Patients presenting for investigation of trauma or painful pathology who may or may not be medicated for that pain.
- Patients suffering acute or chronic pain exacerbated by imaging procedures that may or may not require intervention.
- Patients presenting to the department with a history of acute or chronic pain whose medication for that pain may have an impact on the procedure (e.g., compliance, communication, interactions).
- Patients without pain but in whom the procedure may introduce pain (e.g., biopsy) where anesthesia might be adopted to prevent pain.
- Patients presenting for the management of pain (e.g., palliation).

There is a wide range of medications available to manage pain. The appropriate medication depends on the type of pain, severity, location, and comorbidity. In general, pain tends to result from inflammation associated with tissue damage, chemical agents/pathogens (*nociceptive* pain), or nerve damage (*neuropathic* pain). Pain tends to be undertreated or poorly managed because of the risk and effects of addiction and abuse. With that comes the challenges of assessing pain with different levels of tolerance, perception of scale, and communication barriers. Generally speaking, pain can be classified as follows (see Table 13-1):

- Mild: Respond to acetaminophen (paracetamol), aspirin, nonsteroidal anti-inflammatory drugs (NSAIDs), and nonopioid medications
- Moderate: Short-acting opioids, including codeine, oxycodone, and tramadol, alone or in combination with nonopioid analgesics
- Severe: May require parenteral morphine, meperidine, oxymorphone, or sustained-release transdermal patches such as fentanyl

Universally, a 3-step approach to pain management is used. Step 1, for mild to moderate pain, relies on nonopioid medications such as NSAIDs, acetaminophen (paracetamol), and aspirin. Step 2 is also for mild to moderate pain but uses compound medications generally associated with the combination of codeine with acetaminophen (paracetamol), or ibuprofen. Step 3 is opioid medications for severe pain. In addition, a number of other medications can be used as an adjunct to improve pain management, including but not limited to amitriptyline (tricyclic antidepressant), gabapentin (anticonvulsant), pregabalin (anticonvulsant), and duloxetine (serotonin and norepinephrine reuptake inhibitor). Discussion of the pharmacology of pain management at this point needs to be divided into anti-inflammatory medications (effective for nociceptive pain but less effective for neuropathic pain), opioid analgesic medications (effective for nociceptive pain and neuropathic pain), adjunctive pain medications (ineffective for nociceptive pain but effective for neuropathic pain), and anesthetics.

Pain Management with Opioid Analgesics

Morphine and morphine-like medications (see Table 13-2) act predominantly on the mu (μ)-opioid receptors as agonists. μ-Opioid receptors are responsible for the *analgesic* effects of opioids, sedation, euphoria, respiratory depression, and dependence. In response to chemical, mechanical, or thermal pain stimulus, afferent receptors produce an action potential in the neuron that is subsequently enhanced by mediators and sensitizing agents (Figs. 13-1 and 13-2). Calcium influx potentiates the action potential and release of glutamate, neuropeptides, and substance P into the synaptic cleft where activation of a number of receptors occurs. Glutamate facilitates sodium and calcium influx via α-amino-3-hydroxy-5-methyl-4-isoxazolepropionic acid (AMPA) and *N*-methyl-D-aspartate (NMDA) receptors. Together with activation of the glutamate receptor, neurokinin 1 (NK1) receptor (substance P), and calcitonin gene-related peptide (CGRP) receptor (neuropeptide), the sodium and calcium drive postsynaptic *depolarization*. With the *voltage-gate* sodium channel threshold reached, the action potential drives signal relay and pain. Activation of opioid receptors in the neuron reduces the initial action potential associated with the primary stimulus and reduces calcium influx in the primary afferent neuron. This decreases the action potential and truncates release of neurotransmitters from the vesicle (Fig. 13-2). Activation of the morphine receptor on the secondary afferent neuron increases potassium efflux, which reduces sodium and calcium influx to limit attainment of the voltage-gate potential and, as a result, reduces the action potential relayed and subsequent pain sensation.

TABLE 13-1 Summary of Medication Strategies for Mild, Moderate, and Severe Pain

Pain level	Medication	Form	Dose
Mild	Acetaminophen (paracetamol)	Oral or rectal	1 g 4 times a day to maximum of 4g/d
	Aspirin	Oral or rectal	1 g 4 times a day to maximum of 4g/d
	Celecoxib	Oral	400 mg/d
	Ibuprofen	Oral	400 mg 3 times a day to maximum of 2,400 mg/d
	Naproxen	Oral	1,650 mg/d
	Sulindac	Oral	400 mg/d
Moderate	Codeine	Oral	30–200 mg every 3–4 h
	Codeine combinations	Oral	Variable
	Oxycodone	Oral	5 mg every 3–4 h
	Tramadol	Oral	50–100 mg every 4–6 h to a maximum of 400 mg/d
Severe	Fentanyl	Transdermal patch, intranasal spray, or oral lozenge	25–100 µg/h with new patch at 72 h; 50–200 µg per spray every 48 h; 0.2–1.6 mg per lozenge
	Meperidine	Oral or parenteral	100–150 mg every 3–4 h (oral) or 50–75 mg every 3–4 h (intravenous)
	Morphine	Oral or parenteral	30–60 mg every 3–4 h (oral) or 2–10 mg every 4–6 h (intravenous)
	Oxycodone	Oral	2.5–20 mg every 12 h
	Oxymorphone	Parenteral	0.5 mg every 3–4 h

TABLE 13-2 Comparison of Various Opioid Medications

Medication	Administration	Use	Pharmacokinetics	Adverse Effects
Morphine	Oral, IM, IV, SC, epidural	Acute and chronic pain	2–3.5 h half clearance, metabolized to more active morphine-6-glucuronide	Sedation, respiratory depression, constipation, nausea, itching, euphoria, tolerance, dependence
Buprenorphine	IM, SL, transdermal patch	Acute and chronic pain	12 h half clearance with slow onset; inactive orally due to first-pass metabolism	Same as for morphine but less severe
Codeine	Oral	Mild pain	Prodrug metabolized to morphine	Mainly constipation; fewer issues with dependence
Fentanyl	IV, SC, transdermal patch, lozenge	Palliation, severe acute and chronic pain including in renal impairment	1–2 h with high potency	Same as for morphine
Hydromorphone	Oral, IM, IV, SC	Severe pain	2–4 h with no active metabolites	Same as for morphine with less sedation
Methadone	Oral, IM, IV	Severe chronic pain and addiction management	24 h with slow onset but accumulation may occur due to long half-life	Same as for morphine with minimal euphoria
Oxycodone	Oral, IV, SC, rectal	Moderate to severe acute and chronic pain including in renal impairment	2–3 h	Same as for morphine
Pethidine	IM, IV, SC	Renal and colic pain or in labor	2–4 h with stimulatory metabolite	Same as for morphine with risk of stimulation and convulsions
Tramadol	Oral, IM	Neuropathic pain	4–6 h with good oral bioavailability	Dizziness, potential for convulsions, no respiratory depression

Abbreviations: IM, intramuscular; IV, intravenous; MAOI, monoamine oxidase inhibitor; SC, subcutaneous; SL, sublingual.

Chapter 13 | Pain Management 177

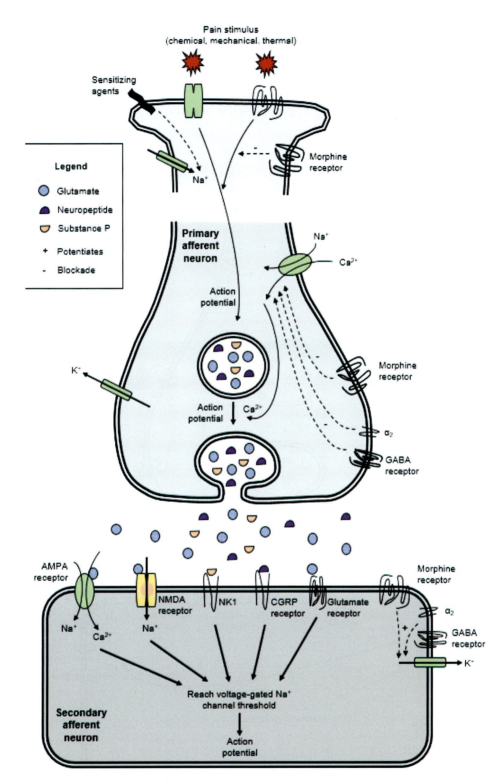

FIGURE 13-1 Schematic representation of the response to chemical, mechanical, or thermal pain stimulus. Afferent receptors produce an action potential in the neuron that is subsequently enhanced by mediators and sensitizing agents. Calcium influx potentiates the action potential and release of glutamate, neuropeptides, and substance P into the synaptic cleft where activation of a number of receptors occurs. Glutamate facilitates sodium and calcium influx via AMPA and NMDA receptors. Together with activation of the glutamate receptor, NK1 receptor (substance P), and CGRP receptor (neuropeptide), the sodium and calcium drive postsynaptic depolarization. With the voltage-gate sodium channel threshold reached, the action potential drives signal relay and pain.

178 Pharmacology Primer for Medications

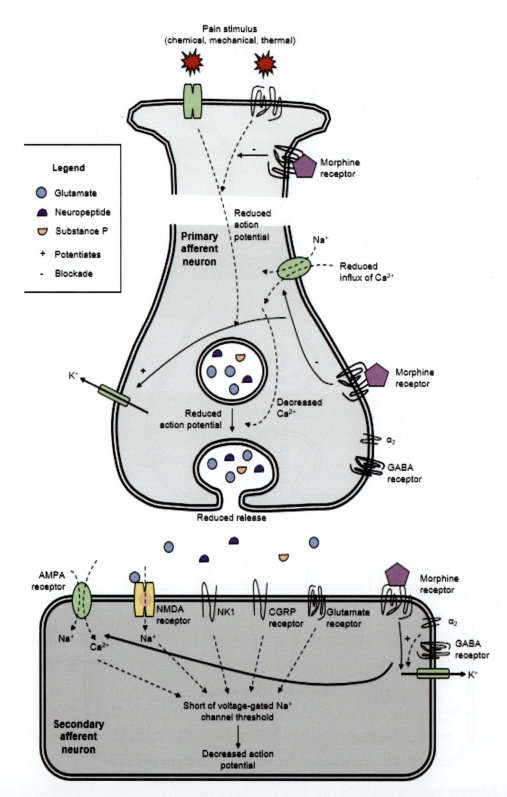

FIGURE 13-2 Schematic representation of the pain stimulus truncated response associated with opioid receptor activation. Activation of opioid receptors in the neuron reduces the initial action potential associated with the primary stimulus and reduces calcium influx in the primary afferent neuron. This decreases the action potential and truncates release of neurotransmitters from the vesicle. Activation of the morphine receptor on the secondary afferent neuron increases potassium efflux, which reduces sodium and calcium influx to limit attainment of the voltage-gate potential and, as a result, reduces the action potential relayed and subsequent pain sensation.

Opioids produce central effects and peripheral effects. Central effects of opioids include analgesia, cough suppression, respiratory depression, sedation, euphoria, dysphoria, miosis, nausea, hypotension, bradycardia, and both tolerance and dependence. Peripheral effects of opioid receptor agonists include decreased gut motility and constipation, sphincter spasm, suppression of spinal reflexes, and histamine release (itching and bronchoconstriction). The most significant adverse reactions from opioids are respiratory suppression, oversedation, dysphoria, constipation, nausea, tolerance, and dependence. Overdose leading to fatality is generally associated with respiratory depression. Interactions between opioid medications and other drugs include the following:

- Alcohol and other CNS depressants increase CNS depression, hypotension, and respiratory depression.
- Opioid agonists or partial agonists cause an additive effect.
- Opioid antagonists can produce withdrawal symptoms if used concurrently.
- Monoamine oxidase inhibitors (MAOIs) enhance the effects of opioids.
- Diltiazem, erythromycin, and fluconazole can inhibit metabolism, increasing concentration.
- Rifampicin can enhance metabolism, decreasing concentration.
- Methadone can have its metabolism enhanced and concentration decreased by a large number of medications, including but not limited to anticonvulsants, antivirals, antifungals, rifampicin, and St John's wort.

A significant issue for opioid medications is potential for developing dependence and tolerance. *Tolerance* means that increasing doses are required to gain the same effect; it can develop within a few days of commencing opioid management and in some cases within 12 to 24 hours. *Dependence* has two components. The first is the physical dependence associated with withdrawal of the medication that produces physiological effects (e.g., irritability, weight loss). The impact of withdrawal depends on the length of opioid use, but signs are apparent even after a short course of pain management (e.g., 2–3 days). The second is the psychological dependence, and this is responsible for addiction. The impact of both tolerance and dependence depend on the treatment regime. For opioid management of acute episodes of pain, tolerance and dependence are a less significant consideration. In chronic pain management, including many patients presenting to the nuclear medicine or radiology department, careful attention needs to be given to these issues. Indeed, the use of radionuclides, such as 89-strontium chloride for palliation of painful bone metastases, is often associated with failure of high doses of mixed opioid medications as a result of tolerance. As doses increase, so do the effects peripherally and centrally; in some cases, the non-pain-related effects are unacceptable to patients. For example, a highly sedated patient may survive to a family milestone event but will not be physically or mentally immersed in the event.

Anti-Inflammatory Mediators in Pain Management

NSAIDs and aspirin (see Table 13-3) have three main effects: reduce inflammation, reduce fever, and reduce some specific types of pain. They also tend to cause gastric irritation, promote bleeding, and pose a risk in renal insufficiency. Among NSAIDs, cyclooxygenase (*COX*) selectivity of medications governs clinical use. COX-1 action is associated with homeostatic functions, gastric irritation, renal effects, and platelet function, while COX-2 action is associated with inflammatory inhibition. This perhaps gives an insight into both usefulness for pain relief and adverse effect profile:

- Ketorolac and flurbiprofen are very selective for COX-1.
- Aspirin, ibuprofen, and naproxen and weakly selective for COX-1.
- Fenoprofen and salicylate are nonselective.
- Diclofenac and celecoxib are weakly COX-2 selective.
- Valdecoxib and etoricoxib are very COX-2 selective.

TABLE 13-3 Comparison of Various NSAID Medications

Medication	Use	Administration/Dose	Precautions	Adverse Effects
All of the below	Mild to moderate nociceptive pain		Allergy, cardiovascular risk, asthma, coagulation disorders, peptic ulcer, gastrointestinal (GI) bleeding, renal impairment, liver dysfunction	Nausea, dyspepsia, GI ulceration, bleeding, headache, dizziness, hypertension
Aspirin (300 mg tablets)	In patients over 12 y	300 mg orally every 4–6 h as required	Gout, pregnancy, breast-feeding; increased risk in elderly; risk of Reye syndrome in children	Tinnitus, skin reactions, bronchospasm, angioedema, urticaria with allergy
Ibuprofen (200 mg tablets)	Osteoarthritis, rheumatoid arthritis, inflammatory pain	400 mg 3–4 times daily to a maximum of 2,400 mg daily; take with food	Low-dose aspirin	
Naproxen (250 and 500 mg tablets or 750 and 1,000 mg controlled-release tablets)	Osteoarthritis, rheumatoid arthritis, inflammatory pain	250–500 mg twice daily or 750–100 mg once daily of controlled-release formulation; maximum of 1,250 mg daily	Take with food	Pseudoporphyria
Meloxicam (7.5 mg or 15 mg capsule)	Rheumatoid arthritis, osteoarthritis	7.5–15 mg once daily	Not for cardiac pain	15 mg has better pain relief but also higher GI adverse effects
Diclofenac (12.5 mg, 25 mg, 50 mg tablets)	Rheumatoid arthritis, osteoarthritis, inflammatory pain	75–150 mg daily in 2–3 doses; maximum of 200 mg daily	Proctitis	
Celecoxib (100 mg or 200 mg capsules)	Rheumatoid arthritis, osteoarthritis, dysmenorrhea, postsurgery; not suitable for coronary pain	200–400 mg daily in 1 or 2 doses; do not use >200 mg daily long term	Heart failure, angina, vascular disease	Dose related
Etoricoxib (30 mg, 60 mg, 120 mg tablets)	Osteoarthritis, gout, acute pain	30–60 mg once daily; 120 mg once daily for maximum of 8 d for gout	Heart failure, hypertension	

TABLE 13-3 Comparison of Various NSAID Medications

Medication	Use	Administration/Dose	Precautions	Adverse Effects
Acetaminophen (paracetamol) (500 mg tablets or 665 mg controlled-release tablets)	Chronic bone pain as in osteoarthritis; no anti-inflammatory effect, so best used with regular and maximal dose	1 g orally every 6 h to maximum of 4 g daily or 1,330 mg every 8 h	Sodium restriction; safe in pregnancy and breast-feeding	Hepatotoxicity
Codeine/aspirin combination (8 mg/300 mg)	Mild to moderate pain	1–2 tablets every 4 h to a maximum of 8 tablets daily	Constipation	Renal dysfunction, pregnancy
Codeine/ibuprofen combination (12.8 mg/200 mg)	Mild to moderate pain	1–2 tablets every 4–6 h to a maximum of 6 tablets daily	Constipation	Renal dysfunction, pregnancy
Codeine/acetaminophen (paracetamol) combination (8 mg/500 mg)	Mild to moderate pain	1–2 tablets every 4–6 h to a maximum of 8 tablets daily	Constipation	Renal dysfunction, pregnancy
Codeine/acetaminophen (paracetamol) combination (15 mg/500 mg)	Mild to moderate pain	1–2 tablets every 4–6 h to a maximum of 8 tablets daily	Constipation	Renal dysfunction, pregnancy
Codeine/acetaminophen (paracetamol) combination (30 mg/500 mg)	Mild to moderate pain	1–2 tablets every 4–6 h to a maximum of 8 tablets daily	Constipation	Renal dysfunction, pregnancy

The bulk of unwanted side effects from NSAIDs are associated with COX-1, especially with long-term use. These include dyspepsia, nausea, vomiting, skin reactions, renal insufficiency, nephropathy, bronchospasm, liver disorders, and bone marrow depression.

Prostaglandins (PGs) do not produce pain but instead enhance pain mediators. PGs are chemical mediators produced by the release of arachidonic acid in response to inflammation and metabolism by COX-2. PG_2 significantly enhances the pain-producing effects of other mediators released in response to tissue injury by macrophages, mast cells, T cells, and neutrophils, including bradykinin (BK), 5-hydroxytryptamine (5-HT), tumor necrosis factor alpha (TNF-α), nerve growth factor (NGF), interleukin, and histamine (Fig. 13-3). This action increases the action potential in the primary afferent neuron to enhance the pain stimulus. NSAIDs and aspirin block the action of COX-2, inhibiting PG formation and reducing the action potential and subsequent pain stimuli (Fig. 13-4). PGs are part of the sensitizing agents depicted in Figure 13-1.

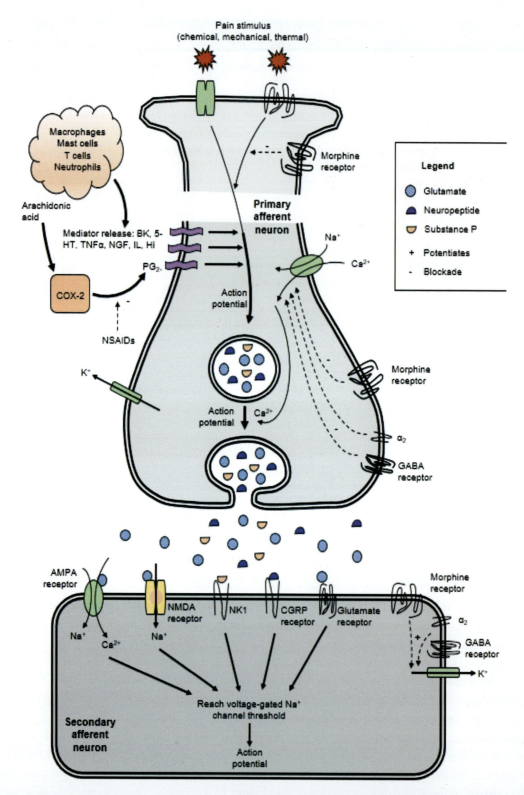

FIGURE 13-3 Schematic representation of the response to chemical, mechanical or thermal pain stimulus. PGs are chemical mediators produced by the release of arachidonic acid in response to inflammation and metabolism by COX-2. PG_2 significantly enhances the pain producing effects of other mediators released in response to tissue injury by macrophages, mast cells, T cells and neutrophils, including BK, 5-HT, TNF-α, NGF, interleukin, and histamine.

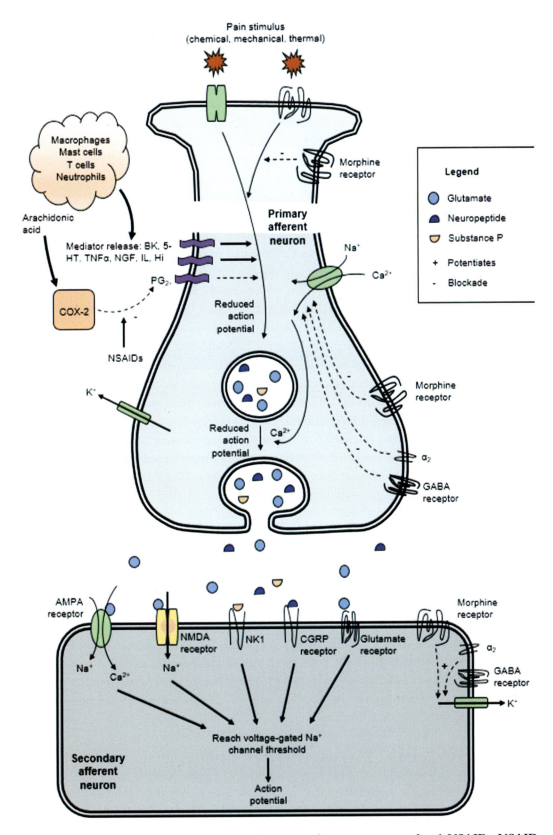

FIGURE 13-4 Schematic representation of the pain stimulus truncated response associated with NSAIDs. NSAIDs and aspirin block the action of COX-2, inhibiting PG formation and reducing the action potential and subsequent pain stimuli.

Aspirin is analgesic, anti-inflammatory, and antipyretic (fever) but also comes in a mini-dose form (81–120 mg) for cardioprotective effects associated with antiplatelet activity. As an analgesic, it is indicated for mild to moderate pain, osteoarthritis, and rheumatoid arthritis. While the additional anti-inflammatory and cardioprotective effects offer an advantage over acetaminophen (paracetamol), the potential adverse effects associated with gastric irritation, nausea, and bleeding risk may be a barrier to more widespread use. Orally administered aspirin is rapidly absorbed from both stomach and intestines with a peak in serum levels at 20 to 40 minutes. Stomach absorption (aspirin is acidic) is an important differentiator and reason aspirin is often taken dissolved in water. Aspirin undergoes metabolism to the active salicylate, which has 50% to 90% plasma protein binding and peak serum levels at 2 to 4 hours after oral administration of aspirin. Salicylate is metabolized by the liver into inactive metabolites. Interestingly, the plasma concentrations required for analgesic (and antipyretic) effects are much lower (28%) than those required for anti-inflammatory effects and just 14% of the toxic concentration levels. The half clearance time of aspirin is dose dependent (by virtue of metabolism) with 3 hours for doses less than 600 mg, 5 hours for 1 g dose, and 9 hours for 2 g. Aspirin has the potential for drug-drug interactions with drugs affecting blood clotting, renal function, and blood glucose. Aspirin also interacts with medication used to manage heart failure and hypertension and specifically with NSAIDs, corticosteroids, and valproate. Aspirin should be used with caution in patients with heart failure, hypertension, renal dysfunction, asthma, peptic ulcer, severe liver disease, bleeding conditions, or during surgery. It should not be used in children under 12 years, and some recommendations suggest it should be used only in adults over 18 years. It should also be avoided in pregnancy (particularly last trimester) and if previous allergy or significant adverse effects have been experienced.

Ibuprofen is an NSAID with analgesic properties indicated for mild to moderate pain, inflammatory pain, osteoarthritis, rheumatoid arthritis, and migraine. Common adverse effects include dizziness, gastric pain, and nausea, but ibuprofen is well tolerated. Orally administered ibuprofen is rapidly absorbed from the duodenum (enteric coated) with a peak in serum levels at 1 to 2 hours (delayed by food), although onset of action occurs within 1 hour. Ibuprofen undergoes extensive metabolism, which leaves virtually no unchanged drug in urine. Ibuprofen has 98% plasma protein binding, and the half clearance time is 1.8 to 2.4 hours. Ibuprofen has the potential for drug-drug interactions with angiotensin-converting enzyme (ACE) inhibitors, angiotensin receptor blockers (ARBs), aspirin, diuretics, H_2 antihistamines, lithium, warfarin, and methotrexate. Ibuprofen should be used with caution in patients with cardiovascular risk, heart failure, edema, hypertension, renal dysfunction, asthma, peptic ulcer, liver dysfunction, bleeding conditions, or coronary artery bypass grafting (CABG). It should not be used in infants under 6 months but has been widely used and recommended in children. It should also be avoided in the 3rd trimester of pregnancy and if previous allergy or significant adverse effects have been experienced.

Acetaminophen (paracetamol) is not technically an NSAID, although it tends to be grouped with them in discussion around pain management. Like aspirin and ibuprofen, acetaminophen (paracetamol) has antipyretic and analgesic effects, but it does not have anti-inflammatory properties. While the mechanism of PG inhibition is via COX-2, the mechanism of action is not fully understood. Acetaminophen (paracetamol) analgesic properties are indicated for mild to moderate, noninflammatory pain such as in osteoarthritis. Acetaminophen (paracetamol) has a superior safety profile compared to aspirin and NSAIDs, with rare allergy and adverse reactions; low risk of gastric irritation or bleeding; minimal potential for drug interactions (low plasma protein binding); and safe use in pregnancy, breast-feeding, and children. Within recommended dosage, adverse effects are rare, but overdose can cause toxicity and acute liver failure (Fig. 13-5). Orally administered acetaminophen (paracetamol) is rapidly and completely absorbed from the gut, with 70% to 90% bioavailability and a peak in serum levels at 10 to 60 minutes (delayed by food). Acetaminophen (paracetamol) undergoes extensive liver metabolism by hepatic microsomal enzymes, including to potentially toxic metabolites (Fig. 13-5). Ninety-five percent is eliminated as metabolites in urine within 24 hours. Acetaminophen (paracetamol) has negligible plasma protein binding, and the half clearance time is 1 to 3 hours. It has low potential for drug-drug interactions but may prolong bleeding times in warfarin use. Acetaminophen (paracetamol) should be used with caution in patients with renal or liver dysfunction.

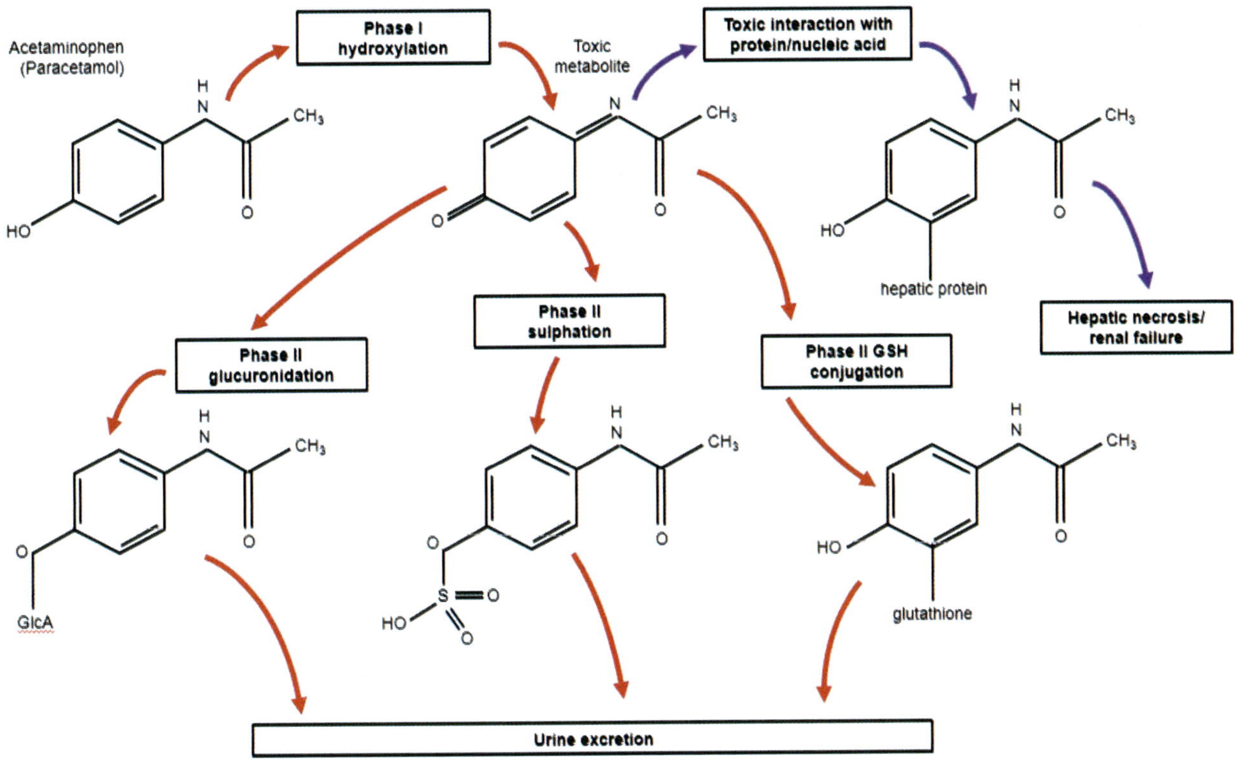

FIGURE 13-5 Phase I and phase II metabolism of acetaminophen (paracetamol). Phase I hydroxylation results in a toxic metabolite with three forms of phase II metabolism converting the metabolite to a form for urine excretion. Toxic interaction can occur, leading to liver necrosis and potentially to renal failure.

Adjunctive Pain Medications

There are a number of other medications that can be used for their analgesic properties. Tricyclic antidepressants such as amitriptyline inhibit norepinephrine reuptake, and as a result, the increased activation of α_2-receptors (Figs. 13-1 and 13-2) decreases calcium influx. The decreased calcium influx, as with opioid agonists, decreases the action potential, neurotransmitter release, and pain. The anticonvulsant medication gabapentin, carbamazepine, and phenytoin have been used for pain management. Carbamazepine and phenytoin act directly on the voltage-gate sodium channels. Gabapentin and pregabalin are GABA analogs that decrease calcium influx via activation of the GABA receptor (Figs. 13-1 and 13-2) to reduce the action potential. This action makes them useful in neuropathic pain such as diabetic neuropathy. Ketamine is an anesthetic that can block the NMDA receptor to inhibit sodium influx and truncate voltage-gate sodium channel and the action potential.

Pain Prevention with Anesthetics

Local anesthetics are used in nuclear medicine and radiology primarily to provide pain prophylaxis for potentially painful procedures (e.g., biopsy or lumbar puncture). Topical local anesthetics are sometimes used in children or those with *trypanophobia* to provide decreased sensation at the injection site. The general mode of action for local anesthetics needs consideration of the action potential and voltage-gated sodium channel discussed previously. As shown in Figure 13-6, under resting conditions (potential), the sodium channel is closed. The internal negative environment and positive external environment also leave the voltage-gated potassium channel closed. In response to pain stimulus, neurotransmitters stimulate the opening of the sodium channel (Fig. 13-7). As sodium moves into the cell, the internal environment becomes less negative and drives complete opening of the sodium channel, allowing sodium to rush in, satisfying the voltage-gate threshold, and causing depolarization. This produces an action potential that is transmitted along the axon. The voltage-gated potassium channel responds to the change to internal charge and opens for potassium outflow and repolarization. To prevent pain transmission, local anesthetic can be injected (Fig. 13-8) which can diffuse across the cell membrane. Pain stimulus will continue to cause the sodium channel to open, but the local anesthetic migrates to the sodium channel and reversibly blocks sodium influx. Consequently, the voltage-gate threshold is not met, depolarization does not occur, and the action potential is not generated. Given that the internal environment does not change charge, there is no driver for opening of the potassium channel or repolarization.

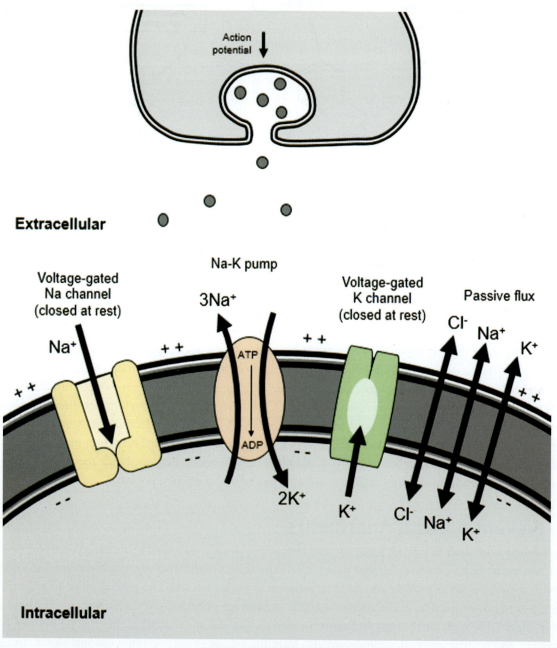

FIGURE 13-6 Schematic representation of the voltage-gated sodium channel at rest.

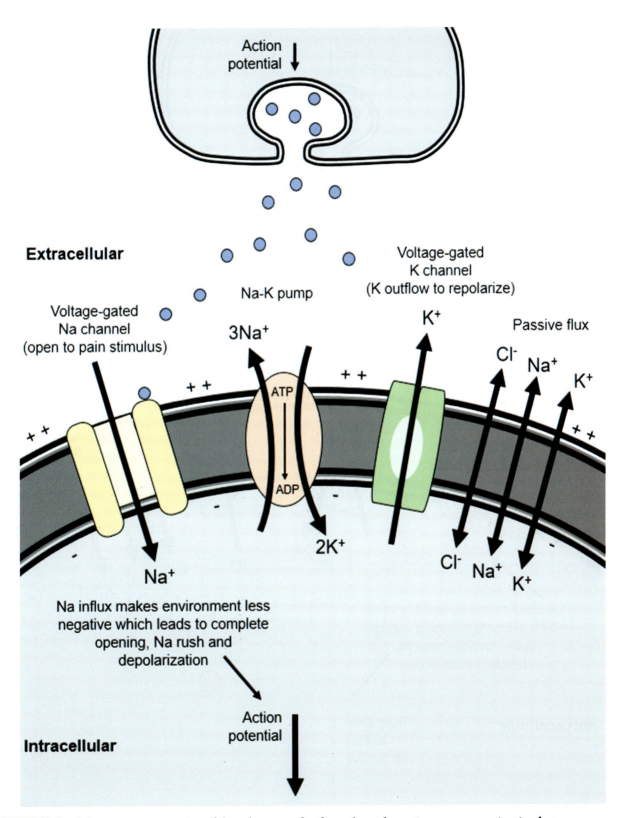

FIGURE 13-7 Schematic representation of the voltage-gated sodium channel open in response to pain stimulus.

188 Pharmacology Primer for Medications

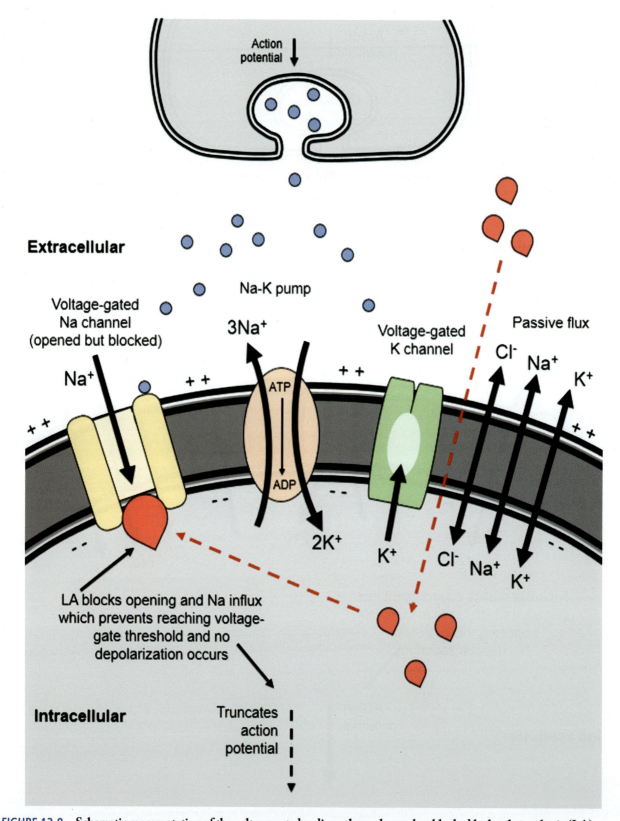

FIGURE 13-8 Schematic representation of the voltage-gated sodium channel open but blocked by local anesthetic (LA).

Lidocaine is the prototype local *anesthetic* designed to reversibly inhibit initiation and conduction of peripheral nerve impulses by blocking sodium channels and preventing depolarization (Figs. 13-6, 13-7, and 13-8). In this capacity, it can be administered parenterally into target tissue, topically, intrathecally, or as an epidural. Onset of action is rapid but dependent on dose (volume and concentration) and route of administration. The duration of effect is generally 1 to 1.5 hours, although it is variable based on total drug dose (rather than volume or concentration). After the drug is absorbed into general circulation (or after intravenous administration), it is metabolized in the liver and eliminated via the kidneys with a half clearance time of 1.5 to 2 hours. Adverse reactions tend to relate to high doses, rapid absorption, or delayed elimination with impacts on CNS, cardiac, and respiratory depression. Clearance can be delayed by β-blockers, cimetidine, erythromycin, and itraconazole. Lidocaine and its cardiac effects can be potentiated by other antiarrhythmic medications, phenytoin, and alcohol. Doses should be reduced in children and the elderly. It should be used with caution in neurological, cardiac, liver, or kidney disease; in known hypersensitivity; and in shock or hypotension. It is contraindicated for use in tissue that is inflamed or septic. Dosage depends on the dose form:

- Up to 200 mg (40 mL of 0.5%, 20 mL of 1%, or 10 mL of 2%) infiltration injection in and around the site requiring local anesthesia (e.g., biopsy site)
- 2% gel applied for urinary catheterization lubrication and anesthesia
- 4% topical liquid applied to a site requiring numbing (e.g., injection site)

For those chemically curious, the resemblance of the lidocaine chemical structure to that of biliary imaging agents (iminodiacetic acid derivatives) can be readily explained. The cardiac effects of lidocaine at some point historically justified radiolabeling with technetium-99m (^{99m}Tc). While the end product was not a useful cardiac imaging agent, biliary excretion was noted. ^{99m}Tc hepatobiliary iminodiacetic acid (HIDA) is essentially 2 analogs of lidocaine chelated to ^{99m}Tc.

There are a number of other local anesthetics generally classified by duration of action. Short-acting local anesthetics have a duration of effect of 0.5 to 1 hours, tend to be ester based (leading to rapid plasma metabolism and shorter duration of action), have potential for toxicity (associated with rapid metabolism), and include benzocaine and cocaine. Long-acting local anesthetics have a duration of effect of 3 to 10 hours, which increases systemic toxicity and potential for cardiac effects; tend to be of higher potency than lidocaine (4- to 5-fold), and include bupivacaine (amide metabolized in plasma) and amethocaine (ester metabolized in the liver). Intermediate-acting local anesthetics have a duration of effect of 0.5 to 4 hours, tend to be amide based (leading to slower liver metabolism and longer duration of action than esters), have lower potential for toxicity, and include lidocaine, prilocaine, and mepivacaine.

Used as an infiltration local anesthetic, lidocaine may be used in combination with epinephrine (adrenaline) in various concentration combinations (e.g., 1% lidocaine, 1:200,000 epinephrine). If combined with epinephrine, it should not be injected into fingers, toes, nose, ears, or genitals. The small region surrounding the key area (e.g., biopsy site) is injected into the skin and progresses to subcutaneous tissue with the dilute lidocaine. A small area may require only a single puncture, while a larger area may need multiple punctures across the region. Repeat injections can be used to extend the duration of effect if required.

Prilocaine is most commonly used in combination (2.5%:2.5%) with lidocaine as cream or patch (eutectic mixture of local anesthetics [EMLA]). EMLA cream is often used to desensitize tissue prior to injection in children or those with a phobia. In some regards, reliance on EMLA reinforces the fear of an impending painful experience. The EMLA has a duration of effect of 0.5 to 2 hours after the cream is removed and can cause local skin irritation, bleaching, or edema.

References

Asperheim K, Favaro J. *Introduction to Pharmacology*. 12th ed. St Louis, MO: Elsevier; 2012.

Block JH, Beale JM. *Wilson and Gisvold's Textbook of Organic Medicinal and Pharmaceutical Chemistry*. 12th ed. Philadelphia, PA: Lippincott Williams & Wilkins; 2011.

Bryant B, Knights K, Salerno E. *Pharmacology for Health Professionals*. 2nd ed. Sydney, Australia: Mosby Elsevier; 2007.

Golan DE, Tashjian AH, Armstrong EJ, Armstrong AW. *Principles of Pharmacology: The Pathophysiologic Basis of Drug Therapy*. 3rd ed. Philadelphia, PA: Lippincott Williams & Wilkins; 2012.

Greenstein B. *Rapid Revision in Clinical Pharmacology*. New York, NY: Radcliffe Publishing; 2008.

Hacker M, Messer W, Bachmann K. *Pharmacology: Principles and Practice*. London, England: Elsevier; 2009.

Jambhekar SS, Breen PJ. *Basic Pharmacokinetics*. London, England: Pharmaceutical Press; 2009.

Katzung BG, Masters SB, Trevor AJ. *Basic and Clinical Pharmacology*. 12th ed. New York, NY: McGraw Hill; 2012.

Rang H, Dale M, Ritter J, Flower R. *Rang and Dale's Pharmacology*. 6th ed. London, England: Churchill Livingston; 2008.

Waller D, Renwick A, Hillier K. *Medical Pharmacology and Therapeutics*. 2nd ed. London, England: Elsevier; 2006.

CHAPTER 14

Chemotherapy

Chapter Objectives

Specific learning outcomes (page ix) of this text addressed in this chapter:

- Apply the pharmacokinetic and pharmacodynamic principles of medications to identify and explain normal and adverse reactions to medications.

After reading, digesting, reflecting on, and reviewing the content of this chapter, readers should be able to

1. Demonstrate command of key pharmacology terms.
2. Demonstrate enhanced understanding of the principles associated with the pharmacology of chemotherapy agents.
3. Demonstrate understanding of the mode of action, pharmacokinetics, risks, precautions, contraindications, adverse effects, interactions, and appropriate dosage of key chemotherapy agents.
4. Apply knowledge of the general principles and concepts in a translational manner to clinical practice.

Key Terms

angiogenesis	anti-inflammatory	cytotoxicity	monoclonal antibody	pyrimidine
antigen	bactericidal	folic acid	multidrug resistance	replication
apoptosis	bacteriostatic	inhibition	mutation	synthesis
antiandrogen	chemotherapy	immunotherapy	proliferation	theranostic
antiestrogen	cytotoxic	metastases	purine	

Introduction

While chemotherapy is generally associated with treatment of cancer (medical oncology), the term actually is more broadly defined as those agents that are selectively toxic to pathogens or tumors. This chapter focuses on chemotherapy in oncology as it relates more closely to the practice of medical radiation science. Nonetheless, the chapter introduces concepts in chemotherapy associated with infective agents, which are also important in the medical imaging patient cohort. The molecular basis of chemotherapy, particularly for pathogens, depends on the type of cell. Bacteria, for example, are prokaryotes (no nuclei); protozoa, fungi, and helminths are eukaryotes (cells with nuclei); viruses are their own special category because they do not meet the definition of a cell; and then there are cancer cells. Since viruses rely on the metabolic mechanisms of the host cells and cancer cells closely resemble the normal cell, selective toxicity can be challenging.

Pathogens

For bacteria, there are a number of effective approaches to chemotherapy:

- Interference with the synthesis or action of folate using sulfonamides or trimethoprim
- Beta (β)-lactam antibiotics such as penicillin and cephalosporins
- Interference with protein synthesis using tetracyclines, aminoglycosides, and macrolides
- Other mechanisms not meeting these categories

Sulfonamides are p-aminobenzoic acid analogs. Since p-aminobenzoic acid is a precursor for folic acid and bacteria need to produce folic acid to replicate, sulfonamides inhibit bacterial growth. This is an important distinction because this class of antibiotic is not bactericidal but rather *bacteriostatic*, slowing replication rather than killing cells. β-Lactam antibiotics inhibit cell wall synthesis, causing bacteria lysis, which means they are *bactericidal*. This is a common class of antibiotic for the medical imaging patient because bactericidal antibiotics are used to treat bone and joint infections, pneumonia, and urinary tract infections, which are common among the radiology and nuclear medicine patient cohort. Antibiotics that interfere with protein synthesis are bacteriostatic and can inhibit protein synthesis using encoding errors, inhibiting transpeptidation, producing premature termination of peptide chains, or inhibiting translocation.

While patients present to radiology and nuclear medicine with viral infections (e.g., HIV or hepatitis B), medical imaging is less directly connected to viral infections. Nonetheless, comorbidity may be a referral point (e.g., secondary lung infections in patients with HIV, liver imaging in patients with hepatitis B). There are a number of chemotherapy approaches to managing viral infections:

- Reverse transcription inhibitors
- Protease inhibitors
- Polymerase inhibitors
- Integrase inhibitors
- Neuraminidase inhibitors
- Immunomodulators

Cancer

Cancer is certainly the most common underlying pathology in the nuclear medicine department and probably across all medical imaging. Therapeutic nuclear medicine and radiation therapy ensure that oncology and medical oncology are important considerations. Some of the mechanisms discussed here are shared between radionuclide therapy and medical oncology and, indeed, with new forms of molecular targeting in diagnostic nuclear medicine. A simple perspective of medical oncology and drug targets in cancer are the hallmarks of cancer:

- Proliferation targeted by epidermal growth factor receptor (EGRF) inhibitors
- Evasion of growth suppression targeted by cyclin-dependent kinase inhibitors
- Avoiding immune destruction targeted by immune activating monoclonal antibodies (MAbs)

- Replication targeted by telomerase inhibitors
- Tumor-promoting inflammation targeted by anti-inflammatory drugs
- Invasion and metastases targeted by human growth factor (HGF) inhibitors
- Angiogenesis targeted by vascular endothelial growth factor (VEGF) signaling inhibitors
- Mutation targeted by poly (ADP ribose) polymerase (PARP) inhibitors
- Resisting cell death targeted by proapoptotic B-cell lymphoma 2 homology 3 (BH3) mimetics
- Deregulation of cellular energetics targeted by aerobic glycolysis inhibitors

These hallmarks are the target of theranostics with localization of diagnostic and therapeutic tracers exploiting molecular changes associated with one or more of these mechanisms, such as targeting receptors overexpressed on the tumor cell surface associated with proliferation or apoptosis. *Theranostics* is perhaps a little simpler given that the target is not to inhibit one of these hallmarks but rather to exploit the hallmark to preferentially accumulate a particle-emitting therapeutic radionuclide for radiation ablation of the cell and, hopefully, cell death. Chemotherapy may utilize similar mechanisms to selectively localize in tumor cells, but chemotherapy agents need to disrupt one or more of the mechanisms driving the hallmarks of cancer. While new chemotherapy agents are being developed regularly, a general summary of major chemotherapy agents includes the following (Table 14-1):

- Cytotoxic agents interfere with tumor cell proliferation or replication. Bone marrow suppression and renal and hepatic toxicity are typical in this class of agent. Methotrexate (Fig. 14-1) and docetaxel (drives apoptosis and inhibits cell survival pathways) are 2 common drugs among many in this class.
- Hormone agents interfere with hormone-dependent tumor growth. Antiandrogen hormone therapy in castrate-resistant prostate cancer is a common example in medical radiation science patients. Somatostatin analogs have emerged more recently and link to theranostics, but the most widely known hormone therapy is the antiestrogen tamoxifen.
- Immunotherapy agents interfere with cell surface antigens to cause a variety of molecular changes such as apoptosis, angiogenesis inhibition, or enhanced immune response against the cancer cell. The MAbs rituximab and trastuzumab are common examples.
- Targeted chemoagents inhibit key cell surface receptors. Gefitinib and imatinib inhibition of tyrosine kinase is a good example.

Methotrexate is a folic acid antagonist (Fig. 14-1) that impairs DNA and RNA synthesis by inhibiting dihydrofolate. This inhibition is why methotrexate is sometimes used for other pathologies with excessive proliferation (e.g., psoriasis). It also has immunosuppressant properties that produce the unwanted side effect in cancer therapy but is a potential therapy for autoimmune disorders. Methotrexate can be administered orally, intramuscularly, intravenously, or intrathecally. After oral administration, peak serum levels occur after 1 to 2 hours, about 50% is plasma protein bound, and almost 100% is eliminated unchanged via the kidneys. Methotrexate is associated with increased risk of hepatotoxicity when used concurrently with other hepatotoxic drugs or medications (e.g., alcohol). Additive effects are noted with other immunosuppressants or bone marrow depressants and other antiplatelet drugs (e.g., NSAIDs). Enhanced toxicity occurs when used with other antifolate drugs (e.g., sulfonamides), and salicylates can prolong excretion of methotrexate, which increases serum levels. The main adverse reactions include bone marrow and immune suppression, hair loss, nausea, vomiting, anorexia, gastrointestinal ulcers, and with longer regimes, hepatotoxicity, pneumonitis, pulmonary fibrosis, and infertility. High doses can also cause severe skin reactions and renal failure.

TABLE 14-1 Summary of the Main Drugs Used for Cancer Treatment (Not an Exhaustive List)

Class	Drug	Mechanism	Type of Cancer Treated	Acute Toxicity
Alkylating	Busulfan	Inhibits DNA synthesis by crosslink formation	CML	Nausea, vomiting
	Mechlorethamine, chlorambucil, carmustine		HD, NHL	
	Cyclophosphamide		Breast, ovarian, NHL, neuroblastoma	
	Melphalan		Multiple myeloma, breast, ovarian	
	Thiotepa		Breast, ovarian	
	Lomustine		Brain	
	Altretamine		Ovarian	
Platinum analog	Cisplatin, carboplatin		NSCLC; SCLC; breast, bladder, ovarian, head/neck	
	Oxaliplatin		Colorectal, pancreatic	
Antimetabolite	Capecitabine	Inhibits DNA synthesis	Breast, colorectal, pancreatic	Nausea, diarrhea, myelosuppression
	5-Fluorouracil			
	Methotrexate		Breast, head/neck, CNS lymphoma, NHL, bladder	Diarrhea, myelosuppression, neutropenia, thrombocythemia
	Cytarabine	Inhibits DNA synthesis and repair	CML, acute lymphoblastic leukemia	
	Gemcitabine		Pancreatic, bladder, NSCLC, ovarian, NHL	Nausea, diarrhea, myelosuppression
	Cladribine		Hairy cell leukemia, NHL	Myelosuppression, nausea, vomiting
Vinca alkaloid	Vinblastine	Inhibits mitosis	HD, NHL, breast	Nausea, vomiting
	Vincristine		HD, NHL, neuroblastoma	Minimal
	Vinorelbine		NSCLC, breast, ovarian	Nausea, vomiting
Taxane	Paclitaxel		Breast, NSCLC, prostate, ovarian, head/neck	Hypersensitivity
	Docetaxel			Nausea, hypotension, arrythmia, hypersensitivity
Cytotoxic antibiotic	Doxorubicin	DNA breaks from free radical binding	Breast, HD, NHL, ovarian, NSCLC, SCLC, neuroblastoma	Nausea
	Mitoxantrone		AML, prostate, NHL	Myelosuppression, neutropenia

TABLE 14-1 Summary of the Main Drugs Used for Cancer Treatment (Not an Exhaustive List)

Class	Drug	Mechanism	Type of Cancer Treated	Acute Toxicity
	Mitomycin		Bladder, breast, NSCLC, head/neck	Nausea
	Bleomycin		HD, NHL, head/neck	Allergy, fever, hypotension
Topoisomerase inhibitor	Etoposide	Inhibits topoisomerase II	NSCLC, SCLC, NHL	Nausea, vomiting, hypotension
	Irinotecan	Inhibits topoisomerase I	Colorectal, NSCLC, SCLC	Diarrhea, nausea, vomiting
	Topotecan		SCLC, ovarian	Nausea, vomiting
Receptor inhibitor	Imatinib	Tyrosine kinase inhibitors	CML, GIST	
	Erlotinib		NSCLC, pancreatic	Diarrhea
	Cetuximab	Epidermal growth factor inhibition	Colorectal, head/neck, NSCLC	Infusion reaction
	Panitumumab		Colorectal	
	Sunitinib	Vascular endothelial growth factor inhibition	Renal cell carcinoma, GIST	Hypertension
	Bevacizumab		Colorectal, breast, NSCLC, renal cell carcinoma	
Hormone modulator	Tamoxifen	Estrogen receptor antagonist	Breast	Thrombosis, endometrial changes
	Flutamide	Androgen receptor antagonist	Prostate	Hepatotoxicity
	Octreotide	Somatostatin receptor antagonist	Neuroendocrine tumor	GIT disorders
	Leuprolide	GnRh receptor antagonist	Prostate and breast cancer palliation	Osteoporosis/bone fractures
	Anastrozole	Aromatase inhibitor	Postmenopausal breast	
Immunotherapy	Rituximab	Tumor-specific MAb (anti-CD20)	NHL	Immunosuppression
	Tositumomab			
	Ibritumomab			
Purine analogs	Pentagastrin	Inhibit purine synthesis	Stomach, hairy cell leukemia	Neurotoxicity
	Fludarabine		CML	

Abbreviations: AML, acute myeloid leukemia; CML, chronic myeloid leukemia; CNS, central nervous system; GIST, gastrointestinal stroma tumor; GIT, gastrointestinal tract; GnRh, gonadotropin-releasing hormone; HD, Hodgkin disease, NHL, non-Hodgkin lymphoma; NSCLC, non–small cell lung cancer; SCLC, small cell lung cancer.

196 Pharmacology Primer for Medications

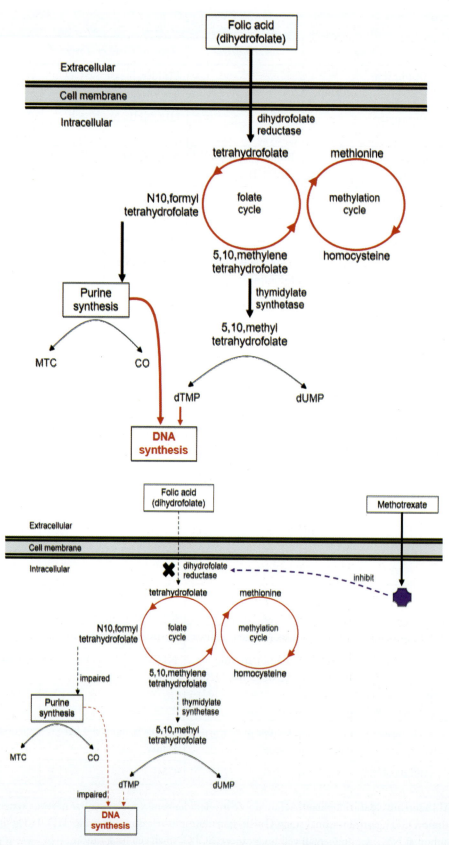

FIGURE 14-1 The folic acid cycle leading to DNA synthesis (top) and the inhibition of proliferation by antagonism of dihydrofolate reductase by methotrexate (bottom).

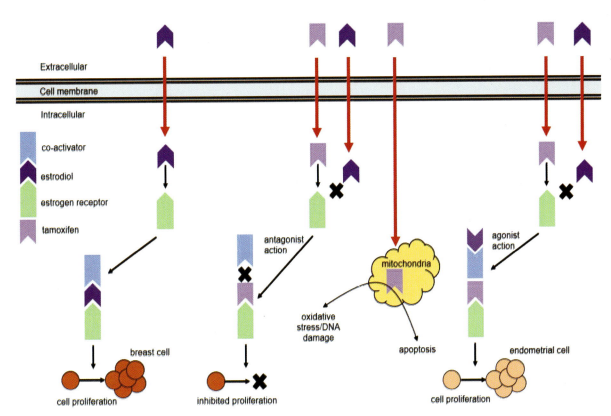

FIGURE 14-2 Schematic representation of the action of tamoxifen as an estrogen receptor antagonist in breast cells (inhibition of cell proliferation). Tamoxifen is cytotoxic via mitochondrial oxidative stress (producing DNA damage) and apoptosis (cell death), and as an agonist in endometrial cells to promote cell proliferation (adverse effect).

Somatostatin analogs warrant a brief discussion because they link closely to theranostics in nuclear medicine. Some types of cancer, such as neuroendocrine tumor, overexpress somatostatin receptors (SSR) on the cell surface. Peptide-receptor principles allow these types of cancers to be preferentially targeted by radiolabeling a diagnostic or therapeutic radionuclide to a peptide that specifically targets that receptor. Indeed, ^{68}Ga-DOTATATE is imaged in positron emission tomography (PET) and is compared to ^{18}F-fluorodeoxyglucose (FDG) PET biodistribution (glucose analog) to tailor therapy. The ^{68}Ga-DOTATATE (octreotate) is specific for SSR_2 (one of 5) and indicates SRR expression. Conversely, ^{18}F-FDG is a marker for proliferation. Thus, high ^{68}Ga-DOTATATE uptake with discordant ^{18}F-FDG results suggests a well-differentiated, slow-growing tumor that is likely to be receptive to either ^{177}Lu-DOTATATE (β-emitting therapy agent) or nonradioactive (cold) octreotide (i.e., hormone therapy). High ^{18}F-FDG uptake in the absence (or discordant) ^{68}Ga-DOTATATE accumulation suggests poorly differentiated, aggressive tumors more suited to molecular agents such as everolimus or sunitinib.

Tamoxifen is an antiestrogen hormone therapy used in estrogen receptor–positive breast cancers. It has both agonist and antagonist activity depending on the receptor (Fig. 14-2). Tamoxifen is administered orally with peak serum levels occur after 3 to 6 hours. A single-dose-per-day regime results in steady state after 4 weeks. It has 99% plasma protein binding and is metabolized in the liver to its active form. Poor metabolism undermines efficacy of therapy. Elimination is via feces, producing a half clearance time of 5 to 7 days. Because tamoxifen is a prodrug, other drugs or conditions that impact liver metabolism can change its metabolism and bioavailability. Cimetidine, terbinafine, fluoxetine, bupropion, paroxetine, and sertraline should be avoided during tamoxifen therapy to avoid increased mortality from breast cancer. Increased bleeding may occur when used with warfarin. Common adverse reactions include hot flushes, endometrial changes, vaginal bleeding, leg cramps, and pneumonitis. If used in a woman of child-bearing age, non-hormone-based contraception should be advised.

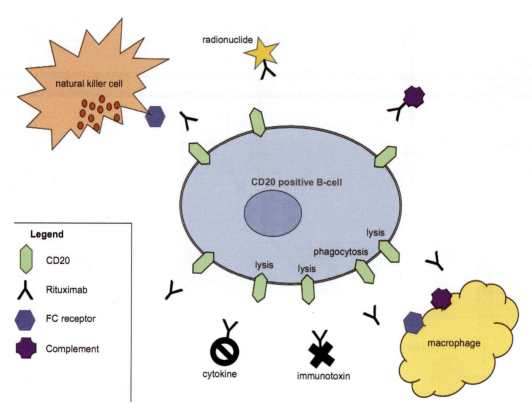

FIGURE 14-3 Schematic representation of a CD20-positive B cell. The CD20 antigen is susceptible to the rituximab Mab, which initiates apoptosis, phagocytosis, and lysis.

Immunotherapy

There are a number of immunotherapy approaches, and once again, immunotherapy shares principles and some agents with radioimmunotherapy (RIT). *Immunotherapy* is a targeting therapy that uses MAbs to target specific cell surface antigens and elicit a response. MAbs can also be labeled to a cytotoxic agent or a radionuclide. The ability for the antibody to specifically bind to a tumor-associated antigen increases the tumor cell targeting while decreasing the impact on normal tissues. The technique requires the tumor cells to express an antigen that is unique to the neoplasm or is inaccessible in normal cells. Some types of cancers, such as follicular non-Hodgkin lymphoma (NHL), have an overexpression of the CD20 antigen. CD20 is a surface molecule expressed on B cells during differentiation and on most mature B-cell cancer cells. CD20 provides an ideal binding site for MAbs such as rituximab and ibritumomab (Figs. 14-3 and 14-4). The antibody-antigen pair produces complement-dependent cytotoxicity, cell-mediated cytotoxicity, and apoptosis. Effectiveness can be enhanced by administering a "cocktail" of MAbs that include the direct-acting "cold" Mab plus MAbs carrying cytotoxic agents, bioactivators, or therapeutic radionuclides. For example, adding a β-emitting radionuclide labeled to a CD20-targeting MAb increases patient response rates from 55% with cold Mab to 83% with the combined therapy. Rituximab has no specific contraindications. A number of potential adverse effects are associated with the infusion: urticaria, hypotension, angioedema, hypoxia, bronchospasm, pulmonary infiltrates, acute respiratory distress syndrome, myocardial infarction, ventricular fibrillation, cardiogenic shock, and anaphylaxis. Severe renal toxicity can develop, and immunological responses can also develop (human antichimeric antibody [HACA]) in 1% of patients.

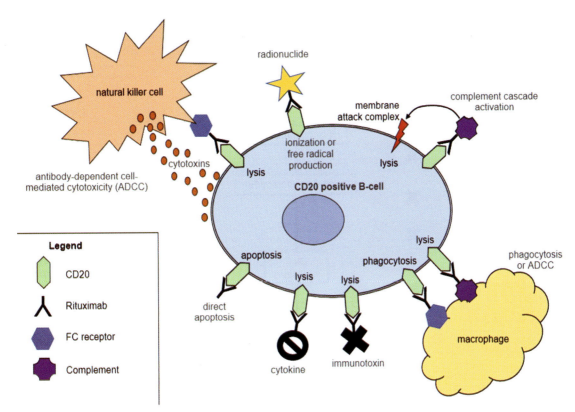

FIGURE 14-4 Schematic representation of a CD20-positive B cell shown in Figure 14-3 after formation of antigen-antibody complexes. Rituximab can produce direct-acting apoptosis, attract natural killer cells to produce cell lysis, attract macrophages for phagocytosis, or activate the complement cascade to cause lysis. Alternatively, Mab can be bound to a radionuclide (therapeutic), immunotoxin, or immunocytokine to initiate cell death.

In medical oncology, it is common for more than 1 drug to be used. Combination therapies are designed to improve response rates, increase cancer cell kill rates, and overcome resistance. Breast cancer, for example, might use a combination of cyclophosphamide, methotrexate, and fluorouracil. An alternative combination regime for breast cancer could be cyclophosphamide, fluorouracil, tamoxifen, and prednisone. Patients may also be prescribed other medications concurrently to help manage adverse effects of the actual treatment. With the exception of immunological agents (MAbs), the major mechanisms for chemotherapy are summarized in Figure 14-5.

Insight

Soft tissue tumors such as parathyroid adenoma, breast cancer, and malignant melanoma accumulate radiopharmaceuticals such as ^{99m}Tc-sestamibi (^{99m}Tc-MIBI). The case (Fig. 14-6) highlights melanoma on resting cardiac imaging that was absent on the stress images performed later the same day. The effects of aminophylline reversal of dipyridamole stress testing was thought to result in rapid efflux of the radiotracer. This requires some consideration within the context of theophylline and caffeine. Phosphodiesterase inhibitors such as sildenafil cause an elevation in intracellular cyclic adenosine monophosphate (cAMP). In normal cells, cAMP plays a role in cell proliferation and differentiation; however, in many cancer cells, cAMP has a negative impact on proliferation. Thus, tumor growth can be retarded in some tumor types by increasing intracellular cAMP with apoptosis within 72 hours and sparing of normal cells. While sildenafil is the more commonly known phosphodiesterase inhibitor, there are a number of other key drugs in this class, including dipyridamole, theophylline, aminophylline, and caffeine. Indeed, theophylline and caffeine have been shown to inhibit cell proliferation and metastatic spread in melanoma. Other studies have shown phosphodiesterase inhibitor tumor proliferation inhibition in lymphoma, lung cancer, spindle cell cancer, breast cancer, and colon cancer.

200 Pharmacology Primer for Medications

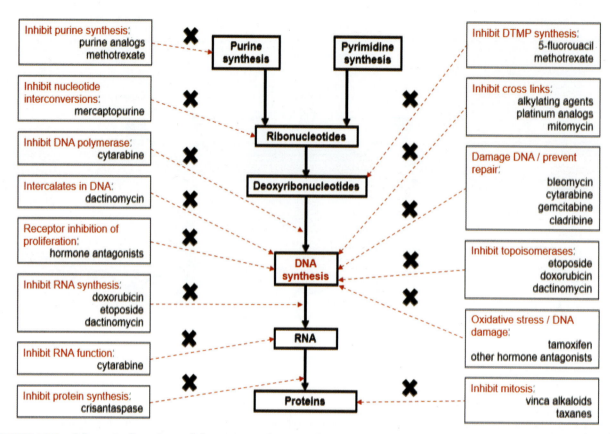

FIGURE 14-5 Schematic flow chart of the main mechanism of antineoplastic activity of the major medications in cancer therapy (excluding immunological approaches). Solid black lines represent the standard pathway in tumor cells for DNA synthesis and proliferation. The red dashed lines identify inhibitory mechanisms.

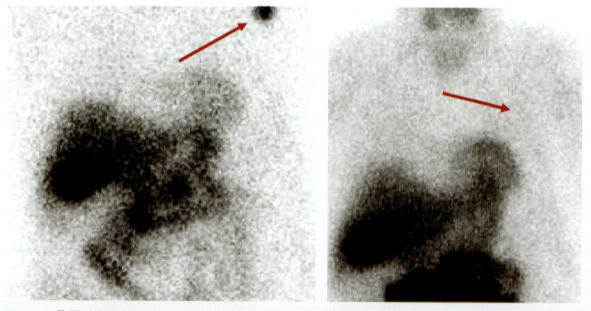

FIGURE 14-6 ^{99m}Tc-MIBI scan at rest (left) and stress (right). On the rest study, incidental extracardiac accumulation was noted and identified as malignant melanoma. The stress study performed later the same day using dipyridamole stress with aminophylline reversal showed absence of both stress dose accumulation and residual rest accumulation due to efflux mediated by dipyridamole.

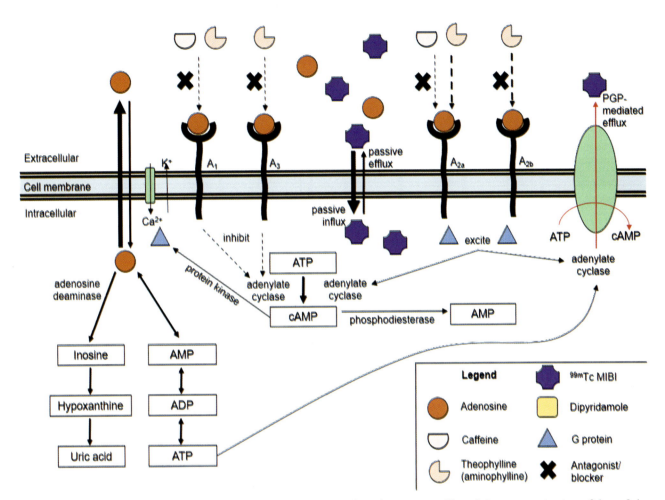

FIGURE 14-7 Schematic representation of ^{99m}Tc-MIBI influx and P-glycoprotein efflux. Adenosine activation of A_1 and A_3 receptors inhibit adenylate cycles while activation of A_2 receptors stimulate adenylate cyclase. With theophylline (all receptors, but higher for A_2) and caffeine (A_1 and A_{2A}) antagonism, there is no upregulation of efflux.

P-glycoprotein and multidrug-resistance protein (MRP1) are overexpressed in some tumors, and this can cause resistance to chemotherapeutic agents, undermining therapy efficacy. ^{99m}Tc-MIBI is a substrate for P-glycoprotein and MRP1, making it useful in evaluating whether tumors are likely to respond to chemotherapy. Tumor cells exhibiting multidrug resistance actively efflux cytotoxic agents from the cytoplasm. P-glycoprotein is part of the adenosine triphosphate (ATP)-binding cassette transmembrane transporter proteins. These have an abundance of ATP-binding sites, and thus, it is possible that increased serum ATP might upregulate P-glycoprotein efflux. Adenosine readily combines with phosphate to form ATP; dipyridamole is a prodrug for increasing serum adenosine levels, and both caffeine and aminophylline competitively inhibit adenosine. While the mechanism for efflux of ^{99m}Tc-MIBI is not known, it was initially suspected to relate to the P-glycoprotein-mediated efflux mechanism known to extend multidrug resistance to some tumors (Fig. 14-7). The elevation of intracellular ATP may upregulate P-glycoprotein efflux, which could be further exacerbated in cells with overexpression of P-glycoprotein.

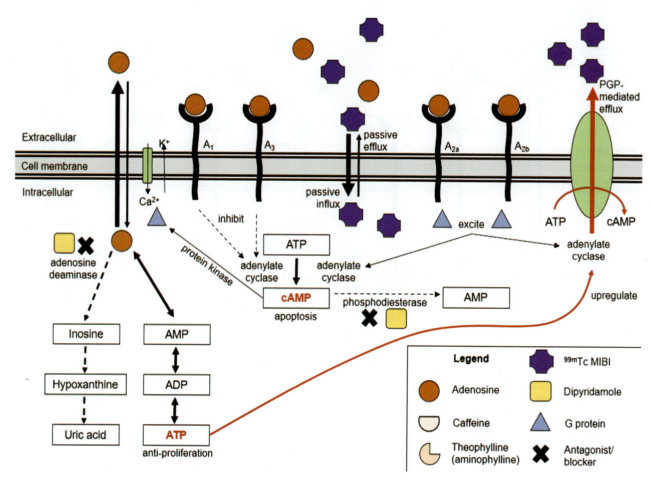

FIGURE 14-8 Schematic representation of ^{99m}Tc-MIBI efflux by P-glycoprotein upregulation resulting from dipyridamole antagonism of adenosine deaminase, increasing intracellular ATP. Phosphodiesterase inhibition also increases cAMP.

Closer consideration of receptor action (Fig. 14-7) revealed that adenosine receptor antagonism by theophylline (all receptors with increase in A_2 inhibition) or caffeine (primarily receptors A_1 and A_{2A}) was unlikely to produce the increase in intracellular ATP to drive increased P-glycoprotein-mediated efflux. As shown in Figure 14-8, dipyridamole itself drives up intracellular ATP and P-glycoprotein-mediated efflux. Indeed, dipyridamole is known for inhibiting tumor growth.

While there has been a history of publications outlining the role of ^{99m}Tc-MIBI in evaluating P-glycoprotein expression in tumors, there is an absence of literature examining the important relationship of purine-mediated ^{99m}Tc-MIBI efflux. The implications are important with the potential for medications altering the relative uptake of MIBI in tumors resulting in false-negative scans in parathyroid adenoma, breast cancer, or metastatic melanoma. Moreover, these same potential confounders could incorrectly stratify on the basis of appropriate therapy.

Case Study

From: "Hormone Therapy in Prostate Cancer: A Case Study" by G. Currie, M. Haase, R. Hashmi, and H. Kiat (*J Nucl Med Technol*. 2013;41(1):49–51).

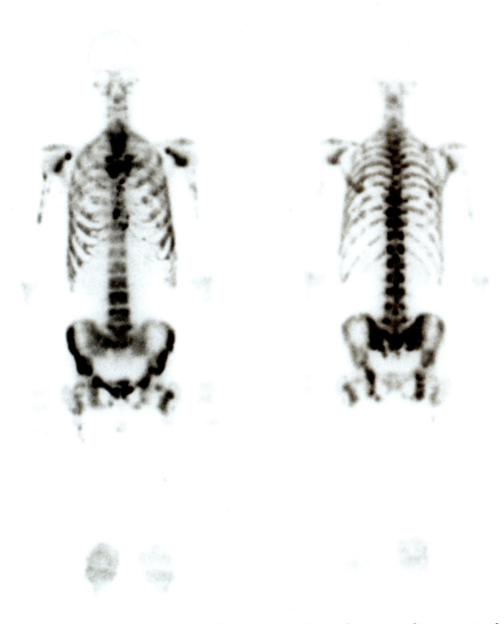

FIGURE 14-9 Baseline nuclear medicine bone scan demonstrating widespread metastatic disease associated with prostate carcinoma.

An 83-year-old male presented for evaluation of reported weight loss and constipation. These symptoms were initially assessed by computerized tomography (CT) of the chest, abdomen, and pelvis. Findings were largely normal, although a left renal staghorn calculus was noted. Despite no previous history of neoplasia, extensive sclerotic lesions were noted throughout the axial skeleton. This finding, combined with the observation of an irregular prostate contour (without enlargement), raised suspicion of previously undiagnosed widespread metastatic prostate carcinoma. Subsequent follow-up revealed a prostate-specific antigen (PSA) of 823 μg/L and nuclear medicine bone scan findings consistent with widespread skeletal metastases (Fig. 14-9). Prostate carcinoma diagnosis was confirmed with histopathology (Gleason score of 9). The patient commenced hormone therapy according to the following:

- 150 mg bicalutamide daily (oral tablet)
- 30 mg leuprorelin depot (intramuscular injection) every 4 months

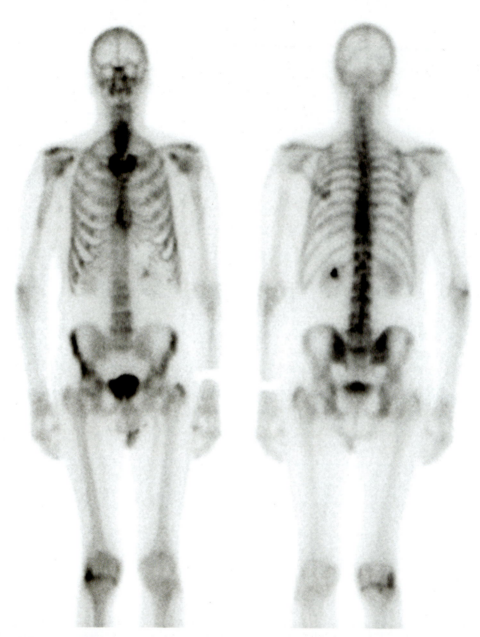

FIGURE 14-10 Follow-up nuclear medicine bone scan demonstrating remission of metastatic disease following hormone ablation therapy.

The patient was reevaluated at 4 weeks postdiagnosis and commencement of hormone therapy. The patient was tolerating bicalutamide well, which was continued at the previously prescribed dosage. In addition, the patient was prescribed and administered 10.8 mg goserelin implant (subcutaneous) every 3 months. Further follow-up at 5 months postdiagnosis and commencement of therapy revealed a PSA of 0.39 µg/L. The PSA dropped further to 0.11 µg/L at 10 months, which corresponded to nuclear medicine bone scan findings demonstrating a remarkable reversal of the previous findings, essentially returning a study within normal limits (Fig. 14-10).

The approach taken in the treatment of prostate cancer depends on a number of factors, including the clinical presentation, Gleason score, and PSA. For patients with metastatic spread of prostate cancer, like the patient in this case, the treatment of choice is androgen deprivation therapy (ADT). ADT has been reported to lead to remission in as many as 80% of patients with advanced prostate carcinoma. ADT is used in advanced prostate cancer to relieve pain, prevent pathologic fractures, and prevent neurologic complications. Typically, androgen deprivation is achieved through 3 mechanisms in prostate carcinoma patients:

1. Gonadotrophin-releasing hormone (GnRH) agonists (goserelin, leuprorelin, and triptorelin) decrease testosterone levels by overstimulation, downregulation, and eventually receptor desensitization. Unfortunately, testosterone suppression also increases the risk of osteoporosis and fracture (loss of bone mineral density), diabetes (altered glucose tolerance), and cardiovascular disease. Some of the more common adverse effects of ADT include weight gain, erectile dysfunction, decreased libido, gynecomastia, insomnia, sweats and chills, and gastrointestinal disturbances.

2. Antiandrogens (bicalutamide, flutamide, and nilutamide) are nonsteroidal inhibitors of androgen receptors. The advantage of this class of ADT medications is that they inhibit conversion of testosterone to dihydrotestosterone (metabolite) and prevent both from binding to the androgen receptor, without suppressing serum testosterone levels.

3. GnRH antagonists (degarelix) can be used prior to the GnRH agonist therapy to block testosterone increases. GnRH antagonists can also be used as an alternative approach to androgen deprivation by inhibiting gonadotrophin production, leading to a reduction in the synthesis of androgens in the testes.

ADT has been shown to result in remission in as many as 80% of patients, and this is reflected in a median period of 12 to 33 months of "progression-free survival." That is, ADT prevents the progression of metastatic spread. Typically, the nuclear medicine bone scan will demonstrate partial improvement or stabilization (nonprogression) of metastatic disease in response to ADT, but it is a rare occurrence for the bone scan to revert to normal. The reversion to normal in this case is remarkable given the advanced stage of disease (Gleason 9) and extent of metastatic disease at the commencement of ADT. Following the progression-free survival period, there will be transformation of the disease to an androgen-independent phenotype that will not respond to ADT (castrate resistant). At this point, alternative therapy (e.g., docetaxel) may be indicated.

References

Asperheim K, Favaro J. *Introduction to Pharmacology*. 12th ed. St Louis, MO: Elsevier; 2012.

Block JH, Beale JM. *Wilson and Gisvold's Textbook of Organic Medicinal and Pharmaceutical Chemistry*. 12th ed. Philadelphia, PA: Lippincott Williams & Wilkins; 2011.

Bryant B, Knights K, Salerno E. *Pharmacology for Health Professionals*. 2nd ed. Sydney, Australia: Mosby Elsevier; 2007.

Cartron G, Blasco H, Paintaud G, Watier H, Le Guellec C. Pharmacokinetics of rituximab and its clinical use: thought for the best use? *Crit Rev Oncol Hemat*. 2007;62:43–52.

Choi S, Lee AK. Efficacy and safety of gonadotropin-releasing hormone agonists used in the treatment of prostate cancer. *Drug Healthc Patient Saf*. 2011;3:107–119.

Currie G, Haase M, Hashmi R, Kiat H. Hormone therapy in prostate cancer: a case study. *J Nucl Med Technol*. 2013;41(1):49–51.

Drees M, Zimmermann R, Eisenbrand G. 3',5'-Cyclic nucleotide phosphodiesterase in tumor cells as potential target for tumor growth inhibition. *Cancer Res*. 1993;53:3058–3061.

Golan DE, Tashjian AH, Armstrong EJ, Armstrong AW. *Principles of Pharmacology: The Pathophysiologic Basis of Drug Therapy*. 3rd ed. Philadelphia, PA: Lippincott Williams & Wilkins; 2012.

Hacker M, Messer W, Bachmann K. *Pharmacology: Principles and Practice*. London, England: Elsevier; 2009.

Hammerer P, Madersbacher S. Landmarks in hormonal therapy for prostate cancer. *BJU Int*. 2012;110(Suppl 1):23–29.

Hanahan D, Weinberg RA. Hallmarks of cancer: the next generation. *Cell*. 2011;144(5):646–74. https://doi.org/10.1016/j.cell.2011.02.013

Hellerstedt BA, Pienta KJ. The current state of hormonal therapy for prostate cancer. *CA Cancer J Clin*. 2002;52:154–179.

Hirose M, Takeda E, Ninomiya T, Kuroda Y, Miyao M. Inhibitory effect of dipyridamole on the growth of various human hematologic malignant cell lines. *Tokushima J. Exp. Med*. 1986;33:51–57.

Huben RP. Hormone therapy of prostatic bone metastases. *Adv Exp Med Biol*. 1992;324:305–316.

Jambhekar SS, Breen PJ. *Basic Pharmacokinetics*. London, England: Pharmaceutical Press; 2009.

Katzung BG, Masters SB, Trevor AJ. *Basic and Clinical Pharmacology*. 12th ed. New York, NY: McGraw Hill; 2012.

Lepor H, Shore ND. LHRH agonists for the treatment of prostate cancer: 2012. *Rev Urol*. 2012;14:1–12.

Michelson S, Slate D. A mathematical model of the P-glycoprotein pump as a mediator of multidrug resistance. *Bull Math Biol*. 1992;54(6):1023–1038.

Rang H, Dale M, Ritter J, Flower R. *Rang and Dale's Pharmacology*. 6th ed. London, England: Churchill Livingston; 2008.

Rossi S (Ed.). *Australian Medicines Handbook 2012*. Adelaide, Australia: Australian Medicines Handbook; 2012: 591–598.

Sandeep G, Bhasker S, Sri Ranganath Y. Phosphodiesterase as a novel target in cancer chemotherapy. *Int. J. Pharmacol*. 2009;7(1). https://doi.org/10.5580/2c8.

Vergote J, Moretti JL, de Vries EG, Garnier-Suillerot A. Comparison of the kinetics of active efflux of ^{99m}Tc-MIBI in cells with P-glycoprotein-mediated and multidrug-resistance protein-associated multidrug-resistance phenotypes. *Eur J Biochem*. 1998;252(1):140–146.

Waller D, Renwick A, Hillier K. *Medical Pharmacology and Therapeutics*. 2nd ed. London, England: Elsevier; 2006.

CHAPTER 15

Issues with Over-the-Counter Medications

Chapter Objectives

Specific learning outcomes (page ix) of this text addressed in this chapter:

- Apply the principles of pharmacology to the safe and effective use of medicines.
- Recognize general, patient-specific, and scenario-specific risks, precautions, and contraindications for use of medicines.
- Apply the pharmacokinetic and pharmacodynamic principles of medications to identify and explain normal and adverse reactions to medications.
- Administer medications safely, effectively, and appropriately according to procedures and within regulatory and statutory parameters.
- Monitor patients for, identify, and manage adverse reactions.

After reading, digesting, reflecting on, and reviewing the content of this chapter, readers should be able to

1. Demonstrate command of key pharmacology terms.
2. Demonstrate enhanced understanding of the principles associated with the pharmacology of over-the-counter medications.
3. Demonstrate critical thinking to effect problem solving related to interventional protocols and procedures.
4. Recognize, explain, and interpret clinical problems and evidence in relation to over-the-counter medications use and application.
5. Demonstrate understanding of the mode of action, pharmacokinetics, risks, precautions, contraindications, adverse effects, interactions, and appropriate dosage of key over-the-counter medications.
6. Apply knowledge of the general principles and concepts in a translational manner to clinical practice.

Key Terms

action potential	antitussive	decongestant	mast cell	self-limiting
analgesic	bronchodilator	demulcent	NSAID	self-medicated
antidiarrheal	bulk forming	expectorant	opioid	stimulant
antihistamine	corticosteroid	fecal softener	osmotic	suppressant
anti-inflammatory	COX-1	laxative	prostaglandin	therapeutic index
antipyretic	COX-2	lubricant	sedation	toxicity

Introduction

A number of medications are considered sufficiently safe that they are available without medical prescription. This availability may vary across regulatory borders. *Self-medication* is useful for mild, chronic, and self-limiting conditions (e.g., pain, headache, hay-fever). The information age associated with the Internet has further empowered individuals to manage their own health. Unfortunately, deciphering information and differentiating evidence-based information from potentially harmful information is generally beyond the average member of the general public. Furthermore, over-the-counter medications, despite their safety profile, can be associated with adverse reactions or interactions with other medications, especially in the presence of comorbidity or polypharmacy. People may turn to self-medication in response to infomercials and marketing or to avoid the cost or inconvenience of visiting a medical practitioner. Patients should keep in mind that over-the-counter medications are generally focused on ameliorating symptoms, and thus, the underlying cause remains unchecked.

Over-the-counter medications are generally thought to be safe and effective for minor symptoms. They have high therapeutic indices and low incidence of adverse reactions. This condition presumes absence or disease, normal conditions, and within the recommended dosage. These medications should not, however, be considered without issues. Adverse reactions, toxicity, and drug interactions do occur. While there are potentially thousands of over-the-counter medications to consider, this discussion focuses on the more common ones that may be encountered in radiology and nuclear medicine. That is, the common medications patients may be taking or that may need to be provided to manage symptoms while patients are in the department's care. The following common conditions and their general medication use are discussed:

- Analgesia
- Antipyretics
- Antihistamines
- Gastric acid reducers
- Laxatives
- Antidiarrheals
- Bronchodilators
- Sympathomimetic decongestants
- Expectorants
- Antitussives

Analgesia

Nonsteroidal anti-inflammatory drugs (NSAIDs) and aspirin have 3 main effects: reduce inflammation, reduce fever, and reduce some specific types of pain. They also tend to cause gastric irritation, promote bleeding, and pose a risk in renal insufficiency. Cyclooxygenase-1 (COX-1) action is associated with homeostatic functions, gastric irritation, renal effects, and platelet function, while cyclooxygenase-2 (COX-2) action is associated with inflammatory inhibition. The bulk of unwanted side effects from NSAIDs are associated with COX-1, especially with long-term use. These include dyspepsia, nausea, vomiting, skin reactions, renal insufficiency, nephropathy, bronchospasm, liver disorders, and bone marrow depression. Prostaglandins (PGs) do not produce pain but instead enhance pain mediators. PGs are chemical mediators produced by the release of arachidonic acid in response to inflammation and metabolism by COX-2. PG_2 significantly enhances the pain-producing effects of other mediators released in response to tissue injury by macrophages, mast cells, T cells, and neutrophils, including bradykinin (BK), 5-hydroxytryptamine (5-HT), tumor necrosis factor alpha (TNF-α), nerve growth factor (NGF), interleukin, and histamine (Fig. 15-1). This action increases the action potential in the primary afferent neuron to enhance the pain stimulus. NSAIDs and aspirin block the action of COX-2, inhibiting PG formation and reducing the action potential and subsequent pain stimuli (Fig. 15-1).

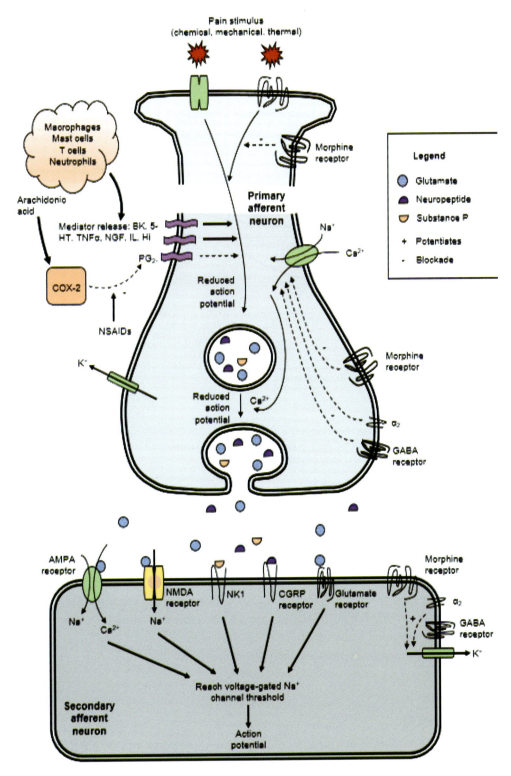

FIGURE 15-1 Schematic representation of the pain stimulus truncated response associated with NSAIDs. NSAIDs and aspirin block the action of COX-2, inhibiting PG formation and reducing the action potential and subsequent pain stimuli.

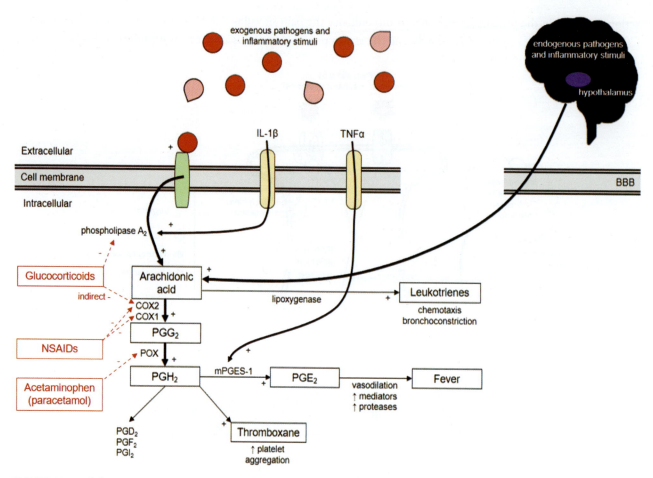

FIGURE 15-2 Schematic representation of the antipyretic actions of over-the-counter medications. Solid black lines represent positive or activation pathways. The red dotted lines represent inhibition pathways. The febrile pathway can be driven from a peripheral cellular level (left) or from a central level (right).

Ibuprofen is an NSAID with analgesic properties suitable for mild to moderate pain and inflammatory pain. Common adverse effects include dizziness, gastric pain, and nausea but is well tolerated. Orally administered ibuprofen is rapidly absorbed from the duodenum (enteric coated) with a peak in serum levels at 1 to 2 hours (delayed by food), although onset of action occurs within 1 hour. Acetaminophen (paracetamol) is not technically an NSAID, as it lacks the anti-inflammatory properties. Acetaminophen (paracetamol) analgesia is indicated for mild to moderate pain and noninflammatory pain. Acetaminophen (paracetamol) has a superior safety profile compared to aspirin or NSAIDs, with allergy and adverse reactions being rare, low risk of gastric irritation or bleeding, minimal potential for drug interactions (low plasma protein binding), and safe use in pregnancy, breast-feeding, and children. Pharmacokinetic information for ibuprofen and acetaminophen (paracetamol) is detailed in Chapter 13.

Antipyretic (Fever)

Fever is the by-product of a number of processes, including but not limited to inflammation and infection. Antipyretic medications include corticosteroids, NSAIDs, and acetaminophen (paracetamol). The mechanism of action of each class of antipyretic acts at different points in the febrile response pathway (Fig. 15-2). Corticosteroids suppress fever by inhibiting the transcription of pyrogenic cytokines and COX-2. They inhibit phospholipase A_2 and prostaglandin synthetic pathways. NSAIDs (including aspirin) inhibit COX-mediated synthesis of inflammatory thromboxanes and prostaglandins. Acetaminophen (paracetamol) is very similar to NSAIDs except that it inhibits synthesis of inflammatory thromboxanes and prostaglandins by inhibiting peroxidase (POX) conversion of the intermediate prostaglandin G2 (PGG_2) to prostaglandin H2 (PGH_2). Properties of aspirin, ibuprofen, and acetaminophen (paracetamol) are discussed in the preceding section.

Antihistamines

Histamine is an amine that has wide dispersion in the body but particularly in mast cells of the lung, skin, and gut. Histamine release from the mast cell is mediated by an interaction between the antigen and the immunoglobulin E (IgE) antibody (Fig. 15-3) or in response to substance P. Antihistamines (H_1) are extensively outlined in Chapters 1 and 9. Histamine antagonists refer to H_2 antagonism by medications such as ranitidine and cimetidine, which are used to treat peptic ulcer.

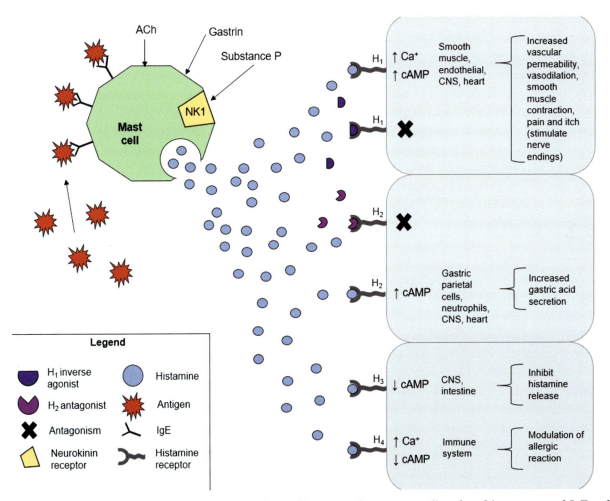

FIGURE 15-3 Schematic representation of the release of histamine from a mast cell mediated by antigen and IgE and substance P activity.

Sedating antihistamines such as diphenhydramine (Benadryl) and promethazine (Phenergan) are used for treatment of allergies, skin disorders, vertigo, motion sickness, and nausea and are used for the sedative effects. Because of their lipophilicity, they cross the blood-brain barrier and cause sedation. Other central effects associated with these first-generation antihistamines include dizziness, dry mouth, cough, blurred vision, urinary retention, constipation, and gastrointestinal disturbances resulting from antagonism of muscarinic, alpha (α)-adrenergic, and serotonin receptors in the brain. Other adverse reactions include fatigue, headache, nausea, and vomiting. Onset of action is generally 15 to 60 minutes after oral absorption. Central nervous system (CNS) depressant effects of first-generation antihistamines are enhanced if taken concurrently with alcohol, CNS depressants, anticholinergic medications, or psychotropics. Concurrent use should be avoided. Antihistamines can also antagonize the effect of levodopa. The adverse effects are more important to consider in older people, especially because of the risk of sedation associated with less-sedating antihistamines. Antihistamine use should be avoided in children, especially under the age of 2 years. Antihistamines have been used safely during pregnancy to manage nausea (antiemetic) or allergy. Sedating antihistamines can result in paradoxical CNS stimulation.

Less-sedating antihistamines such as loratadine, cetirizine, and fexofenadine are generally reserved for allergic responses, hypersensitivity reactions, and hay-fever. The marked reduction in sedation is associated with reduced lipophilicity and reduced blood-brain barrier permeability but improves the safety profile. Less sedating is not nonsedating, and it should be kept in mind that 6% of users experience a sedative effect, in which is increased in the elderly. Antihistamines can interact with other medications. Common adverse reactions for second-generation antihistamines include drowsiness, dry mouth, fatigue, headache, and nausea. The adverse effects are more important to consider in older people, especially because of the risk of sedation associated with less-sedating antihistamines. There is a small risk of cardiac arrhythmia with fexofenadine.

Promethazine is a common first-generation antihistamine that, after oral absorption, has a peak plasma concentration at 1.5 to 3 hours, 25% bioavailability (due to first-pass metabolism), and duration of action of 4 to 6 hours (up to 12 h). Promethazine is 93% plasma protein bound and is metabolized in the liver. The elimination half-life is 12 to 15 hours via urine. A major issue with promethazine is the over-the-counter availability and overuse for child sedation. While an Australian survey revealed 1 in 5 families use promethazine to sedate children on long trips (car, plane), safety advice indicates it should not be used in children under 2 years due to the risk of fatal respiratory depression. Promethazine may also be abused by methadone patients because it may potentiate the high associated with opioids.

Loratadine is a common second-generation antihistamine that, after oral absorption, has a peak plasma concentration at 1 to 1.5 hours (delayed if taken with food), 40% bioavailability (higher if taken with food), and duration of action of 24 hours. Loratadine is 97% to 99% plasma protein bound and in the liver is metabolized into the more active (4-fold increase) metabolite (descarboethoxyloratadine), which has peak plasma concentrations at 3 to 4 hours. The elimination half-life is 10 hours for loratadine and 20 hours for the active metabolite via urine (40%) and feces (40%). One tablet per 24 hours offers convenience, but a common misunderstanding in the general public about its use relates to apparent inaction. When a user is slow to respond symptom-wise, the mantra "1 is good, 2 is better" often sees an increased dose. While some second-generation antihistamines have shorter durations of effect and thus require multiple daily doses, loratadine does not benefit from overdosing in a 24-hour window. The lack of response is more likely to relate to the action of antihistamines. Antihistamines do not reverse receptor agonism and do not block the action of histamines; they are effective only in blocking the release of histamine from mast cells before the histamine is released. Persistence of symptoms after an antihistamine relates to the effects of histamine released prior to taking the medication, and additional doses will not have an impact on that.

Gastric Acid Reducers

Cimetidine is an H_2 histamine receptor antagonist that reduces gastric acidity. Histamine is released from mast cells and stimulates H_2 receptors in the gastric parietal cells to increase gastric acid secretion. Cimetidine is an H_2 histamine antagonist that inhibits histamine stimulation of receptors (Fig. 15-4) and thus reduces both the volume and the concentration of hydrochloric acid in the stomach by as much as 50% to 70%. Cimetidine has an oral bioavailability of 60% to 70%. It has 20% plasma protein binding and is partially (25%) metabolized in the liver, with 50% of the oral dose excreted unchanged in urine. The elimination half-life is 2 hours, but this can be increased in renal dysfunction. After oral administration, onset of action occurs within 30 to 60 minutes, with peak activity seen at 60 minutes if taken on an empty stomach and 120 minutes with food, and effects of significance last 4 to 6 hours. While cimetidine crosses the placenta and is excreted in breast milk, it is safe to use in both situations. Cimetidine is used to treat peptic ulcer disease, gastroesophageal reflux, dyspepsia, and stress ulcers by reducing gastric acid secretion.

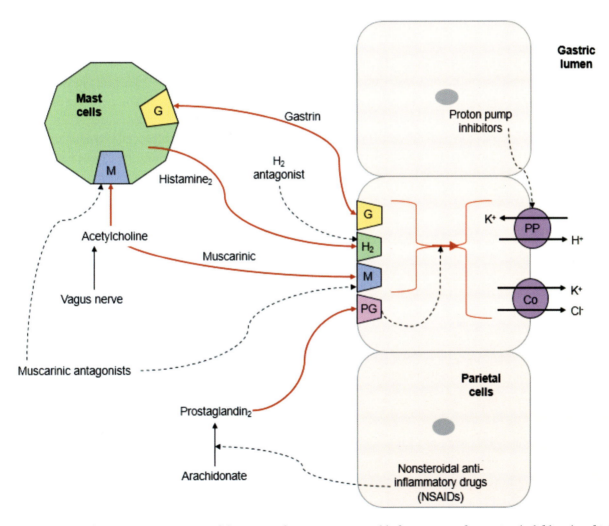

FIGURE 15-4 Schematic representation of the action of receptors responsible for gastric acid secretion (solid lines) and inhibitors of gastric acid secretion (dashed lines).

Ranitidine is an H_2 histamine antagonist that reduces gastric acidity in the same way as cimetidine does. Ranitidine and cimetidine share the same drug class, general information, mode of action (Fig. 15-4), clinical use, contraindications, and precautions. Adverse reactions and common interactions have similarities but also some important differences that should be highlighted. Ranitidine has an oral bioavailability of 50%. It has 15% plasma protein binding and is partially (4% to 6%) metabolized in the liver, with 30% of the oral dose excreted unchanged in urine. The elimination half-life is 2 to 3 hours, but this can be increased in renal dysfunction. After oral administration, onset of action occurs within 60 minutes, with peak activity seen at 2 to 3 hours (independent of fasting) and effects of significance lasting 4 to 13 hours. Ranitidine crosses the placenta and is excreted in breast milk but is safe to use in both situations. Both ranitidine and cimetidine have been discussed in more detail in chapter 9.

Omeprazole is a proton pump inhibitor that inhibits the secretion of gastric acid by inhibiting the proton pump. The proton pump is the enzyme system of hydrogen potassium adenosine triphosphatase (H+/K+ ATPase) in the gastric parietal cell (Fig. 15-3). In essence, when sufficient omeprazole accumulates or binds to the proton pump, the final step in acid production is inhibited, which suppresses acid secretion. The action is irreversible inhibition, which is reflected in the long duration of effect relative to the elimination half-life.

Omeprazole is rapidly but variably absorbed after oral administration, with an oral bioavailability of 30% to 40%. It has 95% plasma protein binding and is extensively metabolized in the liver, with 80% of metabolites excreted in urine and the remaining 20% by feces. The elimination half-life is 0.5 hours, but this can be increased in renal dysfunction. After oral administration, onset of action occurs within 60 minutes, with peak activity seen at 120 minutes and effects of significance lasting 3 to 5 days. Omeprazole has increased bioavailability in the elderly and with liver dysfunction. Omeprazole is used for the treatment of peptic ulcer, NSAID-induced ulceration, esophageal erosion due to acid reflux, and the treatment of Zollinger-Ellison syndrome. It is generally used in conditions in which gastric acid inhibition may relieve symptoms, including aspiration, dyspepsia, gastroesophageal reflux disease, and peptic ulcer.

Laxatives

Laxatives are an important class of over-the-counter medications. While they are intended to treat constipation, they are also frequently abused by individuals trying to reduce energy intake or weight and in individuals with eating disorders. Understanding the action of laxatives debunks the weight loss theory because the resulting evacuation is generally energy depleted, resulting instead in loss of water and electrolytes. Any immediate weight loss is reversed with hydration. In imaging, patients may be investigated for transit issues (radiology and nuclear medicine) where laxatives are being used for therapy; imaging may be required with or without laxatives; and on occasion, laxatives might be used to enhance imaging (differentiate colonic activity on ^{67}Ga-citrate non-Hodgkin lymphoma study).

There are a number of classifications for laxatives (Fig. 15-5):

- Fecal softeners (e.g., docusate) use wetting agents to mix water and fatty substances with the feces, but they have a 1- to 3-day onset of action.
- Bulk-forming agents (e.g., psyllium, methylcellulose) cause water absorption, bowel distention, and reflex bowel activity, with a 12-hour to 3-day lag to onset of action.
- Osmotics (e.g., lactulose, macrogol, glycerol) increase the volume of liquid in the bowel lumen, with onset in 1 to 3 hours.
- Lubricants (e.g., liquid paraffin) coat the surface of the feces to aid passage, with 6- to 8-hour time to onset.
- Stimulants (e.g., bisacodyl, sodium picosulfate, and senna) increase peristalsis via innervation, with onset of 6 to 12 hours.
- Combination therapy (e.g., softener and stimulant) can also be used.

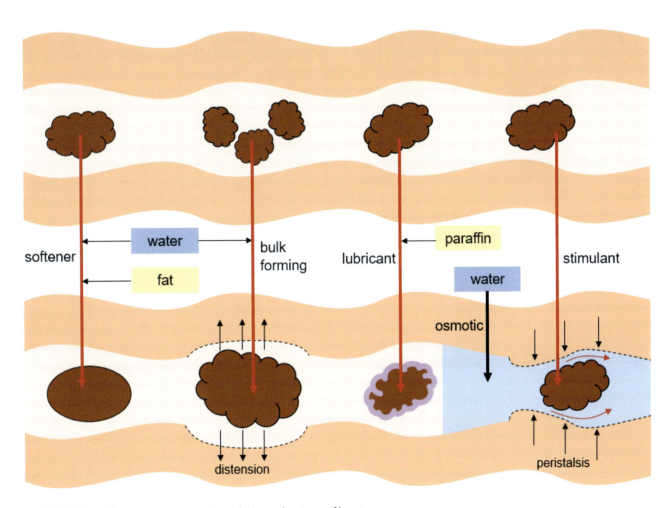

FIGURE 15-5 Schematic representation of the mechanisms of laxatives.

Bulk-forming laxatives are not absorbed from the gastrointestinal tract and therefore have no systemic effects or interactions with medications. They should be taken with ample water, or the risk of obstruction increases. Adverse effects include distension, flatulence, and discomfort. Osmotic laxatives tend to be poorly absorbed from the gastrointestinal tract and cause hypertonic conditions that drive water into the colon to equalize osmotic pressure. Caution should be exercised in severe renal impairment to avoid magnesium ion toxicity. The main adverse effects of osmotic laxatives are nausea and dehydration. Fecal softeners lower the surface tension of stools to drive water and fat penetration, softening the stool for easier evacuation. These are weak laxatives in isolation (hence their use in combination therapy), are not absorbed, and pose no issues of toxicity. Nonetheless, fecal softeners could increase bioavailability (absorption) of some enteral medications. Fecal lubricant such as liquid paraffin is not absorbed but can cause irritation, altered vitamin absorption, and aspiration pneumonia. It should be avoided in children and during abdominal pain or nausea. Stimulant laxatives can cause cramping and electrolyte imbalance with prolonged use. Prolonged use of stimulant laxatives can cause the smooth muscle tone to decrease, which exacerbates constipation, requiring larger doses for effect and further degrading smooth muscle tone. Consequently, stimulant laxatives are recommended only for short-term use.

Bisacodyl is a stimulant laxative that increases water retention in the stool and stimulates peristalsis in the bowel. It acts directly on the mucosal nerve plexus of the large intestine. As such, it is effective for clearing the bowel of fecal content but should not be used regularly for constipation. Bisacodyl has minimal absorption. The small amount that may be absorbed after oral administration has 99% plasma protein binding; it is metabolized in the liver and eliminated via the kidneys. After oral administration, onset of action occurs within 6 to 8 hours. Since bisacodyl causes gastric irritation, it is enteric coated and so should be taken whole (do not crush) and not within 1 hour of antacids. It is worth mentioning sodium picosulfate because it is used for bowel preparation (e.g., colonoscopy). It has a relatively long duration to onset because it is activated by metabolism associated with colonic bacteria. Bisacodyl should not be used when the bowel is obstructed. Caution should be exercised in patients with liver impairment due to liver metabolism of the small fraction absorbed. There are few major adverse reactions other than the expected local reactions that include gastric irritation and cramping. Fluid and electrolyte depletion is possible. Possible interactions with medications that change gastric acidity (e.g., H_2 antagonists, proton pump inhibitors) may alter the effects of bisacodyl.

Antidiarrhea

Diarrhea is an acute but self-limiting condition with a number of potential causes:

- Viruses
- Bacteria
- Parasites
- Medicines (e.g., antibiotics)
- Lactose intolerance
- Food, preservative, or chemical intolerance
- Digestive disorders such as celiac disease and irritable bowel syndrome
- Gastrointestinal bleed
- Stress and anxiety

Diarrhea can lead to dehydration and electrolyte imbalance and can be especially problematic in young children and the elderly. Treatment of diarrhea is an issue of cause and convenience. Under ideal circumstances, hydration therapy and allowing the illness to run its course is the best option. This is consistent with the view that diarrhea is a process of eliminating a toxin from the body, and antidiarrhea medications could slow recovery. There is little evidence that illness is significantly prolonged, but medication provides symptom management, convenience, or comfort. This may permit increased rest during the acute phase (and thus recovery) or allow daily function without inconvenience or embarrassment.

As discussed in Chapter 13, morphine can cause constipation. Activation of morphine receptors on the small and large intestines increases the tone and decreases motility. This, in turn, increases reabsorption of fluids and decreases colonic volume. Loperamide specifically has high-affinity agonism of morphine receptors in the gastrointestinal wall, but absorption results in extensive first-pass metabolism to largely eliminate systemic and central actions. It also acts as a nonspecific calcium channel blocker. While there is no significant absorption of loperamide from the gastrointestinal tract, it has 97% plasma protein binding, liver metabolism, and elimination half-life of 9 to 14 hours. Loperamide should be avoided in severe liver dysfunction, intestinal obstruction, and children. Adverse reactions include abdominal pain, bloating, nausea, vomiting, and constipation.

Bronchodilation

Direct-acting sympathomimetic β_2-agonists such as salbutamol dilate the bronchi by direct action (Fig. 15-6) and have been previously discussed in Chapters 8 and 12. Salbutamol mimics the effects of endogenous norepinephrine by coupling with bronchial smooth muscle cell surface β_2-receptors. Receptor β_2 couples with a G protein, stimulating adenylate cyclase to decrease intracellular calcium. This leads to calcium efflux from the cell and uptake in the sarcoplasmic reticulum, stripping calcium from actin-myosin bridges to produce smooth muscle relaxation and bronchodilation. Short-acting salbutamol is given by inhalation for direct action and symptom relief. Salmeterol is a longer-acting β_2-agonist used regularly as a symptom preventer.

After inhalation, 10% to 20% of the dose reaches the lower airways for direct action on smooth muscle. The direct action and rapid onset combined with the half-life makes salbutamol a short-acting bronchodilator suitable as a symptom reliever. It is not metabolized in the lung but does undergo first-pass metabolism in the liver. Of the remainder not inhaled, that component swallowed is readily absorbed from the gut. Salbutamol and its metabolites are rapidly excreted in urine, with a small amount of fecal elimination. Plasma half-life is 4 to 6 hours. It has rapid onset of action following inhalation (less than 5 min), with peak effect at 1 hour and duration of action lasting 3 to 6 hours. If given orally, onset of action is 30 minutes, peak effect is at 2 to 3 hours, and duration is 6 hours. Salbutamol is a bronchodilator for reversible airways obstruction (e.g., asthma and chronic obstructive airways disease).

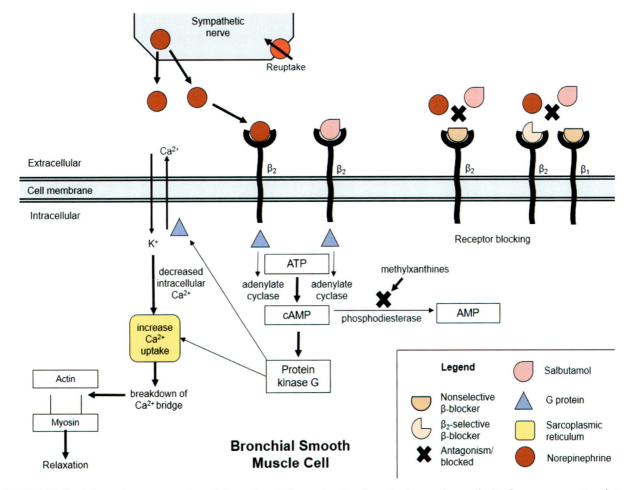

FIGURE 15-6 Schematic representation of the action of β-agonism in a bronchial smooth muscle. Endogenous norepinephrine is released from the sympathetic nerve. In the extracellular space, endogenous norepinephrine and exogenous salbutamol can couple with β_2-receptors. Receptor β_2 couples with an adenylate cyclase, stimulating G protein to produce decreased intracellular calcium through calcium efflux and uptake in the sarcoplasmic reticulum, leading a reduction in actin-myosin bridge formation and producing smooth muscle relaxation and bronchodilation. Inhibition of phosphodiesterase conversion of cyclic adenosine monophosphate (cAMP) to adenosine monophosphate (AMP) by methylxanthines (e.g., caffeine, theobromine, theophylline) further decreases intracellular calcium. This response can be antagonized by a β-blocker either nonselective (e.g., labetalol) or selective for β_2 (e.g., butoxamine).

Sympathomimetic Decongestant

Decongestants are generally associated with treatment of the cold and influenza. The purpose of decongestants is to reduce the swelling associated with mucosa and to provide local constriction of blood vessels in nasal passages. This serves to improve mucus drainage and open the airways. Decongestants can be delivered systemically (oral tablet) or locally (nasal spray). The only decongestant that is effective systemically is pseudoephedrine, but in recent times, over-the-counter availability of products containing pseudoephedrine have been restricted (refer to local regulations) due to diversion and abuse (methamphetamine production). Over-the-counter tablets generally contain phenylephrine, which has poor oral absorption and significant first-pass metabolism. Consequently, the phenylephrine substitutes are significantly less effective as systemic decongestants. Conversely, when delivered locally, phenylephrine provides rapid and potent vasoconstriction. This extends significant advantage because the vasoconstriction also inhibits systemic absorption, reducing adverse effects and potential drug interactions. Local (nasal) decongestants can generally be used when systemic decongestants are contraindicated. Local decongestants remain contraindicated with monoamine oxidase (MOA) inhibitor use (Fig. 15-7). Prolonged use of nasal decongestants can result in rebound effects (congestion, rhinitis).

Ephedrine is an α- and β-adrenergic receptor agonist. It acts directly on α-receptors and indirectly by increasing norepinephrine release (Fig. 15-7). Ephedrine is a racemic drug, which means it is composed of dextrorotatory and levorotatory forms in an equal proportion, or it has equal amounts of left-hand and right-hand enantiomers (structure). Pseudoephedrine is just the L-ephedrine stereoisomer. As shown in Figure 15-7, norepinephrine agonism of $α_1$-receptor in vascular smooth muscle increases the concentration of inositol trisphosphate (IP_3), increasing intracellular calcium, building actin-myosin bridges, and causing contraction. Conversely, $α_2$-agonism inhibits adenylate cyclase to reduce intracellular cAMP, leading to vasoconstriction. Norepinephrine reduces further norepinephrine release via activation of the autoreceptor. Ephedrine and pseudoephedrine provide the same antagonism of $α_1$- and $α_2$-receptors but also stimulate increased release of norepinephrine via the autoreceptor. Pseudoephedrine has lower affinity of β-receptors. Pseudoephedrine has peak serum levels after oral administration of 6 hours, which can be prolonged to 12 hours when taken with food. It has less than 10% plasma protein binding and is eliminated by the kidneys largely unmetabolized (99%), with a 6 hour half-life. Adverse reactions can include dizziness, headache, nausea, vomiting, sweating, thirst, tachycardia, chest pain, palpitations and arrhythmias, difficulty urinating, muscle weakness, muscle tension, anxiety, restlessness, and insomnia. Toxicity can lead to toxic psychosis, circulatory collapse, convulsions, coma, and respiratory failure.

Phenylephrine acts only on $α_1$-receptors to produce vascular smooth muscle contraction (vasoconstriction). Systemically, phenylephrine produces hypertension, pupil dilation, arrhythmia, and bradycardia. Over-the-counter preparations are either oral, which have poor absorption (38% bioavailability) and high first-pass metabolism, or local (nasal) administration, causing potent vasoconstriction. In each case, systemic absorption and adverse reactions are minimized. Systemic phenylephrine is eliminated via the kidneys, with the majority being metabolized to the inactive metabolite. The local vasoconstrictive action of phenylephrine has seen it employed as a "home remedy" for the pain and discomfort of hemorrhoids based on the theory that constriction of vascular smooth muscle will relieve the symptoms associated with swollen and tortuous rectal veins. The lack of vascular smooth muscle of veins (compared to arteries) makes this mechanism unlikely to be helpful.

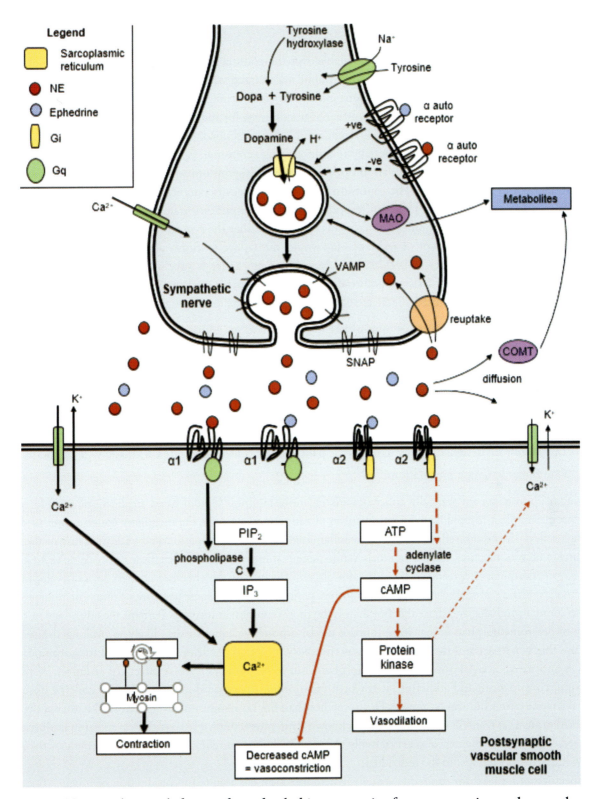

FIGURE 15-7 Norepinephrine, ephedrine, and pseudoephedrine are agonists for α_1-receptors in vascular smooth muscle, increasing the concentration of IP_3, increasing intracellular calcium, building actin-myosin bridges, and causing contraction. They are also agonists for α_2, which inhibits adenylate cyclase and reduces intracellular cAMP, leading to vasoconstriction.

Cough Medicines

There are a number of different medications available over-the-counter for cough, but the most appropriate medication depends on the type of cough. The general public are charged with the responsibility of appropriate use of over-the-counter medications but seldom understand in sufficient detail the pharmacologic principles that could shape use. A general example is antibiotic use. It is not uncommon for individuals to stockpile unused antibiotics from a previous prescription or to have prophylactic antibiotics prescribed. The latter is not uncommon for individuals preparing for an overseas trip, especially to a developing economy. The point to be made is that with this comes inappropriate use, such as taking antibiotics as soon as the symptoms of influenza develop. Influenza is a virus, and antibiotics have no effect. The confusion arises perhaps because, on occasion, when a serious viral infection leads to a secondary bacterial infection (especially in upper respiratory tract infections), antibiotics are prescribed. Inappropriate use of antibiotics not only fails to address either the symptoms or the disease course but also poses a real threat to development of resistance (as would the failure to finish a prescribed course because the symptoms have resolved—sufficient bacteria have been killed to render it subclinical, but the remaining living bacteria are likely to be the most resistant and ready to replicate). Cough medicines may fail to help the individual if the inappropriate medicine is used. There are essentially five approaches to cough medicines:

1. *Suppressants*, or antitussives, are appropriate for dry, irritating, nonproductive coughs. Cough suppression requires inhibition of the cough reflex, which requires CNS activity. These medicines typically include codeine for that purpose.
2. *Expectorants* are for productive (mucus- or phlegm-producing), chesty coughs. The purpose of the medication is not to suppress the cough but rather to make it more efficient at expelling lung contents.
3. *Decongestants* are designed for chesty coughs that are unproductive but associated with chest tightness.
4. *Demulcents* are designed simply to sooth the pain and discomfort associated with any type of cough.
5. Combination cough preparations.

Cough suppressants are generally either opioids or antihistamines. Opioid-based medications include codeine and dextromethorphan (opioidlike). The mechanism of action is to suppress the medullary cough center to depress the cough reflex. The cough reflex is activated by inflammation and irritation associated with the cause of the cough (e.g., foreign object, infection, ACE inhibitor). While there is some evidence of the efficacy of codeine as an antitussive, dextromethorphan is considered by some as a placebo because of the chemical changes in its development to eliminate dependency. Nonetheless, in many countries, codeine-based products have been limited or removed from over-the-counter products, and dextromethorphan is the most common antitussive. Perhaps the advantage of the lost efficacy of dextromethorphan is that inappropriate use in productive coughs is less likely to prolong the course of symptoms that would occur if the cough reflex was effectively inhibited. Codeine is metabolized to morphine, which enhances antitussive activity (over dextromethorphan) but also produces adverse effects of sedation, respiratory depression, constipation, and addiction. It is worth mentioning that typical over-the-counter codeine doses have minimal adverse effects but can be abused. Dextromethorphan has no significant adverse effects. Neither codeine nor dextromethorphan, at over-the-counter doses, has known drug interactions. First-generation sedating antihistamines (discussed earlier in this chapter) also act centrally to suppress the cough reflex, but the biggest benefit of their use is in providing sedation and rest to the individual.

Expectorants are used for productive coughs where infection has resulted in production of mucus. The cough forms part of the necessary process for clearing the mucus, as the mucus is expelled by ciliary action. Not only does the cough expel the pathogen but, by expelling the mucus, it helps keep the airway open. Suppressing this type of cough would be deleterious to the individual's health. Expectorants are also referred to as *mucolytics* and aim to reduce the viscosity of the mucus for more efficient elimination. Expectorants also tend to be emetic agents (promote vomiting) at higher doses. The pathway for stimulation of the vagus nerve is similar to stimulation of the bronchial glands and cilia. As a result, over-the-counter strengths of expectorants are largely subtherapeutic, and there is little evidence for efficacy (or adverse reactions). Preparations that include guaifenesin, ammonium chloride, and ipecacuanha are in this category. More effective expectorants include nebulized acetylcysteine (adverse effects include stomatitis, nausea, and bronchospasm) and bromhexine (adverse reactions include nausea, vomiting, diarrhea, and allergic reaction).

Bromhexine has the highest over-the-counter efficacy but is not available in the United States. Bromhexine is rapidly absorbed after oral administration and undergoes extensive first-pass metabolism to render bioavailability only 20%. It is highly plasma protein bound and is largely eliminated via the kidneys as metabolites with a 12 hour half-life. It is contraindicated in known hypersensitivity and used with caution in those with a history of gastric ulceration, liver dysfunction and renal dysfunction. Adverse reactions include headache, dizziness, sweating, and allergy, but there are no known drug interactions.

There are two main categories of decongestants: sympathomimetics such as pseudoephedrine and methylxanthines such as theophylline. Pseudoephedrine and other sympathomimetics mimic norepinephrine at α- and β-receptors to produce constriction of smooth muscle and vasoconstriction (Fig. 15-7) and bronchodilation (Fig. 15-6). Adverse effects were discussed previously. Xanthine medications (Chapter 8) can cause bronchodilation by antagonism of adenosine receptors (Fig. 15-8) and vascular smooth muscle relaxation by inhibition of phosphodiesterase to inhibit cAMP breakdown (Fig. 15-8). The principle methylxanthine is aminophylline, which is a prodrug ester for the active theophylline. While not an over-the-counter medication, a number of over-the-counter products contain the methylxanthine caffeine, which has been purported to cause bronchodilation but with lower efficacy than theophylline (due to receptor affinity).

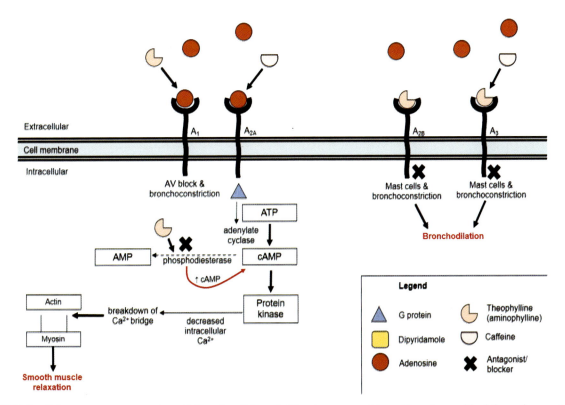

FIGURE 15-8 Schematic representation of the role of theophylline in antagonizing adenosine to block bronchoconstriction and inhibit phosphodiesterase to increase intracellular cAMP to drive smooth muscle relaxation. It is worth noting that caffeine has affinity for receptor A_3, which may offer some bronchodilation.

222 Pharmacology Primer for Medications

As previously outlined, there are four main adenosine receptor subtypes:

1. A_1 blocks AV conduction; reduces force of cardiac contraction (negative inotropic and chronotropic action); and causes decreased glomerular filtration rate, cardiac depression, renal vasoconstriction, decreased CNS activity, and bronchoconstriction.
2. A_{2A} triggers anti-inflammatory response, vasodilation, decreased blood pressure, decreased CNS activity, inhibition of platelet aggregation, and bronchodilation.
3. A_{2B} stimulates phospholipase activity, release of mast cell mediators, and actions on colon and bladder (contributes to bronchoconstriction).
4. A_3 stimulates phospholipase activity and release of mast cell mediators (contributes to bronchoconstriction).

Demulcents provide relief from irritation by coating the pharyngeal mucosa. They are short acting and, some argue, of only placebo value. The only major issue relates to sugar content, and caution should be exercised in people with diabetes. Soothing agents include glycerol mixed with honey or lemon. There are no specific adverse effects or drug interactions that need attention.

Insight

As mentioned previously, oral phenylephrine lacks the efficacy to be an effective decongestant because of poor absorption and high first-pass metabolism. Yet pseudoephedrine has higher restrictions due to diversion to methamphetamine trade. Figure 15-9 provides an insight into this process chemically.

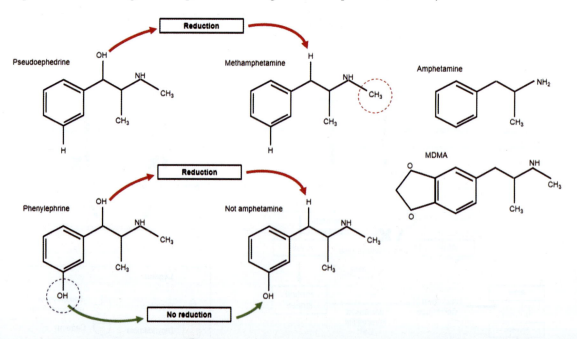

FIGURE 15-9   For pseudoephedrine, a simple reduction step transforms the hydroxyl group (OH) into a hydrogen to produce methamphetamine. Conversely, phenylephrine has two hydroxyl groups. The hydroxyl group OH corresponding to the same position as pseudoephedrine is readily reduced, however, the hydroxyl group in the blue circle (called a *phenolic group*) is chemically unreactive. As a result, phenylephrine is not converted to methamphetamine. The second methyl group (CH_3) on methamphetamine differentiates it from and adds the "meth" compared to amphetamine. 3,4-Methylenedioxy-methamphetamine (MDMA), street named *ecstasy* or *molly*, is similar in structure to methamphetamine but with the additional ring.

References

Asperheim K, Favaro J. *Introduction to Pharmacology*. 12th ed. St Louis, MO: Elsevier; 2012.

Block JH, Beale JM. *Wilson and Gisvold's Textbook of Organic Medicinal and Pharmaceutical Chemistry*. 12th ed. Philadelphia, PA: Lippincott Williams & Wilkins; 2011.

Bryant B, Knights K, Salerno E. *Pharmacology for Health Professionals*. 2nd ed. Sydney, Australia: Mosby Elsevier; 2007.

Golan DE, Tashjian AH, Armstrong EJ, Armstrong AW. *Principles of Pharmacology: The Pathophysiologic Basis of Drug Therapy*. 3rd ed. Philadelphia, PA: Lippincott Williams & Wilkins; 2012.

Greenstein B. *Rapid Revision in Clinical Pharmacology*. New York, NY: Radcliffe Publishing; 2008.

Hacker M, Messer W, Bachmann K. *Pharmacology: Principles and Practice*. London, England: Elsevier; 2009.

Jambhekar SS, Breen PJ. *Basic Pharmacokinetics*. London, England: Pharmaceutical Press; 2009.

Katzung BG, Masters SB, Trevor AJ. *Basic and Clinical Pharmacology*. 12th ed. New York, NY: McGraw Hill; 2012.

Nathan A. *Non-prescription Medicines*. London, England: Pharmaceutical Press; 2010.

Patrick GL. *An Introduction to Medicinal Chemistry*. 3rd ed. New York, NY: Oxford University Press; 2005.

Rang H, Dale M, Ritter J, Flower R. *Rang and Dale's Pharmacology*. 6th ed. London, England: Churchill Livingston; 2008.

Rossi S (Ed.). *Australian Medicines Handbook 2012*. Adelaide, Australia: Australian Medicines Handbook. 2012: 591–598.

Sweetman SC (Ed.). *Martindale: The Complete Drug Reference*. 26th ed. Chicago, IL: Pharmaceutical Press; 2009.

Waller D, Renwick A, Hillier K. *Medical Pharmacology and Therapeutics*. 2nd ed. London, England: Elsevier; 2006.

CHAPTER 16

Lifestyle and Sports Drugs

Chapter Objectives

Specific learning outcomes (page ix) of this text addressed in this chapter:

- Apply the pharmacokinetic and pharmacodynamic principles of medications to identify and explain normal and adverse reactions to medications.
- Monitor patients for, identify, and manage adverse reactions.

After reading, digesting, reflecting on, and reviewing the content of this chapter, readers should be able to

1. Demonstrate command of key pharmacology terms.
2. Demonstrate enhanced understanding of the principles associated with the pharmacology of lifestyle or sports drugs.
3. Demonstrate critical thinking to effect problem solving related to the effects of lifestyle or sports drugs.
4. Recognize, explain, and interpret clinical problems and evidence in relation to lifestyle or sports drugs.
5. Demonstrate understanding of the mode of action, pharmacokinetics, risks, precautions, contraindications, adverse effects, and interactions of lifestyle or sports drugs.

Key Terms

anabolic	gene doping	narcotic	prohibited	toxicity
antidepressant	hormone	obesity	satiety	virilization
cannabinoid	masking agent	peptide	stimulant	WADA
diuretic				

Introduction

A number of drugs are common in sports and lifestyle, but a detailed treatment of those drugs is beyond the scope of this text. Instead, a general overview is provided with specific immersion in drugs or circumstances that may intersect with the radiology and nuclear medicine department experience. A range of drugs in sports are summarized in Table 16-1, and lifestyle drugs are summarized in Table 16-2.

TABLE 16-1 Summary of Key Sports Drugs

Drug Type	Examples	Sport Use	Consideration in Imaging
Anabolic	Testosterone	Increase muscle development and strength	Negligible
Hormones	Erythropoietin	Increase erythrocyte formation and capacity of oxygen transport	Negligible
	Growth hormone	Reduce body fat and increase lean body mass	Negligible
	Insulin	Glucose load muscles	Potentially issue in fluorodeoxyglucose PET. Patients with diabetes are sometimes given insulin, but it would be managed in an athlete.
β-Agonists	Salbutamol	Increase oxygen intake	Negligible issue in inhaled applications.
β-Blockers	Metoprolol	Slow heart rate, tremor, and anxiety in precision sports	Could be used in emergency response but is not banned in most sports.
	Propranolol		
Stimulants	Epinephrine	Enhance performance	Epinephrine could be used in emergency response (e.g., contrast allergy), but it is prohibited only during competition. Potential for abuse to impact interventional medications.
	Ephedrine		
	Amphetamines		
	Caffeine		
Diuretics	Furosemide	Rapid weight loss and to mask use of banned drugs	Used interventionally and potentially in hypertension emergency management.
	Thiazides		Negligible.
	Acetazolamide		Approved for topic dose forms but used interventionally for brain scanning.
Narcotics	Codeine	Mask pain associated with injury	Potential for opioids to be used for pain management or biliary imaging.
	Morphine		

TABLE 16-2 Summary of Key Lifestyle Drugs			
Drug	*Clinical Use*	*Lifestyle Use*	*Consideration in Imaging*
Sildenafil	Erectile dysfunction	Erectile dysfunction	Yes (refer to Chapters 8 and 12)
Contraceptive	Birth control	Birth control and acne	Negligible
Orlistat	Obesity	Weight loss	Unlikely outside gastrointestinal tract transit studies
Bupropion	Nicotine addiction	Nicotine addiction	Possible (refer to Chapter 2)
Methadone	Opioid addiction	Opioid addiction	Yes (refer to Chapters 7 and 13)
Minoxidil	Hypertension	Baldness	Yes (refer to Chapters 6 and 8)
Opiates	Analgesia	Recreational	Yes (refer to Chapters 7 and 13)
Alcohol	Nil	Recreational	Possible at abuse levels
Caffeine	Nil	Recreational	At abuse levels (refer to Chapter 8)
Cannabis	Emerging	Recreational	Possible at abuse levels
Nicotine	Nil	Recreational	Possible at abuse levels
Botulinum toxin	Spasm relief	Cosmetic	Unlikely for cosmetic applications
Nutrients and vitamins	Support health	Support health	Possible in overdose
Herbal formulations	Support health	Support health	Significant potential interactions

Drugs Used in Sports

A number of drugs can produce a competitive advantage in sports. These drugs are regulated and banned by a variety of sports agencies (e.g., World Anti-Doping Agency) for 3 very important reasons:

1. They undermine the integrity of competition, equity, and fairness.
2. Evidence of actual benefit in performance is lacking and likely to be variable across individuals.
3. They pose serious risks to the health and well-being, both short and long term, of users if left unregulated.

While there is a lengthy list of medications whose use in sports is banned, a number of important medications can be approved for use under exemptions on the basis that they provide therapeutic benefit to the individual. Specifically, such exemptions would be granted on the basis that the therapy was necessary and that the benefit to athletic performance from using the medication is not greater than that which would be expected from the individual returning to normal health associated with the treatment. There are also considerations given when the prohibited medication is administered for emergency reasons (refer to Chapter 12).

Given radiology and nuclear medicine departments have a substantial role in imaging the elite amateur and professional athlete, some awareness of medications that could jeopardize their sports career is required. While it is unlikely that adjunctive or interventional medications administered in the medical imaging department would result in sporting sanctions, awareness and education provide a safety net. The World Anti-Doping Agency classifies banned drugs according to the following:

♦ S_0 are nonapproved substances that are not approved for use in humans and, outside research, should not be used in humans. These are of no interest to the medical radiation technologist.

- S_1 are anabolic steroids that are similar in action to endogenous testosterone. These are of no interest to the medical radiation technologist except in a very rare circumstance of interest rather than impact. Virilization in women associated with adrenal pathology is often imaged in ultrasound, computed tomography (CT), magnetic resonance imaging (MRI), single-photon emission computed tomography (SPECT) and positron emission tomography (PET). On occasion, the patient may be a female athlete subjected to such gender scrutiny.
- S_2 peptide hormones, growth factor, and related substances are of no interest to the medical radiation technologist.
- S_3 beta-2 (β_2)-agonists are banned, but in emergency situations, β_2-agonists are likely to be administered via inhalation (inhaler or nebulizer), and such medications in these forms are exempt.
- S_4 hormones and metabolic modulators are unlikely to be associated with medical imaging but could be part of medical oncology.
- S_5 diuretics and other masking agents are banned and are the most likely issue in medical radiation science, as diuretics are used interventionally in renal imaging and could be used adjunctively to manage hypertension in the department. They are used by athletes (and nonathletes) to reduce body fluid and weight quickly and to attempt to mask other classes of banned substances.
- S_6 stimulants come in a wide variety of forms unrelated to a medical imaging department (e.g., amphetamines), but under emergency conditions, banned drugs such as epinephrine (adrenaline) could be used or an EpiPen could be used in allergic response (e.g., to contrast media). Stimulants are banned only during competition.
- S_7 narcotics include illicit drugs, but morphine augmentation in biliary imaging or the use of opioid medications for pain relief are an issue. This class of drug is banned only during competition, so understanding the half-life could be important.
- S_8 cannabinoids, whether natural or synthetic, are of little interest in medical radiation science except in the case of patients who may take medicinal cannabis for seizures or pain.
- S_9 glucocorticosteroids are banned during competition, are not generally of interest in medical radiation science, but some patients may be using glucocorticosteroids to treat inflammation.
- M_1 manipulation of blood and blood components (by any physical or chemical means) includes radiolabeling of red blood cells or white blood cells. In this case, an exemption should be sought. Technically, an in vivo blood label would avoid this classification, but in vitro or in vivtro methods would be classified as banned.
- M_2 physical and chemical manipulation do not relate to medical administrations associated with infusions (contrast, PET auto-injector).
- M_3 gene doping is unlikely to be associated with medical imaging.
- P_1 alcohol is banned only in specific sports and of no interest to medical radiation science.
- P_2 β-blockers are banned only in specific sports where modulation of the heart rate may present an advantage (e.g., shooting). β-Blockers are seldom administered in the imaging department but are a common medication patients may be prescribed. In terms of risk to an athlete, response to an emergency is the most likely scenario.

Lifestyle Drugs

An increasing number of patients are presenting to radiology and nuclear medicine departments with obesity and for investigation of issues relating to obesity (e.g., coronary artery disease). Obesity comes with a raft of other well-documented health risks, including but not limited to cancer, cardiovascular disease, metabolic disorders, bone and joint disease, and diabetes. Obesity can result from endocrine disorders, but the obesity epidemic confronting western civilization is the result of an imbalance between energy intake and energy use: overconsumption. While the pathophysiology of obesity is beyond the scope of this text, it is important to consider 2 processes contributing to obesity. The first occurs when the energy imbalance occurs in childhood, resulting in an increased number of adipose (fat) cells. The second relates to adulthood when the number of fat cells does not necessarily increase but rather the cells get bigger. Obesity is complex and requires careful consideration to manage, but these 2 processes are an important part of those considerations.

Obesity is perhaps best considered like any other disease or disorder. Pathology develops slowly and symptoms emerge. Medications can be used to manage symptoms without changing the underlying cause of the symptoms (pathology). Medications or more invasive interventions (e.g., surgery), could be used to resolve the pathology itself. In obesity, obesity is the symptom, not the cause. Medications tend to be targeted at decreasing food consumption rather than resolving the driver of overconsumption. Norepinephrine-like medications (e.g., phentermine) are designed as appetite suppressants but are contraindicated in cardiovascular or cerebrovascular disease, a very common comorbidity of obesity. Selective serotonin reuptake inhibitors (SSRIs), such as the antidepressant fluoxetine, are effective at short-term weight reduction, but beyond 6 months, even with continued use, SSRIs do not reduce weight. Leptin is a peptide produced in fat cells that stimulates decreased food intake under normal circumstances, but in obesity, leptin resistance causes this negative feedback mechanism to fail. Release of cholecystokinin (CCK) during digestion reduces hunger (increases satiety) to decrease food intake and, given the role of bile in emulsifying fats, should be particularly active during a fatty meal.

Orlistat is perhaps the most commonly used medication for obesity. Orlistat inhibits important lipases required for the breakdown of dietary fat. This reduces absorption of cholesterol and lipid-soluble nutrients (vitamins) by as much as 30%. Clearly, increasing the residual fat content to transit the gastrointestinal tract produces side effects such as fatty stools, flatulence, liquid stools, fecal urgency, abdominal pain, and fecal incontinence.

Substance abuse is another important consideration in the medical imaging department. While illicit drugs are an important consideration, alcohol and nicotine abuse also require discussion. Illicit drugs such as narcotics, cannabinoids, and cocaine have origins of use in medicine. Side effects and interactions are well understood and documented in previous chapters. Of importance to note is the potential interaction between an illicit drug and a medication that could increase or decrease efficacy.

Alcohol is widely consumed, including at abuse levels. Alcohol is a prodrug that is metabolized in the liver to produce acetaldehyde. Alcohol is eliminated following zero-order kinetics, and it can be several days before normal function, particularly of the liver, returns. Alcohol consumption interferes with many drugs, but of particular interest are drugs metabolized in the liver. Some medications, especially those with a sedative effect, are potentiated by alcohol consumption (e.g., antihistamines). As illustrated in Figures 16-1 and 16-2, ethanol activates the GABA receptor to decrease action potential and produce central nervous system (CNS) depression.

Nicotine is a stimulant for peripheral and CNS tissues (Fig. 16-3). Nicotine can increase or decrease the effects of a wide variety of medications by changing the half clearance rate or receptor activity. In Chapter 8, the impact of alcohol and nicotine on altering metabolism of xanthine in the liver was outlined; this alteration leads to increased elimination half-life and thus increases bioavailability and effects of xanthines. Specifically, and recognizing this is not an exhaustive list, nicotine has an impact on the following medications:

- Clozapine and olanzapine show increased metabolism and decreased plasma concentrations with smoking.
- Fluvoxamine and imipramine require higher doses in smokers.

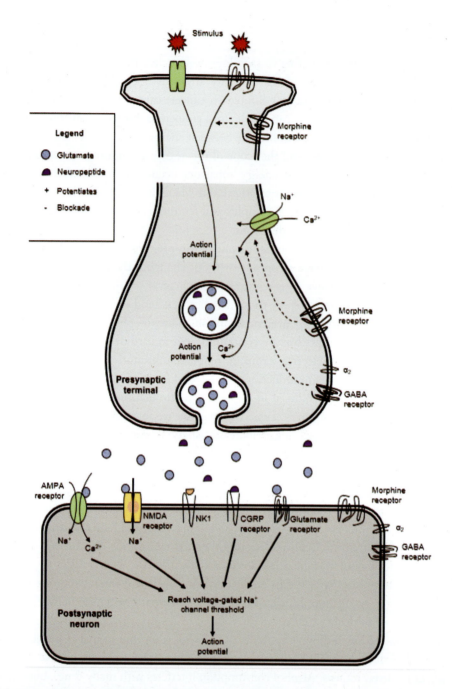

FIGURE 16-1 Schematic representation of the presynaptic terminal and postsynaptic neuron without the effects of alcohol. Glutamate release and receptor activation produce action potential and conduction.

- Warfarin can have increased clearance and decreased plasma concentrations with smoking.
- Prodrugs such as clopidogrel have enhanced metabolism in smoking, increasing plasma concentrations.
- Smoking substantially decreases the plasma concentrations of caffeine, meaning a smoker requires up to 4 times more caffeine to reach the same plasma concentrations as a nonsmoker.
- The sedative effects of benzodiazepines can be reduced in smokers.
- Smoking potentiates the risks associated with the oral contraceptive pill.

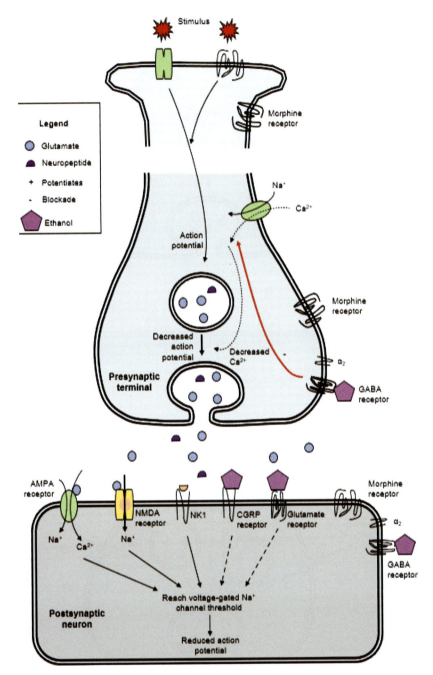

FIGURE 16-2 Schematic representation of the presynaptic terminal and postsynaptic neuron in Figure 16-1 with the effects of alcohol. GABA receptors on the presynaptic terminal decrease calcium influx in a manner similar to morphine on morphine receptors. This decreases the action potential and glutamate release, decreasing activation of postsynaptic receptors. Ethanol also inhibits glutamate and calcitonin gene-related peptide (CGRP) receptors, further reducing action potential.

Caffeine is also a lifestyle drug that, as detailed in Chapter 8 and addressed in Chapter 14, can significantly influence the effects of other medications (e.g., dipyridamole). Specifically, caffeine antagonizes adenosine at adenosine receptors, which can inhibit the vasodilatory effects (Fig. 16-3), the bronchospasm effects, and the CNS inhibitory effects (stimulant).

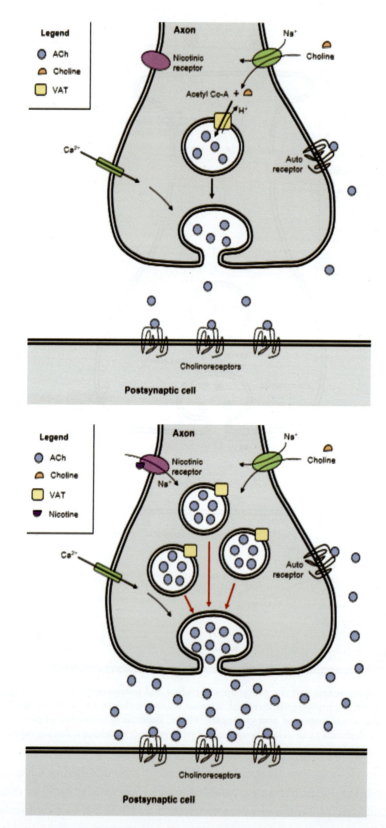

FIGURE 16-3　The effects of nicotine at the nicotinic receptors (peripherally in smooth muscle and cardiac muscles) and acetylcholine (Ach) receptors (CNS) produce stimulation. The top image is without nicotine, and the bottom image represents nicotine activation of the receptor, sodium influx, increased activation potential, increased number of vesicles, and increased release of neurotransmitter to cause stimulation.

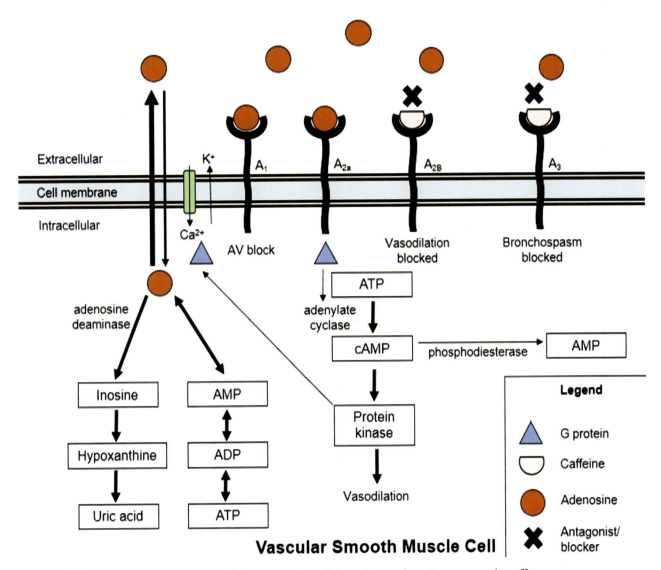

FIGURE 16-4 Schematic representation of the antagonism of adenosine at adenosine receptors by caffeine.

Some consideration should also be given to the widespread use of natural and herbal products. Herbal and natural therapies can have significant effects on the behavior of drugs. St John's wort, perhaps, appears in the most important drug interaction lists (e.g., warfarin, digoxin, theophylline, phenytoin), but natural iodine products (radiopharmaceuticals and contrast) and grapefruit juice (e.g., atorvastatin, fentanyl, loratadine, warfarin, verapamil) are among the natural products that can significantly alter medication pharmacokinetics and thus side effect profiles. While a large number of herbs and natural products are available, few have evidence of efficacy that warrants consideration in this text.

References

Asperheim K, Favaro J. *Introduction to Pharmacology*. 12th ed. St Louis, MO: Elsevier; 2012.

Block JH, Beale JM. *Wilson and Gisvold's Textbook of Organic Medicinal and Pharmaceutical Chemistry*. 12th ed. Philadelphia, PA: Lippincott Williams & Wilkins; 2011.

Bryant B, Knights K, Salerno E. *Pharmacology for Health Professionals*. 2nd ed. Sydney, Australia: Mosby Elsevier; 2007.

Katzung BG, Masters SB, Trevor AJ. *Basic and Clinical Pharmacology*. 12th ed. New York, NY: McGraw Hill; 2012.

Rang H, Dale M, Ritter J, Flower R. *Rang and Dale's Pharmacology*. 6th ed. London, England: Churchill Livingston; 2008.

Waller D, Renwick A, Hillier K. *Medical Pharmacology and Therapeutics*. 2nd ed. London, England: Elsevier; 2006.

CHAPTER 17

Known Interactions with Radiopharmaceuticals

Chapter Objectives

Specific learning outcomes (page ix) of this text addressed in this chapter:

- Recognize general, patient-specific, and scenario-specific risks, precautions, and contraindications for use of medicines.
- Apply the pharmacokinetic and pharmacodynamic principles of medications to identify and explain normal and adverse reactions to medications.
- Administer medications safely, effectively, and appropriately according to procedures and within regulatory and statutory parameters.
- Monitor patients for, identify, and manage adverse reactions.

After reading, digesting, reflecting on, and reviewing the content of this chapter, readers should be able to

1. Demonstrate command of key pharmacology terms.
2. Demonstrate enhanced understanding of the principles associated with interactions between drugs and radiopharmaceuticals.
3. Recognize, explain, and interpret clinical problems and evidence in relation to interactions.
4. Apply knowledge of the general principles and concepts in a translational manner to clinical practice.

Key Terms

adverse reaction	direct action	fluoridated	iatrogenic	pretargeting
biodistribution	DNA break	free radical	indirect action	sensitize
collateral	hypersensitivity	HAMA	myelosuppression	vasovagal

Introduction

While the focus of this text has been on the medications encountered in nuclear medicine and radiology, some consideration should be given to the potential adverse reactions or interactions that occur with radiopharmaceuticals. Adverse reactions to contrast media are detailed in Chapters 10 and 11.

Adverse Reactions to Radiopharmaceuticals

Adverse reactions to the administration of a diagnostic radiopharmaceutical are uncommon (2.3 per 100,000 administrations and zero deaths). This low number of adverse reactions relates largely to the tracer principle: the use of trace concentrations of chemicals at benign levels. Recall that only the dose makes the poison. This includes ^{18}F-fluorodeoxyglucose (FDG), ^{18}F-sodium fluoride, and similar relatively inert tracers. When an adverse reaction occurs, it is likely to be transient, mild, and associated with hypersensitivity. Common reactions include nausea, dyspnea, bronchospasm, decreased blood pressure, itching, flushing, hives, chills, coughing, bradycardia, muscle cramps, and dizziness. Most adverse reactions require no or minimal treatment, but antihistamines are the front-line approach; if this approach fails, aminophylline can be used. In anaphylaxis, epinephrine may be required. A *vasovagal* reaction is often confused with an allergic reaction by patients or their caregivers. While careful management of a vasovagal reaction is important, the reaction is to having an injection rather than to the contents of the injection.

Recent developments in radiochemistry have seen the emergence of immunological imaging (e.g., monoclonal antibodies [MAbs]). A major limitation of MAb use has been the induction of an immune response to the MAb (e.g., human antimurine antibody, or *HAMA*), which can sensitize the patient and result in a severe immunological response to a second administration. In short, the assumption that patients rarely have adverse responses to radiopharmaceuticals generally holds true, but the diverse array of radiopharmaceuticals demands scrutiny of specific risks of each product before use. The adverse reaction rate is generally low, but there is a risk (1%–5%) of more serious symptoms, such as fever, hypotension, chest pain, and angioedema.

Radionuclide therapy comes with a diverse adverse risk profile associated with the particulate radiation over and above those outlined previously. A partially extravasated dose can cause local tissue damage. Normal and altered elimination can produce damaging radiation doses to critical organs (e.g., kidneys or bladder). Collateral tissue damage can produce a raft of adverse reactions (e.g., pulmonary fibrosis, secondary neoplasia development, myelosuppression). Radiation damage occurs through direct action to produce double- or single-strand DNA breaks or by indirect action associated with production of free radicals that damage the DNA. This damage can occur in any tissue exposed to the particulate radiation. It is an important reason to maximize uptake in target tissue and expedite clearance from nontarget tissue. For radiopharmaceuticals with slow localization, the nontarget dose is high, the actual dose needs to be reduced to accommodate dosimetry, and efficacy is undermined. A novel approach to addressing this issue utilizes *pretargeting* in which the "cold" tracer is administered to accommodate the slow localization and is followed by a radionuclide that targets the tracer (e.g., peptide) more rapidly.

Iatrogenic Changes to Radiopharmaceutical Biodistribution

Many drugs have the potential to alter the *biodistribution* of radiopharmaceuticals. As discussed in previous chapters, this alteration can be intentional to facilitate interventional studies. Nonetheless, the risk of unintentional and undesired alterations to biodistribution threatens image quality and diagnostic integrity. Table 17-1 provides a brief insight into the major radiopharmaceuticals and their common drug interactions.

TABLE 17-1 Common Drug Interactions for Frequently Used Radiopharmaceuticals		
Radiopharmaceutical Group	*Medication*	*Adverse Effect*
Bone imaging	Melphalan, actinomycin	Increased bone uptake
	Corticosteroids, phosphorus derivatives, dextrose, nifedipine	Decreased bone uptake
	Meperidine, heparin, iron dextran (in site), aluminium (liver), estrogens (breast), phenytoin (spleen), doxorubicin (cardiac)	Soft tissue uptake
	Chemotherapy agents, dextrose, iron, gentamicin	Increased renal activity
Myocardial perfusion	Dipyridamole, furosemide, isoproterenol, dexamethasone	Increased myocardial uptake
	Beta blockers, glycosides, phenytoin, lidocaine, minoxidil, doxorubicin	Decreased myocardial uptake
Biliary imaging	Cholecystokinin	Increased gallbladder contraction
	Narcotics, phenobarbital	Prolonged transit to duodenum
	Atropine	Prolonged gallbladder activity
	Nicotine	Decreased liver uptake
	Erythromycin	Increased liver uptake
Thyroid imaging	Iodine solutions, iodinated contrast media, antithyroid drugs, iodinated food (cabbage, kelp, soy), amiodarone, antihistamines, bromides, glucocorticoids, benzodiazepines, NSAIDs, cough medicines, antibiotics	Decreased uptake
^{67}Ga citrate	Iron dextran or deferoxamine before ^{67}Ga injection, frusemide (tumor)	Decreased uptake
	Iron dextran or deferoxamine after ^{67}Ga injection	Increased uptake
	Chemotherapy agents, amiodarone	Diffuse lung uptake
	Phenobarbital	Increased liver uptake
	Antibiotics	Colon uptake
	Chemotherapy agents, furosemide, phenytoin, allopurinol, antibiotics, NSAIDs	Increased renal uptake
	Estrogens, amiodarone, busulfan, fluphenazine, reserpine, metoclopramide	Breast uptake
	Gadolinium contrast, methotrexate	Diffuse bone uptake
RBC labeling	Heparin, dextran, doxorubicin, methyldopa, propranolol penicillin, hydralazine, iodinated contrast media, digoxin, nifedipine	Poor label

(continued)

TABLE 17-1 Common Drug Interactions for Frequently Used Radiopharmaceuticals

Radiopharmaceutical Group	Medication	Adverse Effect
Sulfur colloid imaging	Aluminium, iron, virilizing androgens, niacin, magnesium	Increased lung uptake
	Anesthetics, methylcellulose	Increased spleen uptake
	Chemotherapy agents, epinephrine, antimalarials	Decreased spleen uptake
	Nitrosoureas	Increased bone marrow uptake
	Estrogens	Focal increases in the liver
Gastric empty/transit	Antacids, anticholinergics, atropine, levodopa, metoclopramide, morphine, propantheline	Prolonged transit
Renography	Diuretics	Increased clearance
	ACE inhibitors, angiotensin receptor blockers, aluminium, gentamicin	Altered GFR
FDG	Corticosteroids, serum insulin and glucose levels	Altered biodistribution
MIBG	Tricyclic antidepressants, nifedipine, methylphenidate, β-blockers, cocaine, neuroleptics, amiodarone, salbutamol	Altered biodistribution

Abbreviations: ACE, angiotensin-converting enzyme; FDG, fluorodeoxyglucose; ^{67}Ga, gallium-67; GFR, glomerular filtration rate; MIBG, metaiodobenzylguanidine; NSAID, nonsteroidal anti-inflammatory drug; RBC, red blood cell.

Insight

From "Potential Iatrogenic Alteration to ^{18}F Fluoride Biodistribution" by C. Currie, H. Kiat, and J. Wheat (*J Nucl Med.* 2010;51(5):823).

^{18}F-fluoride positron emission tomography (PET) has reemerged as a genuine clinical alternative to technetium-99m (^{99m}Tc)-diphosphonate scintigraphy. In vivo, sodium fluoride (NaF) dissociates into its salts, Na$^+$ and F$^-$ (fluoride). Fluoride is exchanged with OH$^-$ (hydroxyl) ion in the hydroxyapatite matrix of the bone before migrating into the crystalline matrix. Approximately 50% of the injected dose localizes in bone, and bone retention of fluoride continues until bone remodeling. Fluoride has minimal protein binding affinity, allowing more rapid excretion of the fraction not localized in bone and favoring earlier post-administration imaging and low background activity. Elevation in plasma concentrations of unlabeled fluoride may reduce ^{18}F-fluoride uptake because of competition. In vivo competition is likely to increase the ratio of ^{18}F-fluoride excreted to ^{18}F-fluoride bound in bone, decreasing the percentage of the injected dose localizing in the bone. The effects on image quality may include a decrease in target organ count density and an increase in renal and bladder activity. The implications might be even more crucial for quantitation of fluoride bone uptake.

There are several fluoridated hydrocarbon-based general anesthetics that are metabolized to produce fluoride ion, which should be considered a potential confounder of ^{18}F-fluoride bone uptake. Of the fluoridated ethers, the most frequently used inhaled anesthetic agents in developed countries are enflurane, isoflurane, desflurane, and sevoflurane. Enflurane has 2% to 8% oxidative metabolism in the liver to produce fluoride ions to plasma levels as high as 20 to 40 µM. Sevoflurane has about 1% to 5% liver metabolism, with one of the by-products being fluoride ions. Plasma fluoride concentrations in excess of 50 µM are produced; more than 50 µM is associated with renal impairment. Both enflurane and sevoflurane show serum fluoride ion levels peaking soon after completion of surgery (cessation of anesthetic delivery). Nonetheless, elevated serum fluoride ion levels are high beyond 24 hours. The retention of high serum levels after cessation of anesthesia is likely to represent saturation of fluoride on bone and reverse exchange from the bone surface to blood once blood concentration falls below that of bone. The implication for ^{18}F-fluoride PET is that significantly less than the usual 50% of the injected dose may localize to bone if enflurane or sevoflurane anesthesia has been used in the previous 24 to 36 hours, perhaps longer for prolonged general anesthesia or in those with renal impairment.

Although potential competitive interaction between ^{18}F-fluoride and the by-products of inhalation anesthetics may decrease image quality, of greater importance is the potential impact of this competition on bone uptake quantitation. Further qualitative and quantitative research should be undertaken to determine the relationship and time course of interaction between fluoride ion–producing inhalation anesthetics and ^{18}F-fluoride PET image quality.

References

Brunton LL, Lazo JS, Parker KL. *Goodman & Gillman's The Pharmacological Basis of Therapeutics*. 11th ed. Philadelphia, PA: McGraw-Hill; 2006: 353–360.

Currie G, Kiat H, Wheat, J. Potential iatrogenic alteration to ^{18}F fluoride biodistribution. *J Nucl Med*. 2010;51(5):823.

Duffy CM, Matta BF. Sevoflurane and anesthesia for neurosurgery: a review. *J Neurosurg Anesthesiol*. 2000;12:128–140.

Grant FD, Fahey FH, Packard AB, Davis RT, Alavi A, Treves ST. Skeletal PET with ^{18}F-fluoride: applying new technology to an old tracer. *J Nucl Med*. 2008;49:68–78.

Metler F, Guiberteau M. *Essentials of Nuclear Medicine Imaging*. 6th ed. Philadelphia, PA: Saunders; 2012.

Rang HP, Dale MM, Ritter JM, Flower RJ. *Pharmacology*. 6th ed. Philadelphia, PA: Churchill Livingstone; 2008: 526–531.

Saha GB. Adverse reactions to and altered biodistribution of radiopharmaceuticals. In: GB Saha, ed. *Fundamentals of Nuclear Pharmacy*. Cham, Switzerland: Springer; 2018.

Theobald Y. *Sampson's Textbook of Radiopharmacy*. 4th ed. London, England: Pharmaceutical Press; 2011.

ABOUT THE AUTHOR

Dr. Geoff Currie was appointed in Medical Radiation Science at Charles Sturt University in 2002. Geoff has a bachelor's degree in pharmacy, master's degree in medical radiation science (nuclear medicine), a master's degree in applied management (health), a master's degree in business administration (MBA), and a doctor of philosophy (PhD). Geoff has broad research and teaching interests across the medical radiation sciences and, indeed, health generally, with more than 150 peer-reviewed journal papers, 150 conference presentations, 55 invited speaker presentations, and as a reviewer for 25 international journals.

Geoff teaches pharmacology to medical radiation science students at Charles Sturt University and previously developed the pharmacology content for medical students at Macquarie University. Geoff is International Consulting Editor of the *Journal of Nuclear Medicine Technology* (JNMT) and is cofounder of the Rural Alliance in Nuclear Scintigraphy (RAINS). On Australia Day 2020, Geoff was awarded Member of the Order of Australia (AM) in recognition of his contribution to nuclear medicine and medical radiation science. A significant part of that award was his commitment to advanced practice training and continuing education, including initiatives in Australia, Canada, and the United States for pharmacology training through JNMT, Society of Nuclear Medicine and Molecular Imaging Technologist Section (SNMMI-TS), Canadian Association of Medical Radiation Technologists (CAMRT), and RAINS. Other than this book, a summary of his pharmacology-related peer-reviewed journal articles include (non-pharmacology-based outputs excluded):

- Currie G. Pharmacology part 5: CT and MRI contrast. *J Nucl Med Technol.* 2019;47(3):189–202.
- Currie G. Pharmacology part 4: nuclear cardiology. *J Nucl Med Technol.* 2019;47(2):97–110.
- Currie G. Pharmacology part 3B: general nuclear medicine; other interventions and adjunctive medications. *J Nucl Med Technol.* 2019;47(1):3–12.
- Currie G. Pharmacology part 3A: general nuclear medicine; renal and hepatobiliary imaging. *J Nucl Med Technol.* 2018;46(4):326–334.
- Currie G. Pharmacology part 2: introduction to pharmacokinetics. *J Nucl Med Technol.* 2018;46(93):221–230.
- Currie G. Pharmacology part 1: introduction to pharmacology and pharmacodynamics. *J Nucl Med Technol.* 2018;46(2):81–86.
- Cousins J, Czachowski M, Muthukrishnan A, Currie G. Pediatric brown adipose tissue (BAT) on FDG PET: diazepam intervention. *J Nucl Med Technol.* 2017;45(2):82–86.
- O'Loughlin S, Currie G, Trifonovic M, Kiat H. Impact of ambient temperature on cardiac accumulation of FDG. *J Nucl Med Technol.* 2014;42(3):186–193.
- Currie G, Haase M, Hashmi R, Kiat H. Hormone therapy in prostate cancer: a case study. *J Nucl Med Technol.* 2013;41(1):49–51.
- Currie G, Kiat H, Wheat J. Pharmacokinetic considerations for digoxin in older people, *TOCMJ.* 2011;5:130–135.
- Currie G, Wheat J, Wang L, Kiat H. Pharmacology in nuclear cardiology. *Nucl Med Commun.* 2011;32(7):617–627.
- Currie G, Kiat H, Wheat J. Potential iatrogenic alteration to ^{18}F fluoride biodistribution. *J Nucl Med Technol.* 2010;51(5):823.

INDEX

Page numbers followed by an "*f*" refer to figures; those followed by a "*t*" refer to tables.

5-fluorouracil, 194*t*
5-hyroxytryptamine (5-HT), 9–11
^{67}Ga citrate, 237*t*

A

absorption, 27*f*, 28–30, 28*f*, 29*t*, 30
  distribution
    metabolism
      excretion, and toxicity
        (ADMET) of drugs, 26
    and excretion (ADME) of drugs,
      26, 27*f*, 28*f*, 61
    metabolism, and excretion
      (ADME) of drugs,
      age-related changes in, 61
ACE inhibitors. *See*
  angiotensin-converting enzyme
  (ACE) inhibitors
acetaminophen, 33*f*, 174, 175*t*, 180*t*,
  184, 185*f*
  /codeine combination, 181*t*
acetazolamide, 106–110, 107*t*, 109*f*
acetylcholine (ACh), 6–8, 6*f*
  pharmacology of, 156, 157*f*
ACh. *See* acetylcholine (ACh)
active transport, 26
adenosine, 11–13, 84–89, 86–87*f*, 88*t*
  in crash cart, 152*t*
  mode of action, pharmacokinetics,
    adverse reactions, and
    interactions, 166*t*
  pharmacology of, 156
  receptor subtypes, 222
adenosine monophosphate (AMP), 11*f*
adjunctive medications, 68
ADME. *See* absorption, distribution,
  metabolism, and excretion
  (ADME) of drugs
ADMET. *See* absorption, distribution,
  metabolism, excretion, and
  toxicity (ADMET) of drugs
administration. *See* drug
  administration; routes of
  administration
adrenergic (norepinephrine)
  pharmacology, 8–9, 8*f*, 10–12*f*

adrenergic stimulants in crash cart, 151
adverse reactions
  gadolinium MRI contrast, 143–145
  iodinated CT contrast, 127–128,
    129*f*, 130*t*, 131*f*
  radiopharmaceuticals, 236
affinity, 18, 19
aging, effects of, 58–62, 59*t*, 60*f*
agonists, 3–4, 4*f*
  muscarinic, 6
  nicotinic, 7–8
  opioid, 78–80
  α-adrenoreceptors, 9
  β-agonism, 11*f*
alcohol, 227*t*, 229, 230–231*f*
alkylating drugs, 194*t*
α-adrenoreceptors, 9
altretamine, 194*t*
aminophylline, 93–94, 93*t*, 221
amiodarone
  in crash cart, 152*t*
  mode of action, pharmacokinetics,
    adverse reactions, and
    interactions, 167*t*
amitriptyline, 174, 185
AMP. *See* adenosine monophosphate
  (AMP)
analgesics
  in crash cart, 151
  over-the-counter medications, 208
  pain management with opioid,
    174–179, 175*t*, 177–178*f*
  pharmacology of, 161
  See also pain management
anaphylaxis-like symptoms, 133, 146
  crash cart medications for, 151
anastrozole, 195*t*
anesthestics, pain prevention with,
  185–189, 186–188*f*
angiotensin-converting enzyme (ACE)
  inhibitors, 33
  captopril, 69*t*, 71–73, 72*f*
  enalapril, 69*t*, 73
ANS. *See* autonomic nervous system
  (ANS)
antagonists, 3–4, 4*f*
  histamine, 13–14

  muscarinic, 6
  nicotinic, 7–8
  α-adrenoreceptors, 9
antiarrhythmics
  in crash cart, 151
  pharmacology of, 159, 164–165*f*
anticholinergic medications in crash
  cart, 151
anticholinesterase medications, 7–8, 8*f*
anticoagulants, 134
  heparin, 108*t*, 115–116
antidiarrhea medications, 216
antihistamines, 13–14, 133
  in crash cart, 151
  over-the-counter medications,
    211–212, 211*f*
  pharmacology of, 157, 163*f*
antihypertensive medications in crash
  cart, 151
anti-inflammatory mediators, 179–184
  acetaminophen, 184, 185*f*
  aspirin, 179, 184
  comparison of, 180–181*t*
  ibuprofen, 179, 184
  mechanism of action of, 179–184,
    182–183*f*
antimetabolites, 194*t*
antipyretics, 210–211, 210*f*
anxiolytics
  in crash cart, 151
  diazepam, 108*t*, 114
  pharmacology of, 162
aspirin, 134, 174, 175*t*, 179, 180*t*, 184
  /codeine combination, 181*t*
atenolol, 99, 156
  in crash cart, 152*t*
  mode of action, pharmacokinetics,
    adverse reactions, and
    interactions, 167*t*
atrioventricular (AV) block, 12*f*
atropine, 133, 146
  in crash cart, 152*t*
  mode of action, pharmacokinetics,
    adverse reactions, and
    interactions, 167*t*
autonomic nervous system (ANS), 5,
  5–6*t*

B

bacteria and chemotherapy, 192
Benadryl, 133, 146, 212
benzodiazepines
    diazepam, 108t, 114, 133, 146
    lorazepam, 146
beta-blockers, 11f, 98t, 99–100, 134
    in crash cart, 151
    pharmacology of, 156, 159, 159f
β1-receptors, 99–100
β2-receptors, 99–100
β-adrenoreceptors, 9
β-agonism, 11f
    pharmacology of, 160f
β-agonists medications in crash cart, 151
Bevacizumab, 195t
biliary imaging interventions
    introduction to, 76
    key terms, 75
    morphine, 76t, 78–80
    phenobarbital, 76t, 80
    radiopharmaceuticals for, 237t
    sincalide, 76t, 77–78, 77f
binding, drug-receptor, 19, 30
bioavailability, 18, 28, 56
biodistribution of radiopharmaceuticals, 236, 237–238t
biotranformations, 33
bisacodyl, 108t, 115, 215–216
bisoprolol, 99
bleomycin, 195t
blood-brain barrier, 26
bone imaging, 237t
botulinum toxin, 227t
breast milk, 56–57
bromhexine, 221
bronchodilators
    in crash cart, 151
    as over-the-counter medications, 216–217, 217f
brown adipose tissue (BAT), 116–118, 117f
buprenorphine, 166t
    compared to other opioid medications, 176t
bupropion, 227t
busulfan, 194t

C

caffeine, 11f, 12f, 13, 34, 101–102, 227t, 231, 233f
calcium channel blockers, 11f, 98t, 100
    in crash cart, 151
calculations, dosing, 52

cancer
    chemotherapy for, 192-193, 196–197, 194–195f
    immunotherapy for, 197–199f, 198–202, 194–195t, 197f
    main drugs used for, 194–195t
    prostate, case study on, 202–205, 203–204f
cannabis, 227t
capecitabine, 194t
capsules, 48
captopril, 69t, 71–73, 72f
carbamazepine, 185
carbonic anhydrase inhibitors, 68
    acetazolamide, 106–110, 107t, 109f
carboplatin, 194t
cardiac imaging interventions
    adenosine, 84–89, 86–87f, 88t
    adjunctive medications, 92–98, 95f, 96t, 97f
    aminophylline, 93–94, 93t
    beta-blockers, 98t, 99–100
    calcium channel blockers, 98t, 100
    cessation medications, 98–101, 98t
    digoxin, 98t, 101
    dipyridamole, 88t, 89–91, 98t
    dobutamine, 89t, 91–92
    insight on, 101–102
    introduction to, 84
    key terms, 83
    nitrates, 98t, 100–101
    nitroglycerin (glyceryl trinitrate), 93t, 95–96, 95f
    pharmacological stress testing, 84, 85f, 88–89t
    regadenoson, 88t, 91
    salbutamol, 93t, 96–98, 97f
    xanthines, 98t, 99
cardiac myoctye, 11f
cardiovascular emergencies, crash cart medications for, 151
carmustine, 194t
carrier-mediated transport mechanisms, 26
carvedilol, 100
catecholamines, 8
    pharmacology of, 156
catechol-O-methyltransferase (COMT), 10f
celecoxib, 175t, 180t
central nervous system (CNS), 5
central nervous system (CNS) depressants
    chloral hydrate, 113–114
    diazepam, 108t, 114, 133, 146, 153t, 162, 167t

morphine, 76t, 78–80, 161, 166t, 175t, 176t
phenobarbital, 80
cetirizine, 212
cetuximab, 195t
chemotherapy
    for cancer, 192–193, 196–197f
    case study on, 202–205, 203–204f
    insight on, 199–202, 200f, 201–202f
    introduction to, 191–192
    key terms, 191
    pathogens and, 192
    See also immunotherapy
chemotoxic adverse reactions, 130
children, pharmacology consideration in, 57–58
chloral hydrate, 108t, 113–114
chlorambucil, 194t
cholecystokinin (CCK), 77–78, 77f
cholinergic pharmacology, 6–8, 6f
cimetidine, 107t, 110–112
cisplatin, 194t
cladribine, 194t
clearance, 34
CNS. See central nervous system (CNS)
codeine, 166t, 174, 175t
    /acetaminophen combination, 181t
    /aspirin combination, 181t
    compared to other opioid medications, 176t
    /ibuprofen combination, 181t
compartment modeling, 32, 32f
compliance, 61
computed tomography (CT). See CT contrast, iodinated
concordance, 61
conjugation reactions, 33
contraceptive drugs, 227t
contrast agents. See CT contrast, iodinated
coronary flow reserve, 84
cough medicines, 220–222, 221f
covalent bonds, 19
COX-2, 179, 182–183f
crash cart/emergency trolley
    emergency medication pharmacology and, 156–162, 157–165f, 166–170t
    introduction to, 150, 150f
    key terms, 149
    medications on, 151–152
    medication use in emergencies and, 152, 152–155t

CT contrast, iodinated
    adverse reactions to, 128–132, 129f, 130t, 131f
    contraindications and precautions, 134
    extravasation of, 133
    ideal agents for, 122
    interactions of, 134
    introduction to, 122
    key terms, 121
    mechanism of action of, 125f, 126–127
    pharmacokinetics of, 127–128
    properties of, 122–125, 123t, 125f
cyclic adenosine monophosphate (cAMP), 11f, 12f
cyclophosphamide, 194t
cytarabine, 194t
cytotoxic antibiotics, 194t

D

decongestants, 221
diarrhea, 216
diazepam, 108t, 114, 133, 146
    in crash cart, 153t
    mode of action, pharmacokinetics, adverse reactions, and interactions, 167t
    pharmacology of, 162
diclofenac, 180t
digoxin, 62, 62–64f, 98t, 101
diphenhydramine, 133, 146, 212
dipyridamole, 88t, 89–91, 98t
    pharmacology of, 161f
dissociation constant, 19
distribution, 30–32, 31–32f
    in older persons, 61–62
diuretics, 68
    in crash cart, 151
    pharmacology of, 158, 163f
dobutamine, 89t, 91–92
    in crash cart, 153t
    mode of action, pharmacokinetics, adverse reactions, and interactions, 168t
docetaxel, 194t
dopamine
    in crash cart, 153t
    mode of action, pharmacokinetics, adverse reactions, and interactions, 168t
dose forms, 46–50, 47t, 48–49f
    common examples of medications in different, 47t
    introduction to, 46
    key terms, 45
dose-response curves, 19, 21–22f
dose-response relationship, 20, 21–22f

dosing calculations, 52
    for children, 57–58
doxorubicin, 194t
drug action, 18
drug administration
    basic rule of, 51
    dose forms with common examples of medications administered in each form, 47t
    key terms, 45
    See also routes of administration
drug-drug interactions, 23
drug interactions, 23, 23f
drug receptor interactions, 19, 20f, 22f
drugs
    absorption of, 26, 27f, 28–30, 28f, 29ti, 30
    in crash cart contents, 151–152
    defined, 3
    distribution of, 30–32, 31–32f
    elimination of, 34, 35f
    metabolism of, 31f, 33–34, 33f
    over-the-counter (See over-the-counter medications)
    routes of administration of, 29t, 29ti, 30
    schedules and criteria for United States, United Kingdom, Canada, and Australia, 53t
    teratogenic effects of, 56
    used in emergencies, 152, 152–155t
duloxetine, 174

E

efficacy, 18
elimination, 34, 35f
emergency medications, 152, 152–155t
    pharmacology of, 156–162, 157–165f, 166–170t
emergency trolley. See crash cart/emergency trolley
enalapril, 69t, 73
endocrine emergencies, crash cart medications for, 151
ephedrine, 218, 219f
epinephrine, 133, 146
    in crash cart, 153t
    mode of action, pharmacokinetics, adverse reactions, and interactions, 168t
    for pain prevention, 189
EpiPen, 133
    in crash cart, 154t
    mode of action, pharmacokinetics, adverse reactions, and interactions, 169t

EpiPen Junior, 154t
erlotinib, 195t
etoposide, 195t
etoricoxib, 180t
expectorants, 220–222
extravasation
    gadolinium MRI contrast, 146–147
    iodinated CT contrast, 133

F

facilitated diffusion, 26
FDG, 238t
fentanyl, 166t, 175t
    compared to other opioid medications, 176t
fever, 210–211, 210f
fexofenadine, 212
F-fluoride positron emission tomography (PET), 236, 238–239
fibrinolytic medications, 134
first-order kinetics, 34
fludarabine, 195t
fluid or electrolyte emergencies, crash cart medications for, 151
flutamide, 195t
furosemide
    in crash cart, 154t
    mode of action, pharmacokinetics, adverse reactions, and interactions, 169t
furosemide (Lasix), 68–71, 69t, 70f
    labeling of, 150f

G

gabapentin, 174, 185
gadolinium MRI contrast. See MRI contrast
ganglion blockers, 7
gastric empty/transit radiopharmaceuticals, 238t
gemcitabine, 194t
glutamate, 174, 177f
grapefruit juice, 233

H

half-life, 34, 62
heparin, 108t, 115–116
herbal products, 227t, 233
histamine, 13–14, 13f
    benadryl, 133
    Benadryl, 146
    cimetidine, 107t, 110–112
    pharmacology of, 157, 163f
    ranitidine, 107t, 111f, 112

hormone modulators, 195t
hydrogen bonds, 19
hydrolysis, 33
hydromorphone, 166t
  compared to other opioid medications, 176t
hydrophobic effects, 19
hypnotics
  chloral hydrate, 108t, 113–114
  diazepam, 108t, 114

I

ibritumomab, 195t
ibuprofen, 174, 175t, 179, 180t, 184, 210
  /codeine combination, 181t
imaging interventions
  acetazolamide, 106–110, 107t, 109f
  adjunctive medications common in general nuclear medicine, 107–108t, 113–116
  biliary (See biliary imaging interventions)
  bisacodyl, 108t, 115
  cardiac (See cardiac imaging interventions)
  chloral hydrate, 108t, 113–114
  cimetidine, 107t, 110–112
  diazepam, 108t, 114
  heparin, 108t, 115–116
  insight on, 116–118, 117f
  introduction to, 106
  key terms, 105
  for less common interventional studies, 106–113, 107–108t
  omeprazole, 107t, 112–113
  ranitidine, 107t, 111f, 112
  renal (See renal imaging interventions)
imatinib, 195t
immunotherapy, 197–199f, 198–202, 194–195t, 197f
  main drugs used in, 194–195t
  See also chemotherapy
individual variations in pharmacology
  children and, 57–58
  effects of aging and, 58–62, 59t, 60f
  insight on, 62–63, 62–64f
  introduction to, 56
  key terms, 55
  women and, 56–57
inhalation, 29ti, 30
injection (parenteral) administration, 29ti, 30, 47t, 48, 49f
inotropic agents, 84
  in crash cart, 151
interactions
  gadolinium MRI contrast, 147

iodinated CT contrast, 134
interventional (imaging) medications, 68
intra-aural route, 47t
intramucular route, 29ti, 30
intranasal route, 29t, 47t, 50
intraocular route, 47t
intrarespiratory route, 47t
intravenous route, 29ti, 30
iodinated CT contrast. See CT contrast, iodinated
iodine products, natural, 233
ion channel transport, 26
ionic interactions, 19
irinotecan, 195t

L

labetalol, 100
laxatives
  bisacodyl, 108t, 115
  as over-the-counter medications, 214–216, 215f
leuprolide, 195t
lidocaine
  in crash cart, 154t
  mode of action, pharmacokinetics, adverse reactions, and interactions, 169t
  for pain prevention, 189
lifestyle and sports drugs
  introduction to, 226
  key drugs, 226–227t
  key terms, 225
  regulation and bans of, 227–228
  uses of, 226–227t, 229–233, 230–231f
ligands, 22f
local anesthetics, 189
lomustine, 194t
loop diuretics, 68
loratidine, 212
lorazepam, 146

M

mechlorethamine, 194t
meloxicam, 180t
melphalan, 194t
meperidine, 175t
metabolism, 31f, 33–34, 33f
metformin, 134
methadone, 166t, 227t
  compared to other opioid medications, 176t
methotrexate, 193, 196f, 194t
methylation, 13

methylxanthines, 11f, 13, 93–94, 98t, 220
  managing cessation of, 101–102
metoclopramide in crash cart, 154t
metoprolol, 100
  in crash cart, 154t
  mode of action, pharmacokinetics, adverse reactions, and interactions, 169t
MIBG, 238t
minoxidil, 227t
mitomycin, 195t
mitoxantrone, 194t
monoamine oxidase (MAO), 10f
morphine, 76t, 78–80
  compared to other opioid medications, 175t
  for mild, moderate, and severe pain, 175t
  pharmacology of, 161, 166t
morphine sulphate
  in crash cart, 154t
  mode of action, pharmacokinetics, adverse reactions, and interactions, 169t
MRI contrast, gadolinium
  adverse reactions to, 143–145
  classes of MRI contrast agents and, 138–139
  contraindications and precautions, 143, 144f
  extravasation of, 147
  interactions, 147
  introduction to, 138
  key terms, 137
  mechanism of action of, 141, 142f
  nephrogenic systemic fibrosis and, 145–146
  pharmacokinetics of, 141, 142f
  properties of, 138–139, 140t, 141f
mucolytics, 220–222
muscarinic receptors, 6
myocardial perfusion, 237t

N

naloxone
  in crash cart, 154t
  mode of action, pharmacokinetics, adverse reactions, and interactions, 170t
naproxen, 175t, 180t
nasal sprays, 29t, 47t, 50
natural and herbal products, 227t, 233
natural iodine products, 233
nephrogenic systemic fibrosis, 145–146

neurological emergencies, crash cart medications for, 151
neuromuscular blockers, 7
nicotine, 227*t*, 229–230, 232*f*
nicotinic receptors, 6–8
nitrates, 98*t*, 100–101
nitric oxide, 162*f*
nitroglycerin (glyceryl trinitrate), 93*t*, 95–96, 95*f*, 133, 146
   in crash cart, 155*t*
   as emergency medication, 156
   mode of action, pharmacokinetics, adverse reactions, and interactions, 170*t*
   pharmacology of, 156
nonsedating antihistamines, 14
nonsteroidal anti-inflammatory drugs. *See* NSAIDs (nonsteroidal anti-inflammatory drugs)
norepinephrine
   in crash cart, 155*t*
   mode of action, pharmacokinetics, adverse reactions, and interactions, 170*t*
   as over-the-counter medication, 218, 219*f*
   pharmacology of, 156, 158*f*
   synthesis of, 8–9, 10–12*f*
NSAIDs (nonsteroidal anti-inflammatory drugs), 134, 174, 175*t*, 179
   comparison of different, 180–181*t*
   as over-the-counter medications, 208, 210*f*
nuclear medicine, adjunctive medications in, 107–108*t*, 113–116
   bisacodyl, 108*t*, 115
   chloral hydrate, 108*t*, 113–114
   diazepam, 108*t*, 114
   heparin, 108*t*, 115–116
nutrients and vitamins, 227*t*

O

obesity, 229
octreotide, 195*t*
omeprazole, 107*t*, 112–113, 214
opiates, 227*t*
opioid agonists, 78–80, 185
opioids
   pain management with, 174–179, 175–176*t*, 177–178*f*
   pharmacology of, 161, 166*t*
   receptor activation with, 178*f*
oral (enteral) administration, 29*t*, 29*ti*, 30, 46, 47*t*
orlistat, 227*t*, 229

osmolality, 122
OTC medications. *See* over-the-counter medications
over-the-counter medications
   analgesic, 208–210
   antidiarrheal, 216
   antihistamine, 211–212, 211*f*
   antipyretic, 210–211, 210*f*
   bronchodilators, 216–217, 217*f*
   cough medicines, 220–222, 221*f*
   gastric acid reducers, 213–214, 213*f*
   insight on, 222
   introduction to, 208
   key terms, 207
   laxatives, 214–216, 215*f*
   sympathomimetic decongestant, 218, 219*f*
oxaliplatin, 194*t*
oxidation, 33
oxprenolol, 100
oxycodone, 166*t*, 175*t*
   compared to other opioid medications, 176*t*
oxymorphone, 175*t*

P

pain management, 175*t*
   adjunctive, 185
   anesthetics for pain prevention and, 185–189, 186–188*f*
   anti-inflammatory mediators in, 179–184, 180–181*t*, 185*f*
   introduction to, 174
   key terms, 173
   with opioid analgesics, 174–179, 175–176*t*, 177–178*f*
   See also analgesics
panitumumab, 195*t*
paracetamol (acetaminophen), 33*f*
parasympathetic receptor actions, 5–6*t*
passive diffusion, 26
pediatric pharmacology, 57–58
pentagastrin, 195*t*
percutaneous administration, 29*ti*, 30
peripheral nervous system (PNS), 5
pessary, 50
pethidine, 166*t*
   compared to other opioid medications, 176*t*
pharmacodynamics, 2, 2*f*
   defined, 18
   dose-response relationship, 20, 21–22*f*
   drug action, 18
   drug interactions, 23, 23*f*
   drug receptor interactions, 19, 20*f*, 22*f*
   key terms, 17

   relationship between pharmacokinetics and, 27*f*
pharmacokinetics, 2, 2*f*
   absorption, 26, 27*f*, 28–30, 28*f*, 29*ti*, 30
   distribution, 30–32, 31–32*f*
   elimination, 34, 35*f*
   gadoliunium MRI contrast, 141, 142*f*
   insight on, 34–43, 35–36*f*, 35*f*, 35*t*, 36*f*, 38*f*, 38*t*, 40–43*f*, 40–43*t*
   introduction to, 26, 27–28*f*
   iodinated CT contrast agents, 127–128
   key terms, 25
   metabolism, 33–34, 33*f*
   relationship between pharmacodynamics and, 27*f*
   summary of useful formulae and definitions in, 35*t*
pharmacological stress testing, 84, 85*f*, 90*f*
pharmacology
   adrenergic (norepinephrine), 8–9, 8*f*, 10–12*f*
   cholinergic, 6–8, 6*f*
   considerations in children, 57–58
   considerations in women, 56–57
   definitions of terms in, 3*t*
   effects of aging on, 58–62, 59*t*, 60*f*
   emergency medicine, 156–162, 157–165*f*, 166–170*t*
   introduction to, 2–3, 2*f*, 3*t*
   key terms, 1
   of other important receptors, 9–14, 10–13*f*
phenobarbital, 76*t*, 80
phenylephrine, 218
phenytoin, 185
pindolol, 100
pinocytosis, 26
plasma protein binding, 30–31
platinum analogs, 194*t*
pNS. *See* peripheral nervous system (PNS)
poisoning and overdose, crash cart medications for, 151
polypharmacy, 23, 59–60, 61–62
pore transport, 26
positron emission tomography (PET), 238–239
potassium-sparing diuretics, 68
potency, 3, 18
pregabalin, 174, 185
prilocaine, 189
procainamide
   in crash cart, 155*t*
   mode of action, pharmacokinetics, adverse reactions, and interactions, 170*t*

prodrugs, 33, 93–94
promethazine
  in crash cart, 153t
  mode of action, pharmacokinetics, adverse reactions, and interactions, 167t
  as over-the-counter medication, 212
propranolol, 100
prostaglandins, 181
prostate cancer, 202–205, 203–204f
proton pump inhibitors, omeprazole, 107t, 112
pseudoephedrine, 219f, 220, 222f
purine analogs, 195t

R

radioimmunotherapy (RIT), 197
radiopharmaceuticals
  adverse reactions to, 236
  biodistribution of, 236, 237–238t
  dosing of, 51
  insight into, 238–239
  introduction to, 236
  key terms, 235
radiopharmacy, 31
ranitidine, 107t, 111f, 112
rBC labeling, 237t
receptor inhibitors, 195t
receptors
  action of, 5, 5–6t
  defined, 3
  drug interactions, 19, 20f, 22f
  pharmacology of other important, 9–14, 10–13f
  principles of, 3–4, 4f
rectal route, 29ti, 47t, 50
reduction, 33
regadenoson, 88t, 91
renal imaging interventions
  captopril, 69t, 71–73, 72f
  enalapril, 69t, 73
  furosemide (Lasix), 68–71, 69t, 70f
  insight on, 73–74
  introduction to, 68
  key terms, 67
  summary of, 76t, 80
  table of, 69t
renin-angiotensin-aldosterone system (RAAS), 71–73, 72f
respiratory emergencies, crash cart medications for, 151
rituximab, 195t
routes of administration, 29ti, 30, 48f
  defined, 46
  See also drug administration

S

salbutamol, 93t, 96–98, 97f, 133, 146
  in crash cart, 155t
  mode of action, pharmacokinetics, adverse reactions, and interactions, 170t
saliva, 61
sedating antihistamines, 14
selective serotonin reuptake inhibitors (SSRIs), 10
selectivity, 3, 18
self-medication, 208
serotonin, 9–11
sildenafil, 227t
sincalide, 76t, 77–78, 77f
somatostatin analogs, 197
sotalol, 100
specificity, 18
sports drugs. See lifestyle and sports drugs
SSRIs. See selective serotonin reuptake inhibitors (SSRIs)
St John's wort, 233
stress testing, 84, 85f, 88–89t
subcutaneous route, 29t, 30
sublingual route, 29t, 47t
substance abuse, 229
sulfonamides, 192
sulfur colloid imaging, 238t
sulindac, 175t
sunitinib, 195t
suspensions, 46
sympathetic receptor actions, 5–6t
sympathomimetic decongestants, 218, 219f
synaptosome-associated proteins (SNAPs), 8f, 10f

T

tablets, 48, 49f
tamoxifen, 195t, 197, 197f
taxane, 194t
teratogenic effects, 56
theobromine, 13
theophylline, 11f, 12f, 13, 34, 93–94
  role in antagonizing adenosine, 220, 221f
theranostics, 193
therapeutic index, 18, 61
therapeutic range, 26
thiazide diuretics, 68
thiotepa, 194t
thyroid imaging, radiopharmaceuticals for, 237t
tonicity, 122
topical medications, 29ti, 30, 47t, 50, 50f
topoisomerase inhibitors, 195t
topotecan, 195t
tositumomab, 195t
tramadol, 166t, 175t
  compared to other opioid medications, 176t
transdermal administration, 29ti, 30, 50, 50f
trauma, crash cart medications for, 151
tricyclic antidepressants, 185
trypanophobia, 185
tyrosine, 10f, 156, 158f

U

urethral route, 47t, 50

V

vaginal route, 47t, 50
van der Waals forces, 19
vascular smooth muscle cell, 12f
vasoconstrictor medications in crash cart, 151
vasodilation of arteries, 84, 85f
vasodilators
  in crash cart, 151
  pharmacology of, 161f
verapamil
  in crash cart, 153t
  mode of action, pharmacokinetics, adverse reactions, and interactions, 168t
vesicle-associated membrane proteins (VAMPs), 8f, 10f
vesicle-associated transporter (VAT), 8f
vesicular monoamine transporter (VMAT), 10f
vinblastine, 194t
vinca alkaloids, 194t
vincristine, 194t
vinorelbine, 194t
viscosity, 122
vitamins and nutrients, 227t
volume of distribution (V), 31–32, 37, 56, 61

W

women, pharmacology considerations for, 56–57

X

xanthines, 93, 98t, 99, 220

Z

zero-order kinetics, 34